CREATIVE MASTERY IN HYPNOSIS AND HYPNOANALYSIS

A Festschrift for Erika Fromm

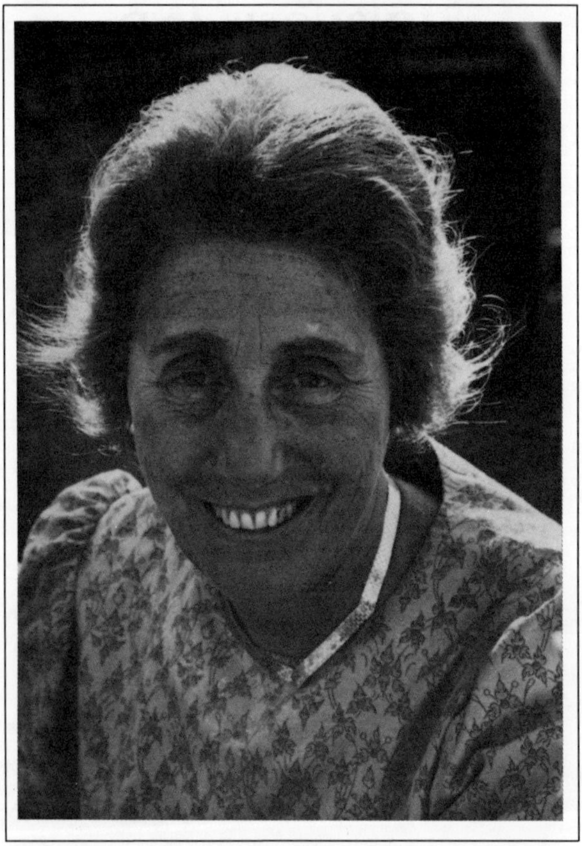

CREATIVE MASTERY IN HYPNOSIS AND HYPNOANALYSIS

A Festschrift for Erika Fromm

Edited by
Margot L. Fass
Clifton Springs Hospital, NY
Daniel Brown
The Cambridge Hospital

LAWRENCE ERLBAUM ASSOCIATES, PUBLISHERS
1990 Hillsdale, New Jersey Hove and London

Cover art is an original lithograph by Margot L. Fass, inspired by Erika Fromm

Lawrence Erlbaum Associates, Inc., Publishers
365 Broadway
Hillsdale, New Jersey 07642

Library of Congress Cataloging-in-Publication Data

Creative mastery in hypnosis and hypnoanalysis : festschrift for Erika Fromm / edited by Margot L. Fass, Daniel Brown.
p. cm.
Includes indexes.
ISBN 0-8058-0832-9 (c)
1. Hypnotism—Therapeutic use. 2. Psychoanalysis. 3. Fromm, Erika. I. Fromm, Erika. II. Fass, Margot L. II. Brown, Daniel P., 1948–
RC495.C74 1990
615.8′512—dc20 90-3792
CIP

Printed in the United States of America
10 9 8 7 6 6 4 3 2 1

To the furtherance of growth, mastery, and creative interaction between guide and follower, therapist and patient (or client), teacher and student, for all of our mutual enhancement and enlightenment.

CONTENTS

PART II
THE NATURE OF HYPNOSIS

PART III
THE CLINICAL RELEVANCE OF HYPNOSIS

PART IV
THE MECHANISMS OF CHANGE IN THERAPY

PREFACE

This book was written in response to a need we recognized in ourselves, and after inquiries among Erika Fromm's students, colleagues, and friends. On the occasion of her 80th birthday, a Festschrift seemed to be the most appropriate way to pay homage to her personal and professional influence on all of us. The fact that proceeds from the sale of the book will go to an Erika Fromm Scholarship Fund to assist students with an interest in hypnosis, will ensure that her wide-ranging effects on others will continue into posterity.

Ideally, a Festschrift would be made up entirely of original scientific and scholarly papers. However, to adequately represent authors who have been close to and profoundly influenced by Dr. Fromm, a few selections are revisions or reprints of already published papers.

It should be clear from the breadth and depth of the contributions to this volume that she has had a seminal and profound influence on the clinical and research literature in hypnosis and related areas. The book's contents are written by persons who have worked closely with and/or have been significantly influenced by her. The authors have refined, expanded upon, revised, and conducted research in many areas that Dr. Fromm has explored in her more than 100 publications on the subjects of hypnosis, self-hypnosis, hypnotherapy, and hypnoanalysis.

Professional therapists with an interest in personal growth, self-awareness, and creative mastery, whether or not they already have an interest in hypnosis, should be well rewarded for reading this book. If the reader has previously eschewed hypnosis, the integrity of the authors is so clear that the book might well stimulate an initial interest that can only enrich clinical practice or research.

The scope and treatment of the subject matter and organization of the book are evident from the table of contents. The subject matter ranges from a detailed accounting of Erika Fromm's professional biography and personal observations from friends and colleagues, to creative synthetic expandings of awareness about process and well-controlled research analyses of biopsychosocial hypnotic phenomena. Applications of scientific theory and principles of treatment to particularly difficult clinical situations are also explored. All are on the cutting edge of advances in the field.

The student might derive the most comprehensive sense of the development of Dr. Fromm's career, which in turn has influenced the maturation and fruition of the work of others, by reading the book from beginning to end. Alternatively, the reader might effectively browse through it, focus on a particular area of interest, and then allow him or herself to be led from one fascinating chapter to the next.

The collection is unique in that it represents the contributions of those persons who write in the area, and were most touched by our request for papers. They responded quickly and cooperated with tight deadlines. We have found them all to have been dedicated, responsible, and motivated to join in this labor of love—a demonstration of their affection for Dr. Fromm and respect for her achievements.

There are friends, colleagues, and students of Dr. Fromm who would have liked to have contributed to this Festschrift, but because of the need to prepare the final product by the fall of this year, we were unfortunately unable to include their offerings. We are nevertheless grateful to them for their warm response.

It is impossible to think of one of our own family members, therapists, patients, teachers, students, employers, employees, friends, or colleagues who has not helped in some way, large or small, to realize this project. The process of working on it has enriched us personally in terms of new positive relationships. One result has been a mutual expansion of affection and respect that now includes a larger "family" for us all. It is intriguing to be a participant observer in the midst of the powerful effect Dr. Fromm has in magnetically mobilizing healing energy that leads to self-actualization. This in turn results in an urge to contribute to the actualization of others, and thus of course, in further benefits to ourselves in the ever widening networks in which we develop.

ACKNOWLEDGMENTS

This project grew out of the enthusiasm, creative energy, and willingness to work hard that Erika Fromm inspired in her many students and colleagues.

We would like to thank the many individuals who supported the idea of the Festschrift with constructive suggestions and original or reprinted contributions.

Publishing this book in time for Erika Fromm's birthday required considerable devotion. The editors would like to thank each author for submitting their excellent chapters and responsibly responding to editorial queries, both often on very short notice, and being patient with and accepting the sometimes significant changes needed to bring each chapter into a consistent volume.

Each publisher who gave us permission to reprint, adapt, and/or translate material deserves not only recognition but an expression of our appreciation as well. It was easiest to obtain permission to republish a modified version of the "Foreword," by Ernest Hilgard from Daniel Brown and Erika Fromm's book *Hypnotherapy and Hypnoanalysis,* one of Lawrence Erlbaum Associates' most successful technical publications. Given that Father Greeley has been a best selling author since his hypnotic experience with Erika Fromm, it also is not surprising that Simon & Schuster, publisher of Andrew Greeley's *Confessions of a Parish Priest,* has given permission to use a portion of the "Prologue" of that book. Guilford Press published Erika Fromm and Stephen Kahn's book *Self Hypnosis: The Chicago Paradigm* in this year. Dr. Kahn used parts of this for his chapter, with*out* telling Dr. Fromm about it! Guilford Press was good enough to keep the secret from her, overlooking protocol for the sake of the surprise. The translated and slightly modified chapter by Germain Lavoie, first published in *Psychiatrie Clinique: Approche Bio-Psycho-Social,* Gäetan Morin Editeur, was well received in its original version in French. Jean Holroyd's chapter "How Hypnosis May Potentiate Psychotherapy" was first published under the same title by the American Society of Clinical Hypnosis in their own journal (Vol. 29, No. 3) in January 1987. Dr. Holroyd selected this as being most representative of the frequent correspondence between hers and Dr. Fromm's thinking. A considerably modified version of Peter Bloom's "The Art of Medical Hypnosis and Therapy" appears with the permission of the Swedish Society of Clinical and Experimental Hypnosis, who originally published it in HYPNOS (Vol. XVI, No. 2, 1989). It is fitting that it should appear here, as this was Dr. Bloom's first published paper. He tells us that Dr. Fromm greatly encouraged him to present and write this material. The Analytic Press gave permission for reprinting the chapter entitled "On Silence and the Holocaust: A Contribution to Clinical Theory" as it was written by Arnold Wilson in *Psychoanalytic Inquiry* (Vol. 5, No. 1, 1985). Drs. Wilson and Fromm collaborated in 1982 on a paper on this subject.

Our thanks go also to a number of people who submitted excellent material that we were unable to include in the Festschrift. Among these individuals are some of Erika Fromm's long-standing friends and colleagues: Sidney Blatt, Richard Horevitz, Campbell Perry, and Erika Wick. Some of these individuals submitted quite original works, which clearly would have been included under normal circumstances, were it not for our tight publication date.

We particularly thank our secretaries, Margaret Norton and Joan Marconi, for their devoted hours spent moving correspondence along, typing, making phone calls, checking references, gathering materials for the volume, and entering substantial information into the computer. Most importantly they provided cheerful moral support and kept us organized.

There were colleagues who relieved us of other responsibilities, including William Swingly, Rashmikant Sangani, and Denish Nanavati, without whose support we would not have had the time to devote to meeting our stringent deadlines.

Larry Erlbaum and Robin Weisberg of LEA both personally orchestrated the production of this book, and saw to its making a production schedule in order to be ready for Erika Fromm's 80th birthday party. We especially thank them for this. Without the considerable assistance of everyone involved, it is hard to imagine that this book would have been in print less than a year and a half after its conception.

With profound and fervent passion, we would like to thank our families for their considerable patience and understanding as we developed this volume. They probably knew better than we did how much time and energy it would take to prepare and complete it. Although the work may have decreased the quantity of time we are used to and prefer spending with them, hopefully our involvement increased the quality of that time. The privilege of working on the book with one another and with the fine ideas and persons that have become a part of it has further enhanced our own sense of Creative Mastery, by which we hope our families, friends, and patients may benefit.

Finally, we thank you, our readers. If you merely read this book, we hope you, too, will further *your* sense of Creative Mastery, and the already wide ranging beneficial effects and influences of Erika Fromm's lifetime to date will be felt even more profoundly. Your purchase of this book will further her work more, as all proceeds will be donated to the Erika Fromm Fund of the Society for Clinical and Experimental Hypnosis (SCEH), of which she was a founding member. This fund will be used to further scholarship and research in hypnosis.

Without the psychological support of the SCEH, particularly from Martin Orne, Kenneth Bowers, and Marion Kenn, this book would not have happened in quite this same way. Please feel free to join, participate in, and support this fine organization!

Margot L. Fass
Daniel Brown

FOREWORD

It is a rare honor to be asked to write a Foreword to the Festschrift for Dr. Erika Fromm, on the occasion of her 80th birthday. Let me digress a bit and remind you of the now classic film by Frank Capra entitled *It's a Wonderful Life,* in which the viewer is shown what life might have been like for the people of a small town had a decent man (played by Jimmy Stewart) never existed. As in this film, it often proves illuminating, when considering the contributions of someone's life work, to ask rhetorically what might be the present reality if the person had not been involved. I posed this question as I pondered the celebration marked by this Festschrift for my long-time friend, colleague, and intellectual provocateur, Professor Erika Fromm. The answer is a testament to the extraordinary person she is and to the lasting contributions she has made to the study of the human mind during the 57 years since she received her doctorate.

By any standard, Erika Fromm has charisma—the charisma born of a strong sense of self, of a commitment to honesty and standards, of dedication to helping as many people as possible. Throughout her life as a teacher, observer of human behavior, and therapist, she has used her charisma to help empower students, colleagues, subjects, and most especially, patients. Above all else, she has provided overwhelming evidence for the importance of empowerment in healing—empowerment through an understanding of psychodynamic ego-psychology, through phenomenological self-knowledge, through the application of hypnoanalysis, and through the teaching of permissive hetero-hypnosis and self-hypnosis. The seminal ideas and practices she articulated in these areas have stood the test of time.

In perhaps no other area of the many contributions she has made is her insight and creative potential more evident than in her use of hypnotic imagery. Possessing what can only be described as an extraordinary ability, Erika can quite literally and metaphorically lead a patient by the hand down a winding spiral staircase covered in a soft, thick, deep purple carpet, to reach a point at which the patient can examine at his or her own pace the many treasures buried deep in the psyche. The point is that she is capable of helping the patient gain mastery over an imagery that empowers the patient to explore deep-seated conflicts in a context that is enriching and forward-looking. Even for a patient who is not endowed with the skill to be a hypnotic virtuoso, hypnosis becomes a very special experience as the patient follows Erika's lead down a path of rich imagery, which can uncover new avenues and approaches for the patient to try yet again in a more creative way to gain insight, and to solve problems. One has to witness her work in this most personal of domains to fully appreciate the immediate and intimate rapport she can establish by her skillful use of imagery.

Similar to the way in which the Hilgards resurrected the field of hypnosis through the development of the behavioral, standardized scales of hetero-hypnotizability and the ensuing systematic research program, Erika Fromm has pioneered a rich self-hypnosis paradigm for the laboratory and clinical contexts that points the way for future researchers and serious clinicians to revitalize the field and allow the impact of the therapeutic alliance to travel with the patient into his or her everyday life. Her innovative work on self-hypnosis and subjective experience has been a tour-de-force in addressing fundamental questions, including investigations of the phenomenological differences between hetero- and self-hypnotic experiences, and the manner in which self-hypnosis is most effectively used in therapy.

This volume highlights the many areas in which Erika Fromm's interests, ideas, and contributions have made a major difference. She has been a pioneer, not only in the clinical and empirical understanding of human behavior through hypnoanalysis, but also in the establishment of reasonable standards and practices with regard to the therapeutic use of hypnosis and self-hypnosis. As a leader among her peers, she has set important and lasting standards as Clinical Editor of the *International Journal of Clinical and Experimental Hypnosis* and as a Past President of the Society for Clinical and Experimental Hypnosis. Most importantly, her life and her work have been an inspiration to her students and colleagues alike, and reminiscent of the character played by Jimmy Stewart, she has made a lasting difference to those who have been fortunate to know her and her work.

Martin T. Orne, MD, PhD
Professor, University of Pennsylvania
Director, Unit for Experimental Psychiatry
The Institute of Pennsylvania Hospital

I

THE WORK AND INFLUENCES OF ERIKA FROMM

The first section of this Festschrift provides an overview of the work and influence of Erika Fromm. Daniel Brown(chapter 1), one of Fromm's students and colleagues for nearly 20 years, traces the development of Fromm's ideas and significant contributions over nearly six decades. He places particular emphasis on her evolving ego-psychoanalytic perspective and its relevance to her understanding of dreams, hypnosis, self-hypnosis, and other altered states of consciousness and also to her humanistic values orientation in treating patients in hypnotherapy and hypnoanalysis. Fromm consistently emphasizes a few themes in her work: receptivity to preconscious and unconscious processes as manifested primarily in imagery; creative coping and mastery; the active problem-solving efforts of the individual; and the here-and-now reality-based relationship between patient and therapist, subject and experimenter, and teacher and student. These themes all reflect her belief in the ability each individual has to discover and master life problems when provided with the right kind of supportive relationship.

A modified version of Ernest R. Hilgard's foreword to *Hypnotherapy and Hypnoanalysis* (chapter 2), Fromm's main clinical textbook (Brown & Fromm, 1986), written by a leading authority on hypnosis, stands as a testimony to "the substantive nature of Erika Fromm's contributions to the field of hypnosis, and to the quality of clinical work done by a practitioner who has become one of the leading hypnoanalysts in the world.

We have also included a more personal reflection by another seasoned hypnoanalyst on how Erika Fromm influenced the development of her own ideas. In "Reflections on Hypnosis and Related Topics"(chapter 3), Doris Gruenewald discusses her ideas and personal observations about the domain of hypnosis, which she sees as a multidimensional continuum that includes such factors as suggestibility, imagery capacity, memory alteration, role playing, and dissociation. This personal account indicates how Erika Fromm influenced the development of another hypnoanalyst's own thinking.

The last section is an even more personal account of Erika Fromm's influence. We have included (chapter 4) an excerpt from Andrew M. Greeley's *Confessions of a Parish Priest.* He opens this autobiography with an account of his first experience with hypnosis. Through an hypnotic age regression facilitated by Erika Fromm, Greeley learned to appreciate the richness of the memories, images, and feelings that hypnosis made available to him. According to his own account, the personal experience was so compelling that it opened an inner world of creativity to him—a world that he has tapped productively ever since through the many novels he has written. He is one of many persons profoundly affected by the quality of relationship Erika Fromm can establish with others and her ability to enable them, through hypnosis, to discover and explore their own rich worlds of inner resources.

Chapter 1

ERIKA FROMM: AN INTELLECTUAL HISTORY

DANIEL BROWN
The Cambridge Hospital / Harvard Medical School

EARLY INFLUENCES

In a recent professional autobiography, Erika Fromm described two themes she considered most important in shaping the development of her professsional career (Fromm, 1987a). First, she always considered herself a "rebel against orthodoxy" (p. 207). Just as she rebelled as an adolescent to the very strict orthodox German Jewish household, throughout her adult life she has always actively questioned and challenged the status quo of society. Whether it be with respect to religion, science, psychoanalysis, or politics, as a scientist and clinician, Erika Fromm has never adhered to an approach or established set of ideas without first questioning its basic assumptions. Much in the spirit of a pioneer she applied this attitude as a useful means of forging new directions in many areas of inquiry.

Second, as a refugee from Nazi Germany, she had watched the Nazis gain power during her adolescence. Her deep distrust of the empty rigidity of the religious orthodoxy of her childhood was compounded by her horror of watching the development of her fellow countrymen's blind allegiance to the new and far more irrational and destructive orthodoxy of Naziism. Her profound disillusionment in the followers of this new and insidious movement left its lasting mark. Erika Fromm fled from Germany to Holland shortly after finishing her doctorate degree, and to this day she considers Holland, not Germany, her home country. Since adolescence she has not spoken a word of German, while delighting in the chance to visit Holland and speak Dutch again.

Erika Fromm studied psychology at The University of Frankfurt under the Gestalt psychologist, Max Wertheimer, and psychopathology with Kurt Goldstein. Training in the Zeitgeist of Gestalt psychology clearly affected Fromm's way of thinking and approaching problems. For example, Wertheimer (1945) was quite interested in "productive thinking." Based on Gestalt principles, productive thinking was a departure from traditional logic and also from associationism. Productive thinking is an attempt to overcome the influence of habitual conceptions and routinized ways of approaching a problem. The productive thinker is aware of the relationship between elements and strives to restructure the elements into some new organization or new way of asking a question about the subject, until all the elements fit together into a new Gestalt. This approach must have had appeal for a young Erika Fromm.

Kurt Goldstein (1963) most influenced Fromm's approach to clinical psychology, especially to psychological testing. Goldstein emphasized the "organism as a whole." When a variety of psychological tools are used to study individual traits, the individual is viewed in a piecemeal fashion as a collection of various capacities and deficiencies. Goldstein emphasized the study of the total personality of the patient. Goldstein's work focused on patients with organic brain conditions. He was particularly interested in the "concreteness" of brain damaged patients, (i.e., the loss of abstract ability). He also focused on the brain damaged patient's disorganized performance on selected tasks caused by what he called the "catastrophic anxiety" experienced by such patients. While focusing on these particular attributes of brain damaged patients, Goldstein continued to emphasize the importance of keeping sight of the total person.

Fromm first became aware of Freud's work when she was 15. She discovered a number of Freud's works hidden behind a row of other books in her father's library. She secretly poured through the pages of these seemingly forbidden works. From her early reading she developed an understanding of unconscious motivation and of the operation of impulses and defenses. Her interest in dynamic psychology continued throughout her graduate training, her clinical work in Holland, her externship under Samuel Beck at Michael Reese Hospital in Chicago in the late 1930s, and her formal psychoanalytic training in the late 1940s and early 1950s.

THE INTEGRATION OF ORGANICITY AND PSYCHODYNAMICS

From these disparate intellectual roots Erika Fromm faced the formidable task of integrating the Gestalt psychology of Wertheimer, Goldstein's views of psychopathology, and Freud's classical psychoanalytic theory. Much in the spirit of Gestalt psychology Fromm strove to integrate biological and psychodynamic perspectives on psychopathology into an understanding of the total personality. Dynamic and biological theories represented different perspectives on the organism as a whole. However, Goldstein himself had rejected drive theory. Although he believed in unconscious processes—what he preferred to call "nonconscious phenomena"—he did not believe that these phenomena were the result of persistent childhood experience. In that sense, Goldstein's theory was nondynamic. Fromm could never accept this part of Goldstein's thinking.

THE INTERFACE OF ORGANICITY AND PSYCHODYNAMICS

Some of Fromm's earliest professional writing reflects Goldstein's interest in organic brain conditions. She attempted to discriminate between and to integrate psychodynamic and biological perspectives on psychopathology. Her earliest works in Holland, for example, concern themselves with mental retardation (Oppenheimer, 1936), infection-induced dementia (Oppenheimer, 1937), and a case of deaf-muteness (Fromm, 1946). In this latter case study of an invalid 10-year-old, she was able to elucidate the complex interaction between organic determinants (complications from a middle ear infection) and psychodynamic determinants (selective inattention to fearful sounds in the service of self-preservation)

Some of her later papers in America reflect continued interest in this area. She devised a battery of psychological tests to assess organic and psychological sequelae to anoxia during labor and delivery (Benaron, et al.,1960). Following the development of her interest in hypnosis in the early 1960s, she devised a series of hypnotic experiments to distinguish between the effects of organic and psychological factors contributing to brain damage (Fromm, Sawyer, & Rosenthal, 1964; Gruenewald & Fromm, 1967). She used the hypnotic state to "suggest" brain injury to hypnotizable subjects. The responses of the hypnotic subjects simulating the brain condition were compared to various control conditions and scored by criteria for assessing organicity. Fromm and her colleagues concluded that hypnosis could be used to produce all of Goldstein's classic signs of organicity (catastrophic anxiety, concreteness, and fatigability) in the absence of brain damage in hypnotizable subjects. The implication of these studies is consistent with what is relatively recently well known (i.e., that seemingly organic signs sometimes can be produced by psychological means).

PSYCHOLOGICAL TESTING: INTELLECTUAL ABILITY AND PSYCHODYNAMICS AS AN EXPRESSION OF THE TOTAL PERSONALITY

For the first two decades of her professional life, Fromm was one of a number of psychologists who pioneered the use of psychological testing. Because of her early interest in Gestalt theories of perception, it is no accident that Fromm became particularly interested in the Rorschach as a psychological instrument. She learned the Klopfer method of scoring in Europe. Later she studied the Beck scoring system with Dr. Beck in Chicago. In the 1940s and early 1950s she worked primarily as a child psychologist. She administered scores of psychological test batteries to children and, to a lesser extent, to adults within the greater Chicago area.

At the time that Fromm first arrived in Holland (1934/1935), psychologists did not hold positions in hospitals, which were run by psychiatrists. She worked as a research associate at The University of Amsterdam and was able to convince an influential psychiatrist at a large state hospital of the valuable contribution that psychological testing could make to diagnosis. As a result, a number of hospitals in Holland began to hire psychologists (Fromm, 1987a). In America, other Nazi refugee psychologists like David Rapaport were destined to make a similar impact and to contribute to the growing appreciation of psychological testing and the role of the psychologist in the mental health profession.

Fromm's interest in psychological testing reached maturity in her book, *Intelligence—A Dynamic Approach*, co-authored with Lenore Hartman (Fromm & Hartman, 1955) This volume, and similar works, represent a continuation of her ongoing attempts to integrate organic and dynamic theory (Fromm, 1960; Fromm, Hartman, & Marschak, 1954, 1957). Many of the psychological tests she administered to children in the 1940s consisted of age-specific intelligence and aptitude tests. Since Binet's introduction of standardized intelligence tests in the early 1900s, intelligence was viewed in American psychology as a genetically determined ability. Fromm brought to the American tradition of intelligence testing not only her background in Gestalt psychology, but also in dynamic psychology. Her perspective on psychological testing again called for an integration of the presumed organically determined notion of intelligence as a genetic trait and dynamic personality functioning, both aspects of the total Gestalt of the person. In a manner akin to Rapaport, Gill, and Schafer's classic *Diagnostic Psychological Testing* (1945/1946), Fromm and Hartmann (1955) in their book, also argue for an appreciation of the dynamic significance of individual items on the various intelligence tests. Their work suggests that the psychologist needs to look beyond the objective pass–fail response to a given test item to the possible dynamic variables involved, including the idiosyncratic nature and meaning the item may have to the respondent.

In a systematic study, Fromm and her associates outlined about 50 variables that could affect responses to intelligence test items. Although Rapaport convincingly had shown the dynamic significance of WAIS subtest scores and responses to individual items in each subtest, Fromm and her colleagues applied this analysis to about 18 standardized intelligence tests commonly used by psychologists at the time. According to her view, a variety of impulses, ego functions, and superego variables potentially influence responses to children's intelligence tests at every age level, from infancy through adolescence. Any given item on an intelligence test can tap a wide variety of personality dimensions. In this sense, Fromm's work, much like Rapaport's, stands as an important contribution to the evolution of psychological testing practice in America and especially to the value and credibility psychological testing has achieved within the clinical disciplines.

PSYCHOANALYTIC INFLUENCES

Short-Term Psychoanalytic Psychotherapy

Erika Fromm received her formal psychoanalytic training at the Chicago Institute for Psychoanalysis during the days of Franz Alexander and Thomas French. In those days, the Chicago Institute was unique among American psychoanalytic institutes in its departure from psychoanalytic orthodoxy. Fromm again thrived in the "rebellious" atmosphere of the Chicago Institute. The pioneering spirit of Alexander and French is best captured in a ground breaking volume entitled, *Psychoanalytic Therapy: Principles and Application* (Alexander & French, 1946). This book was the result of a clinical research study that focused on a search for a shorter and more efficient treatment than psychoanalysis had heretofore allowed, by attempting to extract from analysis its basic therapeutic principles. The volume, which marked the beginning of the psychoanalytic psychotherapy movement, was not well received by many psychoanalysts, who did not believe that quick therapeutic results could yield lasting changes in the dynamics and character structure of the patient, and were also likely to have been threatened by the book's economic implications. Momentum developed within the psychoanalytic profession to influence the Chicago Institute to curtail distribution of the volume if the Institute wished to retain its association with the American Psychoanalytic Association.

Although the book's professional market was lost, its ideas were not. Fromm was deeply influenced by its socially responsible and ethical message, namely, to provide the quickest, least expensive, and yet most effective treatment possible, as an expression of the clinician's assertion of the primacy of the patient's welfare. Later, she would take these ideas to a greater extreme that made some members of the Chicago Institute's orthodoxy uncomfortable: Hypnoanalysis could provide a means of treatment that is quicker and as effective than even psychoanalytic psychotherapy. She came to believe that what could be done in 3 years of psychoanalysis could be done in 3 months, sometimes even 3 hours of hypnoanalysis (Brown & Fromm, 1986).

Dream Interpretation

At the Chicago Institute, Fromm developed a fruitful collaboration with Thomas French, the outcome of which was a new approach to dream interpretation. In the 1950s, French (1952-1958) embarked on an ambitious three volume treatise entitled *The Integration of Behavior*. Although there is much wisdom in these volumes they never received widespread recognition, probably because they require the reader to sift through many complicated analyses of clinical examples to find the essential points. One of these volumes, *The Intrepretation of Dreams* (Vol.2, 1954), describes a genuinely innovative approach to dream analysis. Erika Fromm worked closely with Tom French to rework the ideas contained in this volume and to make them more accessible to a professional audience. Fromm again drew on her background in Gestalt psychology for the collaboration. She resonated with French's ego-psychological view of dreaming and dream organization, as well as with his search for a method that accounted for the "pattern of interrelated meanings" of any given dream. French was influenced by Fromm's emphasis on articulating a method to approach dream interpretation. The product of this collaboration, *Dream Interpretation: A New Approach* (French & Fromm, 1964), greatly simplifies French's earlier work, elaborates his earlier basic ideas, and outlines the method of dream interpretation in greater detail.

Like Freud (1900) in his *Interpretation of Dreams*, French and Fromm believed that dreams are expressions of conflict. However, they also viewed them as reflecting current real-life problems that may reactivate past conflicts. Unlike Freud, they believed that people do not dream directly about the past. The past is relevant to the dream only insofar as it is activated by a current emotional situation. Dreams are, as importantly, manifestations of ego functioning more than mere derivatives of id impulses. Dreams represented the ego's problem-solving activity to which defensive operations are subordinate. Drawing on a botanical metaphor they describe dream activity as representing the "cambium layer of the mind . . . [a] . . . level where active growth, problem-solving, and learning all take place" (p.188).

French and Fromm defined a "focal conflict" as a specific conflict that is activated in the current context of the dreamer's life and represents the dreamer's present attempt to solve current life problems. Although a dream may allude to a number of subfocal conflicts associated with early childhood, it is not overdetermined in that the central conflict in a particular dream represents the dreamer's commitment to resolving one conflict, as it is played out in the current context of the dreamer's life. Every dream thus has a precipitating stimulus, or real-life event that activates the ego's problem-solving activity.

Two sides of the focal conflict are what French and Fromm called the "disturbing wish" and the "reactive motive." The disturbing wish arises from a current problem, and the reactive motive represents the dreamer's reaction to this wish (i.e., why the wish was perceived as disturbing to the dreamer).

French and Fromm also conceptualized the dream's "cognitive structure." They viewed the dream from the Zeitgeist of Gestalt psychology in contrast to Freud's Zeitgeist of associationism. From the Gestalt perspective, the cognitive structure of a dream is a specific "pattern of interrelated meanings" (French, 1954, p.4). A given dream, although fleeting, is a total and particular solution to a current emotional situation so that each element in the dream sequence, and every association to each element, makes perfect sense exactly as it is reported by the dreamer.

Scientific Intuition

Dream Interpretation: A New Approach exemplified Fromm's longstanding interest in developing a scientific approach to intuitive interpretation in psychology. Her interest in what she called "scientific intuition" traces its roots to Wertheimer's "productive thinking" (1945). Scientific intuition also is a method for overcoming habitual ways of interpreting material, testing hypotheses, and discovering the structural organization underlying the material.

Fromm showed her own skill in scientific intuition, which integrated principles of scientific method, dynamic, and Gestalt psychology with the previously mentioned deaf-mute boy (Fromm, 1946). She devised a series of ingenious practical tests to determine under what conditions the boy might react to sounds. For example, she presented the boy with chirping noises coming from a wind-up toy bird that was out of his sight. The boy did not react to the sound. After he played with the toy, it was taken away. Then, when the bird was kept out of sight, the boy reacted to the chirping noises. In subsequent sessions she used sounds from a toy cap pistol, a tuning fork, and a piano. In a systematic manner she was able to test her hypothesis that the boy was not deaf, but reacted to sounds only under very specific conditions, then developed a dynamic explanation for the boy's selective deafness to unpleasant sounds.

Later, Fromm described and recommended a scientific/intuitive method for interpreting projective test data, especially from the Rorschach (Fromm, 1958). She saw responses to projective material like dreams, as a manifestation of the patient's ego activity in solving current reality situations. She suggested that the psychologist attempting to interpret projective material begin by developing intuitions about the projective responses. He or she then should check and recheck these hypotheses by quantitative, qualitative, content, and sequence analyses of each projective test, until finally arriving at the total Gestalt of the patient's focal conflict.

Fromm's methodology of scientific intuition reaches its maturity in *Dream Interpretation: A New Approach* and later in the application of her method of interpreting art (Fromm, 1969). According to Fromm, interpretation in psychoanalysis is intuitive but needs to be balanced by an "objectively critical approach" (p.22). Interpreting dreams, the language of the unconscious, is like reading the Rosetta stone. Dream interpretation is not simply a matter of decoding symbols, but of capturing the spirit or central meaning of the message conveyed by the symbols. The disciplined clinician begins by allowing his or her intuitive imagination to respond to the patient's dream report. Through intuition the clinician tries to find the central problem expressed in the dream. He or she develops a working hypothesis.

The second stage in dream interpretation entails "critical analysis" of these intuitions. In a deductive manner the interpreter sifts through the dream and its associations to look for clues and parallels that might allow some elaboration of the working hypothesis. He or she continuously checks and rechecks the working hypothesis against the evidence. He or she also pays special attention to gaps in the evidence and material that does not fit. The skilled interpreter is disciplined enough to drop the working hypothesis and begin again when elements do not fit. In Fromm's words, the process of beginning again, checking and rechecking, is "painstaking." Yet, the persistent and disciplined dream interpreter finally arrives at an accurate understanding of the total gestalt of the dream. Fromm believed there is only *one* correct interpretation for each dream. The interpreter must account for all the evidence of the elements in the dream, *all* the associations to each element, and *all* the process material from the clinical session in which the dream was reported. The skilled dream interpreter is able to reconstruct the cognitive structure of the dream and explain each and every element in the exact sequence in the dream as an illustration of a specific problem solving attempt by the patient.

Although Fromm clearly wished to emphasize that something as seemingly undisciplined as dream interpretation could be subject to disciplined scientific method, she also believed that valid interpretation sometimes, albeit rarely, occurred by a different mechanism, namely by what she called an "aesthetic experience" (Fromm & French, 1962). Much like the scientist who intuitively resolves a scientific puzzle (like Kukule and the benzene ring) in a single vision, the dream interpreter sometimes correctly grasps the total gestalt of a dream in a single instant. Fromm believed that an aesthetic experience was a legitimate means to understand a dream, However, she warned that such an approach can go astray when the interpreter gets carried away with the "aha" experience and fails to critically test the intuition against the evidence.

Psychoanalytic Ego Psychology

In her psychoanalytic training, Erika Fromm was especially influenced by psychoanalytic ego psychology. Psychoanalystic ego psychology began as a reaction against Freud's narrow view that the ego's main function was to tame drives. The first departure came with Anna Freud's (1936/1946) classic volume, *The Ego and the Mechanisms of Defense*, in which defenses were seen as ego functions. A short time later, Heinz Hartmann's (1958) classic volume, *Ego Psychology and the Problem of Adaptation*, appeared. Hartmann's central concepts were the "relative autonomy of the ego" and the ego's "adaptive function." He departed from Freud's classical libido theory and emphasized the ego's role of adaption to and mastery of reality and the ego's role in the defenses against drives that associate ego with conflict. Although early ego development may be associated with defense against conflict, the ego later achieves a position of relative autonomy from the vicissitudes of impulse life. This conflict-free sphere of the ego contains a number of ego apparatuses such as perception, memory, motor functioning, language, thinking, and decision making.

Fromm was particularly impressed by the themes of coping and mastery in the ego-psychoanalytic writings. Ives Hendrick (1942) first described an "instinct to master." Robert White (1963) posited a third independent ego energy in addition to Freud's notions of libido and aggression that he called "effectance." He believed effectance could be readily observed in the child's playful exploratory activity and developing social competence. Lois Murphy (1962) elaborated on the child's age-specific coping abilities. Rapaport (1953b) first developed the concept of ego orientation in his essay on ego activity and passivity. He saw the former as showing relatively more ego autonomy, actively asserting control over drives, and the later a manifestation of relatively less ego autonomy, and lacking control over drives. He also distinguished between ego and behavioral activity. Fromm accepted the basic tenets of Rapaport's theory of ego orientation, but Rapaport's model was limited to the ego's orientation toward drives or impulses. Fromm expanded the concept to include the ego's orientation toward the environment (Fromm, 1972a) and the superego (Stolar & Fromm, 1973, 1974).

Moreover, Fromm blended Rapaport's concept of ego activity/passivity with Hart's (1961) work on the "feeling of choicelessness" as the subjective experience of ego passivity. In other words, Fromm was not just interested in the metapsychological functioning of the ego but its implications for the subjective experience of hypnotized subjects and patients. Fromm's theory of ego orientation consists of two essential ingredients. She emphasized first the decision-making function of the ego, and its subjective counterpart, the feeling of choice or choicelessness.

The second ingredient, derived from Murphy (1962), is the creative coping function of the ego. The ego is said to be active when it maintains relative autonomy from the demands of the id, superego, and/or environment and when it manifests autonomous decision-making and coping functioning. The subjective experiences associated with ego activity are the capacity for choice and the pride of mastery. Conversely, the ego is said to be passive when it loses relative autonomy to demands from the id, superego, and/or the environment, and also loses its decision-making and coping functions. Such an individual experiences being overwhelmed and helpless in the face of such internal or external demands.

The concepts of ego orientation and coping came to hold a central place in the decades of Fromm's professional career. They are critical to any understanding of her approach to patients. As her clinical ideas evolved, she came increasingly to appreciate the patient's coping resources. She conceived of two kinds of coping: creative and defensive (Fromm, 1981). It is certainly true that patients manifest defensive operations. Fromm, like Anna Freud, saw defenses as a function of the (active) ego. The sensitive clinician supports this ego activity. Pushing the patient would have the unfortunate effect of shifting the patient from a position of ego activity to ego passivity, and in turn, from a sense of control to the sense of being overwhelmed. On the other hand, supporting creative over defensive ego function leads to mastery over the id, ego, superego, and/or environmental demands.

Such an approach potentially has profound implications for the patient. Through ego activity, the patient learns, discovers, develops confidence in, and strengthens his or her own inner coping resources. The therapist sets the context for the patient's often creative discovery and exploration of inner coping resources. The patient in turn directly experiences mastery of the presenting problem, and along with it, feels a sense of pride, competence and/or self-efficacy. Coping, in the form of creative mastery, is at the very heart of Erika Fromm's clinical practice and teaching.

THE NATURE OF HYPNOSIS

The Hypnotic State

Erika Fromm's interest in hypnosis began in the 1960s, shortly before she took a faculty position at The University of Chicago. Like most psychoanalytically trained clinicians, she was initially quite skeptical about hypnosis and hypnoanalysis. Since Freud, the master, had rejected hypnosis in favor of free association, analysts after Freud had essentially dismissed hypnosis as a clinical tool. In 1960 Fromm was asked to participate in an APA program on hypnosis. She originally declined the offer. However, she was persuaded to participate as the voice of healthy scientific reason in an area about which she knew little, except for negative stereotypes attributed to hypnosis. To her credit, she participated with an open mind and left the program convinced of the merits of hypnosis as a legitimate area of scientific and clinical inquiry. Totally converted after participating in a workshop in which hypnotic phenomena were demonstrated with an hypnotic "virtuoso," her research and clinical interests in hypnosis and hypnoanalysis would span the next three decades of her professional career at The University of Chicago up to the present. Over these years, Fromm has emerged as one of the leading figures in hypnoanalysis in the world. Her contributions in this field of inquiry include a theory of hypnosis and self-hypnosis as an altered state of consciousness, and as clear a statement as can be found anywhere about the theory and practice of hypnoanalysis from an ego-psychological perspective.

Fromm brought her background in psychoanalytic ego psychology to her understanding of hypnosis. Gill and Brenman's (1959) classic work, *Hypnosis and Related States*, was the first major post-Freudian ego-psychoanalytic contribution to understanding hypnosis and hypnotherapy. Fromm extended the application of these principles, further elaborating the nature of the hypnotic state. She viewed hypnosis as a context for regression in the service of the ego; the hypnotic state, or trance, as a manifestation of altered ego functioning.

Over the years Fromm described a number of important parameters of the hypnotic state. These include: ego receptivity/activity, attention cathexis, fading of the generalized reality orientation, deautomatization, shift from secondary to primary process, access to imagery and fantasy and adaptive regression (Fromm, 1979, 1981).

In a series of works beginning with "Ego Activity and Ego Passivity in Hypnosis," Fromm (1972a) developed a theory of ego orientation that served as the basis for her ego-psychoanalytic theory of altered states of consciousness in general, and hypnosis in particular (Brown & Fromm, 1986; Fromm 1976, 1977, 1979, 1981, 1984b, 1987b; Fromm & Hurt, 1980; Stolar & Fromm, 1973, 1974).

Fromm added a third orientation to her understanding of a continuum of ego activity/passivity in states of consciousness. From Deikman's (1971) essay on "Bimodal Consciousness," she came to describe subjects in an altered state of consciousness as ego receptive. Ego receptivity is characterized by the relative suspension of strict reality orientation, critical judgment, and goal-directed thinking. In such a state, individuals become more receptive to unconscious and preconscious material that floats into the awareness of the relaxed alert subject. Just as the elements of choice and coping are essential in understanding ego activity, the element of attention is critical in understanding ego receptivity. Ego receptivity can be intentionally cultivated by an individual by adopting a particular attentional posture (Fromm, 1979; Fromm & Hurt, 1980).

Theories of ego orientation help us to understand the nature and experience of hypnosis. Fromm came to see ego activity and ego receptivity as continuua along which the hypnotized subject's experience varied. Hypnosis begins by focusing attention. Once the hypnotic state is induced, the subject may shift at times to a mode of unfocused free-flowing attention. During this condition of ego receptivity, the subject is more open to suggestions and also to the events occurring in the stream of consciousness (i.e., to unconscious and preconscious material and to coping resources and solutions to problems not readily available to waking consciousness). At other times the hypnotized subject actively explores coping resources and attempts solutions to problems. During this condition of ego activity, the hypnotized subject retains the capacity for choice and the ability to shape the unfolding experience. The skilled hypnotherapist supports the ego-receptive and ego-active orientation, and carefully avoids challenging the subject's defenses and thereby overwhelming the individual. In this approach to hypnosis, the hypnotized subject experiences mastery, discovers inner resources, and delights in functioning at a new and more creative level.

Attention Cathexis

Fromm's appreciation of the pivotal role of attention was derived partly from Rapaport's (1959) theory of attention cathexis and Brown's (1977), cognitive/structural model of altered states of consciousness. Among the variety of attentional skills that individuals draw on in altered states of consciousness, Fromm focused on a continua of focused, concentrated versus free-flowing attention, and of restricted versus an expanded range of attention. Hypnosis requires facility in accessing the full range of both (Fromm, 1979, 1981; Fromm & Hurt, 1980). The former pertains to relative selectivity or lack of selectivity of attention. It allows the hypnotized subject to shift voluntarily from an ego orientation of receptivity to activity, respectively. The latter refers to the span of attention (i.e., how much of the total stimulus range comes into awareness at any given moment). For example, the hypnotized subject may be receptive to one event in the stream of consciousness at a given moment (restricted range) or be receptive to a great variety of events at any given moment (expanded range). Fromm's development of a theory of attention brings her basic theory of ego orientation even further into the arena of the subject's own capacity. This theory again underscores the subject's voluntary control and free will in the exploration of states of consciousness and the discovery of unconscious and preconscious coping resources.

The Fading of the Generalized Reality Orientation

Fromm and Shor (1972a, 1979) elaborated on the mechanisms by which the hypnotized subject achieves adaptive regression. From a cognitive perspective, Shor (1959) developed the concept of the generalized reality orientation (GRO), by which he meant the stable frame of reference an individual in the waking state uses to maintain an orientation to external reality. Fromm and Shor felt that the GRO fades in hypnosis. In Fromm's ego-psychological terms, the active ego temporarily suspends its concern with external reality and shifts its concern to the events in the stream of consciousness.

Deautomatization

Fromm understood the induction of hypnosis in terms of deautomatization (Fromm, 1977b, 1979; Fromm & Hurt, 1980). The concept of deautomatization was first applied to hypnosis by Gill and Brenman (1959) and its application was extended to other altered states of consciousness by Deikman (1971) and Van Nuys (1973). *Deautomatization* has been defined as "an undoing of the automatizations . . . directed toward the environment" (Gill & Brenman, 1959, p. 178). The individual in the normal waking state develops automatized or habitual modes of perceiving, thinking, or acting with respect to the demands of reality. These occur largely outside of conscious awareness. These habitual processes are deautomatized through the redistribution of attention in hypnosis and are brought into the arena of conscious awareness. This reinvestment of such processes with attention disrupts the patterning of normal waking consciousness and results in quasi-stable new organization of ego functions. This new Gestalt allows access to an altered state of consciousness like the hypnotic trance.

The Shift Along the Continuum of Primary and Secondary Process

Fromm developed Freud's description of primary and secondary process operations and their manifestations in thinking and mental functioning (Freud, 1900) as a way of understanding the content occurring in the stream of consciousness in hypnosis (Fromm, 1981; Fromm, Oberlander, & Gruenewald, 1970). Primary process manifestations represent a form of largely unconscious mental activity dominated by impulses, wishes, or symbolic expressions that strive toward immediate gratification. Secondary process manifestations represent largely conscious mental activity dominated by reality orientation, verbal expression, and the capacity for delay. Fromm believed that these two processes coexist and interact. Induction of a hypnotic trance represents a shift along the continuum in the direction of increased primary process mental activity. Hypnosis is a means to recover a primary process mode of functioning and thereby gain greater access to unconscious and preconscious material.

In an attempt to test the concept of primary/secondary process mental activity, Fromm and her colleagues (Fromm et al., 1970; Oberlander, Gruenewald, & Fromm 1970) devised an experiment in which Rorschach inkblots were administered to highly hypnotizable subjects in the normal waking and hypnotic condition in a counterbalanced design. Rorschach protocols were scored using the Holt (1963) system for scoring levels of primary process manifestations and defensive operations. As predicted, hypnotized subjects experienced significant primary process mental activity relative to the waking state. However, an unexpected finding was that there was no significant increase in defensive operations in trance relative to the waking state. An implication of these findings is that the greater access to unconscious and preconscious material in hypnosis occurs by a mechanism relatively autonomous from waking defensive operations. In other words, unconscious and preconscious material seems to just float into awareness during trance without necessarily evoking significant defensive reactions.

The Role of Imagery

Fromm became particularly interested in the role of imagery in hypnosis and later in other states of consciousness. Holt (1964) wrote a seminal paper on how imagery had returned from ostracism in the post-behavioral Zeitgeist. Fromm understood imagery in terms of two central themes: voluntarism and demand source. Gordon's (1949) distinction between bidden and unbidden imagery is based on voluntarism. Bidden imagery is voluntarily produced; unbidden imagery arises by itself. Two kinds of imagery also exist according to the demand source. Reality-oriented imagery is directed toward the demands of external reality and represents a kind of cognitive problem-solving activity. It is usually unbidden and associated with ego activity. Symbolic imagery is associated with drive demands and is a form of expression of unconscious wishes. The symbolic fantasy is usually unbidden and associated with ego receptivity (allowing the imagery to arise) or ego passivity (becoming overwhelmed, as in a nightmare). This "psychodynamic structure of imagery" illustrates its variation in hypnosis and other states of consciousness (Fromm, 1979). In hypnosis, for example, imagery serves as a vehicle *both* for uncovering unconscious wishes and fantasies and for the active exploration of coping ability through rehearsal in fantasy (Brown & Fromm, 1986; Fromm, 1977b). Moreover, imagery plays a vital role in creative acts and intuitive interpretation. The skilled patient and clinician alike find imagery to be a medium for exercising healthy primary process mental activity (Fromm, 1977b).

Regression

Erika Fromm's earlier understanding of the role of regression in hypnosis was related to Gill and Brenman's (1959) application of Kris' concept of "regression in the service of the ego" to hypnosis. Fromm (1981) saw hypnosis as a temporary return to earlier forms of thinking.

As more research and clinical studies on hypnotic age regression appeared, Fromm expanded her concepts. She came to see regression as a partial reinstatement of earlier modes of functioning. These would include a shift to earlier modes of physiological and cognitive/perceptual functioning, and earlier developmental levels of self-and object representations and associated affective experiences (Brown & Fromm, 1986). Work that further influenced Fromm's reformulation of the concept of adaptive regression in hypnosis included Rieff and Scheerer's (1959) experimental studies of cognitive and perceptual functioning of hypnotized age-regressed subjects; Watkins' (1971) clinical work studies with the affect bridge method; and Nash, Johnson, and Tipton's (1979) work on self-and object relations in hypnotic age regression.

As usual, the interplay between theory, research, and clinical material powerfully motivated Fromm. Her interest in age regression was sparked by her treatment of a highly hypnotizable Japanese-American young man (1970). Don was born in the United States immediately after the Japanese attack on Pearl Harbor. He lived with his farmily for the first 4 years of his life in a relocation camp and spoke mainly Japanese. Upon release, Don quickly became assimilated into American culture. He completely repressed his Japanese heritage and with it the ability to speak Japanese. During hypnotic age regression he was able to recover the ability to speak Japanese. Subsequent linguistic analysis of the treatment transcripts demonstrated that he had recovered a child's version of the Japanese language that could not have been confabulated. She found this case to be convincingly illustrative of hypnotic age regression as a reinstatement of earlier modes of functioning.

Hypnosis As an Altered State of Consciousness

These parameters of hypnosis—ego orientation, attention cathexis, GRO fading, deautomatization, shift to primary process mental activity, increased primacy of imagery and adaptive regression—essentially justify Fromm's ego psychoanalytic view of the hypnotic trance as an altered state of consciousness. Her perspective traces its roots to Rapaport's (1951) essay on " States of Consciousness." Rapaport defined consciousness: (a) as an ego function, (b) which represents a complex organization of various ego functions, and (c) exists in a variety of states with (d) its variations associated with the distribution or redistribution of attention cathexis. Fromm integrated Rapaport's ego-psychoanalytic theory with Tart's (1969, 1975) definition of altered states of consciousness. Tart saw a discrete state of consciousness as a "unique, dynamic pattern or configuration of psychological structures" (Tart, 1975, p.5). This concept of a unique organization resonated with Fromm's emphasis on the total Gestalt of ego functions.

Fromm's state definition of hypnosis also is situated within a tradition of other significant contemporary works on the nature of the hypnotic state, notably Orne's description of the "essence" of hypnosis as characterized by the ability to produce significant cognitive/perceptual distortions that are experienced by the hypnotized subject as convincing and real (1959), and Hilgard's neodissociative theory (1977).

TOWARD A PSYCHOANALYTIC THEORY OF ALTERED STATES OF CONSCIOUSNESS

Although some of Erika Fromm's work in the 1970s focused on developing an ego-psychological model for hypnosis, she then expanded this model to include a variety of other states of consciousness. This move toward a general ego-psychoanalytic theory of altered states of consciousness grew out of her collaboration with Daniel Brown (1977) and also out of her attendance at a series of invited conferences in the early 1970s that were sponsored by the Menninger Foundation on the Voluntary Control of Internal States. She became increasingly familiar with research on other altered states of consciousness, such as drug-induced states and meditation. Consistent with her earlier work on hypnosis, Fromm continued to view a given altered state of consciousness as a quasi-stable reorganization of ego function or cognitive structures. Moreover, she emphasized focus of and redistribution of attention as defining the ego-active and/or ego-receptive orientation of and shifts to given states of consciousness. She saw the ego function of decision making and the capacity for voluntary control over particular states, as paramount (Fromm, 1977, 1978/1979, 1981; Fromm & Hurt, 1980).

Fromm expanded the number of axes or continuua along which states of consciousness can vary incorporating her parameters of hypnosis. Thus, she was able to develop a topology of specific altered states of consciousness according to variations along the continuua of ego receptivity/activity; unfocused, free-flowing versus focused, concentrated attention; automatization/deautomatization; shift in primary/secondary process mental activity; and fantasy/reality orientation. Thus, she came to describe and define altered states of consciousness in very specific terms, for example, hypnosis as primarily an ego-receptive state of focused attention with a relative shift toward primary process dominance. Imagery increases along with trance depth. Nocturnal dreaming is a state alternating between ego activity and ego receptivity, characterized by a somewhat expanded range of attention and an extreme shift toward primary process mentation, and therefore greater access to the unconscious. Altered states of consciousness induced by psychedelic drugs are primarily ego-receptive states characterized by a greatly expanded range of attention and a marked shift toward primary dominance. Attention in meditative states can be either focused or expansive, depending on the type of meditation practice, and a similar shift toward primary process dominance occurs in some meditative states (Fromm, 1979).

THE ORGANIZATION AND PHENOMENOLOGY OF HETEROHYPNOSIS AND SELF-HYPNOSIS

Fromm and her students at The University of Chicago conducted extensive studies on the comparison of heterohypnosis and self-hypnosis in the 1970s and 1980s. In these studies she maintained her interst in delineating the comparative structures of these two similar altered states of consciousness. In the first edition of *Hypnosis: Research Developments and Perspectives* (1972a), Fromm and Shor first addressed the phenomenological investigation of hypnosis as a cutting edge of hypnosis research. Always integrating her new knowledge and formulations with earlier foundations, Fromm emphasized a phenomenological approach to the inquiry on hetero-and self-hypnosis, which came to be known as the Chicago Paradigm. Her extensive hypnoanalytic work and her collaboration with Ron Shor were the basis of this interest.

This work began in 1972. Thirty-six subjects were given one experience each with heterohypnosis and self-hypnosis in a counterbalanced sequence. A taped version of the Harvard Group Scale of Hypnotic Susceptibility (Shor & Orne, 1962) was used for the heterohypnosis experience and a taped version of the Inventory of Self-Hypnosis (Shor, 1970) was used for self-hypnosis. A comparison of the similarities and differences between heterohypnosis and self-hypnosis was made using structured interviews. The least hypnotizable subjects (about one third of the sample) were not able to distinguish heterohypnotic and self-hypnotic experiences. The most hypnotizable subjects reported a greater quantity of and richer quality of imagery in self-hypnosis than in heterohypnosis. In self-hypnosis they also reported a greater number of ego splits, between ego states such as speaker, listener, experiencer, and voice of doubt (Fromm, 1975).

In 1973 the Fromm group reformulated their approach to the comparison of heterohypnosis and self-hypnosis. Earlier research (Johnson & Weight, 1976; Ruch, 1975), including her own study (Fromm, 1975), was limited to self-directed responses to a taped version of standard hypnotic inventories. A question arises as to whether such experiences are genuinely self-hypnotic. In order to investigate a purer form of self-hypnosis in comparison to heterohypnosis, the Fromm group devised a way to assess the experience of relatively unstructured self-initiated self-hypnosis. Thirty highly hypnotizable subjects were given heterohypnotic experiences with standard inventories to use as guidelines to generate ideas for self-initiated self-hypnosis. Then, subjects were asked to practice self-hypnosis daily over a 4-week period in a standard setting. The instructions encouraged subjects to initiate their own self-hypnotic suggestions through creative discovery in trance. A series of phenomenological questionnaires were given to subjects as a means to compare self-hypnosis with their experiences on the standard heterohypnotic inventories.

In their analysis of the questionnaire responses, the Fromm group found both similarities and differences between heterohypnosis and self-initiated self-hypnosis (Fromm et al., 1981). Both heterohypnosis and self-hypnosis were characterized by increased absorption, fading of the GRO, and skillful attention deployment. The reported differences between heterohypnosis and self-hypnosis were divided into three categories of structure, content, and context. With regard to structure, or the overall organization of ego functions, self-hypnosis was characterized by greater ego receptivity, free-flowing attention and significant fluctuation in trance depth. By contrast, heterohypnosis was characterized by greater ego activity, focused, concentrated attention, and constancy of trance depth. With regard to content, more vivid idiosyncratic imagery, spontaneously emerging personal memories and time distortions were reported in self-hypnosis. By comparison, there was a greater capacity to successfully experience age regression and positive hallucinations in heterohypnosis. With regard to context, there was greater awareness of the presence of and influence of the hypnotist in heterohypnosis.

The Chicago group also studied what the evolution of self-hypnotic experiences over time were. According to results from a longitudinal questionnaire, subjects in self-hypnosis reported increased skill in adapting to their inner world, greater trance depth and increased confidence in their ability to establish and maintain the self-hypnotic trance as they gained experience during the weeks of practice. A subsequent phenomenological investigation of the self-hypnotic diaries kept by the subjects detailed the idiosyncratic and richly varied experiences of these skilled self-hypnotic subjects (Fromm, Boxer, & Brown, 1985).

In subsequent papers, the Fromm group devised coding systems to test the validity of an ego-psychoanalytic theory of self-hypnosis. Fromm, Skinner, Lombard, and Kahn (1987/1988) scored the diary entries for the presence or absence of a particular ego orientation such as ego receptivity, ego activity, or ego passivity. They found that self-hypnosis is *both* an ego-active and ego-receptive state. They emphasized that even when ego acitivity occurs, ego receptivity is at the very heart of self-hypnosis. They also found a strong positive correlation between ego receptivity and the degree of absorption, trance depth, and the quantity and quality of both reality-oriented and symbolic imagery. Another study by Lombard, Fromm, and Kahn (in press) and Kahn, Fromm, Lombard, and Sossi (in press) further elaborated on the central role of imagery in self-hypnosis. More recent studies have focused on personality variables associated with self-hypnotic experience. Subjects whose self-hypnosis was rated as significantly more ego receptive than others had a need for independence, were self-reliant, and tended to trust in their own unconscious. Subjects whose self-hypnosis was rated as significantly more ego active were characterized by a need for structure, certainty, and control.

A recent book by Erika Fromm and Steve Kahn (1990) describes the Fromm group's nearly two decades of research on self-hypnosis, a synopsis of which is included in this volume. Other recent studies have also emphasized the clinical significance of self-hypnosis (Eisen & Fromm, 1983; Fromm & Elsen, 1982).

THE THEORY AND PRACTICE OF HYPNOANALYSIS

Theory

Erika Fromm's (1965,1968a,1984b) theoretical elaborations of ego psychology served as the basis for the development of a general theory of hypnoanalysis. The hypnoanalyst facilitates an ego-active/ego-receptive orientation in the patient during the treatment hour, and helps the patient learn to shift between these modes as indicated by the unfolding process. The patient's skills are directed as necessary, either toward uncovering (an ego-receptive mode) or problem solving (an ego-active mode), both required in successful hypnoanalysis.

The hypnoanalyst further helps the patient shift between utilization of symbolic fantasy and practical reality-oriented imagery fostering the patient's ability to creatively discover unconscious and preconscious inner coping resources and to learn mastery. He or she provides reassurance that the patient can resort to a protective coping mode when creative coping resources are unavailable.

In addition to her theory of the importance of ego activity and coping, Fromm clarified the nature of the therapeutic relationship in hypnoanalysis. In her paper on transference and countertransference in hypnoanalysis (Fromm, 1968b), Fromm expands on earlier descriptions of the hypnotic transference (Gill & Brenman, 1959; Ferenczi, 1909; Kubie & Margolin, 1944). The hypnotic state is characterized by the activation and reinstatement of self-and object representations, memory impressions, and associated affects from earlier points in the patient's developmental history. These are transferred to the hypnoanalyst. The perception of the hypnoanalyst is thus distorted and the affects experienced toward the therapist are significantly intensified. Although similar to transference that occurs in psychoanalysis over time, the very induction of the hypnotic state activates and intensifies transference reactions even in early stages of the developing therapeutic relationship.

In a later work (Brown & Fromm, 1986), Fromm enumerates on three major types of transferences occurring in hypnoanalysis according to the level of psychopathology of the patient. The three major types of transference are arranged along a continuum from more to less severe psychopathology. These are borderline and psychotic, self-object, and neurotic transferences. The latter are further subdivided into dependent, oedipal, and sibling transferences.

Fromm also emphasized the patient's here-and-now reality-based perception of the therapist in the hypnotic relationship. She deeply believes that patients, irrespective of transference reactions, have the capacity to accurately perceive qualities of caring or insensitivity in the hypnoanalyst. The therapeutic alliance or misalliance is highly dependent on the way the therapist treats the patient. The hypnoanalyst who offers a patient a series of successful experiences and leaves the patient with the impression that the patient's gains are a function of his or her own inner coping resources will significantly increase a healthy collaboration (Eisen & Fromm, 1983; Fromm & Eisen, 1982).

Clinical Practice

Fromm has made numerous contributions to the practice of hypnotherapy and hypnoanalysis. She applied the four classical psychoanalytic methods of free association, dream interpretation, interpretation of defenses, and the analysis of transference to hypnoanalysis. Fromm felt that hypnotically suggested associations and dreams allowed the patient greater access to unconscious and preconscious material for uncovering work. Hypnosis thus becomes another "royal road to the unconscious" (Fromm, 1987a, p. 209).

Because the patient is less defended against spontaneously emerging unconscious and preconscious material, the hypnoanalyst respects more than circumvents defenses. This may mean enhancing the patient's need for protective coping, and/or facilitating a search for unconscious and preconscious coping resources.

Fromm has contributed a variety of fantasy-based hypnotic inductions such as the beach induction, the boat technique, induction while imagining strolling through a museum, and the deep sea induction (Brown & Fromm, 1986). She also has created several scene visualization techniques such as the cloud technique and the old picture visualization (Brown & Fromm, 1986). Her Ideal Self Technique is a particularly useful method for modifying the patient's self-representation (Fromm, 1965). Moreover, she has articulated a number of ways to work with affect during hypnotherapy and hypnoanalysis (Brown & Fromm, 1986). Her clinical textbook, *Hypnotherapy and Hypnoanalysis* is devoted to a detailed discussion of the wording and rationale of these methods.

Values Orientation

Erika Fromm's ego-psychoanalytic work has served as the basis of a values system with respect to the treatment of patients in hypnoanalysis as well as to teaching hypnotherapy and hypnoanalysis to mental health professionals. These values are implicit in all of Fromm's clinical papers, developed particularly in a paper entitled "Values in Hypnotherapy" (Fromm, 1980). The primacy of patient welfare and respect for the client as a person, and her image of the "permissive hypnotherapist" stand at the heart of her clinical values. Hypnosis is a relatively easy state to induce in a hypnotizable patient. Because hypnotherapy entails clinical practice while the patient is in an altered state of consciousness, in which unconscious material is more readily accessible and less defended, the hypnoanalyst must always be watchfully protective and guard against too rapidly uncovering material or otherwise challenging the patient's defenses. The permissive hypnoanalyst gives very open-ended suggestions and refrains from introducing his or her own fantasy content into the patient's unfolding process, mindful of the patient's increased suggestibility and tendency to accept suggestions uncritically (Brown & Fromm, 1986; Eisen & Fromm, 1983). Further, the hypnoanalyst must

1. draw on a sophisticated understanding of the therapy process and the transference;
2. facilitate the patient's creative coping efforts and active problem-solving attempts;

3. leave the patient with the belief that his or her experiences in hypnosis and gains in hypnotherapy are a product of his or her own resources;
4. help the patient discover and choose his or her own goals for treatment;
5. allow the patient the joy of discovery, the wonder of the inner world, the trust in his or her own coping capacities, and the pride of accomplishment; and
6. enhance the patient's belief in the self over the magic of the therapist.

New Clinical Directions

In the last decade Erika Fromm has expanded the scope of her original outline for the theory and practice of hypnoanalysis to include approaches for a number of new patient populations. She has pioneered the use of hypnoanalysis with at least three new groups:

1. hypnoanalysis with severely disturbed patients;
2. hypnoanalysis with patients suffering from post-traumatic stress disorder (PTSD); and
3. hypnobehavioral medicine, with patients suffering from psychophysiological and habit disorders.

In each area she has made a major contribution by articulating a theoretical basis for her work with the patient population in question as well as by developing new methods for working with these special populations.

The 1970s were characterized by a virtual renaissance in contemporary psychoanalytic thoery, that included the convergence of, in particular object relations theory (Jacobson, 1964; Kernberg, 1975, 1976; Modell, 1968), self-psychology (Bach, 1985; Kohut, 1971; Lichtenberg, 1975; Tolpin, 1971), and affect development theory (Lewis & Rosenblum, 1978). During the same decade, outside of psychoanalytic circles, researchers were carefully scrutinizing the stages of child development with much greater clarity than had been achieved previously. The synthesis of contemporary psychoanalytic theory and the data from empirical child development studies seemed inevitable. Works integrating child developmental observations with self-psychology (Stern, 1985) and affect theory (Brown, 1985) began to appear. Within psychoanalysis a new paradigm was emerging for the study of severely disturbed psychiatric patients heretofore neglected by psychoanalysis. Exciting new theories and methods began appearing for the treatment of the severely disturbed patient. Severe psychopathology was seen along a continuum from schizophrenia to borderline to narcissistic pathology. Severe disturbance was being viewed as a manifestation of earlier developmental failures along an ideal model of the phase-specific tasks of normal human development toward "progressive structuralization" of the psyche (Gedo & Goldberg, 1973). This new psychoanalytic theory came to be known as developmental psychoanalysis (Stolorow & Lachmann, 1980) or structural psychoanalysis (Baker, Chapter 20, this volume). Erika Fromm became quite interested in this literature as it applied to understanding the patients she was treating. It was simply a matter of time before she was to develop a theory and method of hypnoanalysis for severely disturbed patients.

For several decades hypnoanalysts avoided using hypnosis with severely disturbed patients. One popular misconception was that patients with serious psychopathology were not hypnotizable. Studies began to appear in the 1970s and 1980s demonstrating that no significant differences existed between severely disturbed patients and normals with respect to hypnotizability. Another popular misconception was that hypnosis was dangerous and could precipitate psychotic episodes in severely disturbed patients (Abrams, 1964). Pioneers in the use of hypnosis with severely disturbed patients in the 1970s had reported just the opposite. Hypnosis rarely precipitated fragmentation when done sensitively. In some cases it actually helped contain and strengthen the patient against vulnerability to fragmentation. Fromm had become convinced of the efficacy of hypnosis with such patients from the work of Baker (1981). Baker devised a series of structured hypnotic visualizations to facilitate increased object constancy, primarily in borderline patients. Fromm applied these methods in her own work (Brown & Fromm, 1986). She modified and extended Baker's approach (Fromm, 1984a), for example, adding some additional methods to help the borderline patient gain control over splitting. Moreover, she described in careful detail an exemplary case illustration of the successful hypnoanalytic use of these methods with Jessica, in *Hypnotherapy and Hypnoanalysis* (Brown & Fromm, 1986).

The goal of treatment of the severely disturbed patient is "restructuralization" (Fromm, 1984a, p. 73). The hypnoanalyst presents the patient with a systematic series of visualizations designed to help the patient master the phase-appropriate tasks of child development along the line of development of stable, integrated, and differentiated self-and object representations. Hypnosis serves as a useful tool because structured visualizations can be presented to the patient in a relaxed comfortable state wherein the patient has greater access to imagery and affects—the building blocks of healthy internalization. The hypnoanalyst is able to actively structure the experience to foster the development and stabilization of healthy internal representations more quickly than is possible in nonhypnotic psychotherapy (Fromm, 1984b).

The protocol entails eight steps (Fromm, 1984a). The first five visualizations are designed to facilitate the internalization of a representation of the therapist as a "good object." The therapist first suggests that the hypnotized patient image him or herself in some pleasant activity in the presence of the hypnotist. This exercise is designed to help the patient overcome the fear of engulfment. Next, the patient is instructed to open his or her eyes, take in the hypnotist's presence, close his or her eyes, and attempt to maintain the image of him or herself. This visualization is designed to lay the groundwork for the separation of self-and object representations. The patient next visualizes the therapist alone, then the therapist and patient in the same scene, as separate but together, and finally, therapist and patient in interaction. The scenes often disappear or fragment early in the work. With persistence the patient develops stable internal representations for the self and the therapist without diffusion of boundaries.

The patient learns to differentiate and integrate these developing internal representations in the next three visualizations. The patient is instructed to visualize previously pathological introjects as external to the self, the self and therapist with both positive and negative qualities, and an actual merger of the good and bad self. Through these exercises the patient overcomes splitting and achieves a realistic representation of self and other.

The eight steps are designed to enable the patient symbolically to proceed along the normal developmental line of self-object differentiation toward greater object constancy (Baker, 1981; Fromm, 1984a). This may speed up the therapeutic task of developmental repair, but Fromm is careful to remind us that hypnotic imagery alone, although helpful, is not in itself curative. She believes that a successful outcome is more a function of the quality of the relationship between therapist and patient than of the visualization per se. The patient's images are the result of an active, engaging but not threatening therapeutic stance that provides the context for healthy internalization.

Post-traumatic stress disorder (PTSD) was perhaps to the 1980s what borderline and narcissistic conditions were to the 1970s. There was an enormous proliferation of research and clinical studies on the assessment and treatment of PTSD. Within this emerging trend during the last decade, Erika Fromm became quite interested in patients suffering from PTSD. This interest and the development of most of her ideas were sparked through her long-term hypnoanalytic treatment of Jessica, a 38-year-old woman traumatized early in her development by sibling incest (Brown & Fromm, 1986; Fromm & Brown, in press).

Contemporary clinical studies on the hypnoanalytic treatment of PTSD, especially the treatment of incest, are rare (Miller, 1986b). Historically, the literature on the treatment of trauma advocates abreaction. In such cases hypnosis is used to rapidly uncover and encourage the expression of intense feelings associated with traumatization. Contemporary clinicians have warned that this use of hypnosis is dangerous. The patient may become overwhelmed, shift to ego passivity, and experience the therapeutic relationship as retraumatizing instead of as emotionally corrective (Brown & Fromm, 1986). Most contemporary treatment of trauma advocates some sort of stage model for treatment in which the patient's coping resources are enhanced prior to uncovering, and in which uncovering proceeds in a slow indirect manner. Fromm's study of Jessica is exemplary of this approach to treatment.

In the study of Jessica, Fromm outlined 11 stages in the overall treatment of Jessica. The first 6 pertained to the internalization of a good object and the consolidation of object constancy as described earlier. The remaining 5 stages addressed symbolic and direct uncovering of traumatic memories and feelings associated with a forceful sibling incest incident. Fromm was careful to point out that internalization and consolidation of the patient's representational world must occur *prior* to uncovering to protect the patient from fragmentation. She also advocated a stage model to allow the patient to work through the trauma symbolically and then literally. Dreams, guided fantasy, anagrams, and automatic writing also may be used for symbolic working through. Screen memories often provide early symbolic material. In Jessica's case, a "soldier" visiting the family allegedly traumatized her. Later in the treatment, at a time she when she was able to accept direct uncovering of these memories and feelings without fragmentation, Jessica was able to recognize that her brother had been the perpetrator.

The case of Jassica elegantly illustrates how to provide a holding environment in which the patient can recover at a safe speed. Jessica required a treatment plan that addressed both her symptoms of post-traumatic stress and her borderline/narcissistic psychopathology, a commonly seen dual diagnosis in severely traumatized patients.

CONCLUSION

Fromm has distinguished herself as a scientist, clinician, and educator of national and international reputation. Her career is marked by continuous productivity. She serves as a role model for current and future generations of young scientists and clinicians.

Fromm has become one of the foremost authorities in the world on the theory, methods, and applications of clinical hypnosis. She has contributed much to the current humanistic view that hypnosis is an ability of the patient more than of the hypnotist. The invaluable contribution of the therapist is to provide a safe relationship within which the patient can discover and explore coping resources toward mastery and growth. Fromm has provided a consistent theory of the operations of the patient's experience, the manifestations of associative processes, and the nature of the hypnotic relationship during trance. Freud's rejection of hypnosis did much to limit its popularity as a clinical method for the first half of the century. Fromm's work over the past three decades has done much to reestablish hypnosis within the modern repertoire of clinical procedures, and perhaps is largely responsible for the remarkable concurrent resurgence of interest in its techniques even by some psychoanalytically oriented clinicians.

Fromm was one of the founders of the Society of Clinical and Experimental Hypnosis and served as its president from 1975 to 1977. As clinical editor of the *International Journal of Clinical and Experimental Hypnosis* since 1969, she has put her stamp of excellence on the clinical literature in this field. She has also contributed two major texts on clinical hypnosis: *Hypnotherapy and Hypnoanalysis* and *Hypnosis and Behavioral Medicine*. The former has been described in a recent review as "a scholarly, clinically sophisticated reference that sets new standards for our field." The latter is the only textbook currently available that integrates the fields of clinical hypnosis and behavioral medicine.

Fromm has made progressive contributions to research on the nature of hypnosis, the nature and phenomena of self-hypnosis and a theory of altered states of consciousness. In 1972 she co-authored with Ronald E. Shor a major text on experimental hypnosis, *Hypnosis: Research Developments and Perspectives* (Fromm & Shor, 1972a). This book, since its second edition in 1979, has become established as a standard for the field of experimental hypnosis. It received the "best book on hypnosis" award by the Society of Clinical and Experimental Hypnosis.

Moreover, Erika Fromm has played the role of overseer for the evolving field of experimental and clinical hypnosis. On three separate occasions she wrote reviews of the state-of-the-art in the hypnosis field (Fromm 1987b; Fromm & Shor, 1972b, 1979). These reviews not only describe the current state of hypnosis research but also predict future trends. A survey was sent to members of the Society of Clinical and Experimental Hypnosis in 1970 regarding the "growing edges" of research in the field. From the results, Fromm and Shor were able to assess and predict future trends for the field. In 1978 Fromm conducted a computerized library search of all hypnosis articles published from 1971 through 1978. Through a content analysis and by enumerating those areas in which research publications on hypnosis actually appeared between 1971 and 1978, Fromm was able to confirm their 1972 predictions. She has contributed close to 100 articles to the literature and to seven out of nine growing edges identfied in 1970.

Although Erika Fromm's contributions as a clinician and researcher have been impressive, her major and most important contribution, in her eyes, is as an educator. She has dedicated more hours to training graduate students and established professionals in hypnosis and hypnotherapy than any other individual I know. I know her well in this sense, because I have taught with her for 18 years. She is well known for the enthusiasm she brings to her work and especially for her ability to inspire confidence in students and established clinicians to learn about hypnosis and then to apply it to their own clinical work with some sense of mastery. She has taught countless courses and workshops for nearly three decades throughout the United States and the world. She is enormously popular as a teacher and her course evaluations are consistently positive. I recently read through the Directory of the Society of Clinical and Experimental Hypnosis and recognized the names of numerous individuals initially taught by Erika Fromm. She has trained over 4,000 beginning and established professionals in hypnotherapy or hypnoanalysis, probably far more individuals in hypnosis than any other contemporary. Those of us that have had the privilege of working closely with her know that she takes a Platonic view that genuine teaching has more to do with the development of inspiration and character in students than it does with imparting information or technical skills. Many of those inspired by her teaching have subsequently made significant contributions in their own right to the field. The range and depth of contributions to this Festschrift are but a small representation of the dedicated inquiry she has inspired.

Chapter 2

ERIKA FROMM AS CONTRIBUTOR TO HYPNOSIS, HYPNOTHERAPY, AND HYPNOANALYSIS*

ERNEST R. HILGARD
Stanford University

I am pleased to join in the celebration of Erika Fromm for her many contributions to psychology, hypnosis, hypnotherapy, and hypnoanalysis on the occasion of her 80th birthday. She has long been a good friend and colleaque.

In recognition of the substantive nature of her contributions, I am offering here a slightly modified verison of the Foreword that I wrote to one of her more recent books,*Hypnotherapy and Hypnoanalysis* (Brown & Fromm, 1986).

About it, I said:

> [This] book by seasoned practitioners of clinical hypnosis should be welcomed by all who are already using hypnosis in their clinical practice, as well as by graduate students. Their searches for and summarizations of the variety of methods available have been thorough, and the voice of experience shows in their recommendations for practice. For those not entirely familiar with the possibilities offered by hypnosis, the many detailed accounts of what actually is done will serve as an invitation to obtain training in the use of hypnosis. Indeed, the experiences reported here will provide a head start on accumulating the kinds of hands on knowledge that otherwise would require years of practice with patients in all their variety.

*Reprinted from Hilgard, E. (1986). *Foreword.* In D. Brown & E. Fromm, *Hypnotherapy and hypnoanalysis* (pp. xiii–xiv). Hillsdale, NJ: Lawrence Erlbaum Associates.

Scientfic hypnosis has made great advances particularly since World War II, both as part of basic psychological science concerned with the understanding of brain, mind, and personality, and as a professional skill in which knowledge of hypnosis is used to serve human welfare by enhancing the quality of life for those who have the good fortune to benefit from hypnotherapy and the related practice of hypnoanalysis.

The reader is brought abreast of these developments, with the authors' description of hypnosis as an altered state of consciousness interpreted theoretically from several points of view, the therapeutic relationship, the depth of hypnosis and the alterations within hypnosis as perceived by the hypnotized person, the art of hypnotizing, and the most widely used induction and deepening techniques. One without wide acquaintance with hypnotic lore may well be surprised by the variety of approaches that are available to match the preferences, abilities, and needs of the subject or patient. The authors have introduced the reader to the major aspects of hypnosis and how hypnotic procedures are carried out. The reader learns about selecting patients for hypnotic treatment (because it is not appropriate for all who come), how to plan the treatment, what techniques are available in therapeutic practice and finds a full-length case history of hypnoanalysis.

Because hypnosis *per se* is not psychotherapy, the authors wisely distinguish various ways in which hypnosis can be used in therapies based on different perspectives. The authors make important distinctions among three perspectives on the use of hypnosis in therapy. Briefer hypnotherapy includes two of these: the first decribed as *hypnobehavioral* perspective, the second as *dynamic hypnotherapy*, or psychoanalytically oriented psychotherapy. The third is hypnoanalysis.

The hypnobehavioral therapy is appropriate to some of the simpler conditions in which symptom relief restores the patient's ability to cope, without the therapist's delving into such issues as the emotionalized transference between patient and therapist. Therapy using the hypnobehavioral perspective is treated in detail in another volume by the authors (Brown & Fromm, 1987).

Dynamic hypnotherapy uses hypnosis in the context of brief psychotherapy as practiced by psychoanalytically oriented psychotherapists and requires that the therapist be sensitive to transference. Here, though, working through the transference may not be essential as it is in hypnoanalysis, the other perspective considered.

Hypnoanalysis is the utilization of hypnosis in connection with the long-term treatment that is usually associated with psychoanalysis. It may use hypnosis as an uncovering technique, taking advantage of the hypnotic condition to supplement the more typical free association technique of psychoanalysis; or it may use hypnosis to advantage as it facilitates ego strengthening in cases of character problems or maladaptive human relationships. Here working through the transference becomes essential to provide the corrective emotional experience upon which therapeutic success depends.

> The orientations of dynamic hypnotherapy and hypnoanalysis—central to this book—are avowedly based on contemporary psychoanalytic theory, and the practitioner must understand and be able to use approaches essential to these therapies, independent of hypnosis. That is, hypnosis is an adjuvant, often a highly favorable one, but not always to be recommended. The theoretical background not only includes classical psychoanalysis but shows the influence of many psychoanalytic thinkers since Freud, such as influences deriving from Franz Alexander and Thomas French, the later ego psychology within psychoanalysis of Heinz Hartmann, Anna Freud, and Erik Erikson, and the emphasis on narcissism by Heinz Kohut—to mention but a few of the many cited.
>
> It comes as no surprise that the thorough documentation is shared between the references citing many workers in the field of hypnosis whose work is directly relevant and those who are writing in the context of psychoanalytic theory and practice with little or no mention of hypnosis. The originality of the authors rests in the manner by which they integrate psychoanalytic understanding with the advantages in treatment that hypnosis provides for those already committed to psychoanalytic psychology. The old taboo of psychoanalysis against hypnotic therapy, a taboo initiated by Freud when he turned from hypnosis to free association, has of course been broken from time to time by his followers. In this book we find an able case made for the advantages of integrating hypnosis and psychoanalysis in clinical practice.
>
> Those already committed to therapies based on psychoanalytic assumptions will be prepared to assimilate the new teaching most readily, but at the same time there is much wisdom in this book to appeal to the practicing clinician who is uncommitted to psychoanalytic theory.

I believe that I have made it clear from my sentiments in this foreword that over the years I still value her contributions as both profound and original.

Chapter 3

REFLECTIONS ON HYPNOSIS AND RELATED TOPICS

DORIS GRUENEWALD
Laguna Hills, CA

Erika Fromm and I met in the Autumn of 1961. I had recently been admitted to the University of Chicago's doctoral program in psychology—reluctantly on the part of the powers that be as they did not think very highly of women, and older women at that, as students likely to do well or to "stick with it." I did both. That I gained a dear friend in the process was a delightful extra dividend.

Erika Fromm's hypnosis seminar, which I joined to learn what this thing called *hypnosis* was all about, proved to be very important to me. Several years earlier I had observed a demonstration of hypnosis at a meeting of the Chicago Dental Association, to which I had been invited. What I saw there was intriguing, but I put it aside as "one of those things" one comes across here and there. When the opportunity presented itself later, under the aegis of the University of Chicago, to study the phenomenon of hypnosis, I thought it worthwhile to look into it some more. Little did I then think that theory, research, and clinical use of hypnosis would come to occupy a good part of my professional life. I ascribe it to Erika Fromm's enthusiasm and involvement that I did engage seriously in what I had considered little more than a fringe phenomenon. Along with the pursuit of some of the questions inherent in the field of hypnosis, a solid friendship developed between us that I treasure to this day.

Hypnosis has come to represent for me a major facet of the entire human mind–body entity. I think of hypnosis as falling into a broad, multidimensional continuum that includes phenomena such as suggestibility, compliance, and multiple personality. The latter eventually became a topic of special interest to me.

Elsewhere (Gruenewald, 1984) I have presented a model of hypnosis and multiple personality that was more or less limited to such issues as dissociation, memory, and role taking. Not unlike the parable of the elephant and the blind men, it is quite possible to delineate the bio-psychosocial phenomenon called *hypnosis* in many different ways. Some of these are thoroughly dissimilar, some of them overlap with others, but none so far represent the totality of the phenomenon itself. These remarks are certainly not going to fill in what is still missing. My main purpose is, rather, to reflect on some of my thoughts that have evolved over the years to understand what I have personally observed.

For the novice, and even for some seasoned practitioners, hypnosis can have a seductive influence. It is as though the hypnotist brought about what had been suggested. One's narcissism is inevitably an issue, and with it whatever remains of one's latent grandiosity and sense of omnipotence. I well remember my early incredulous, elated reaction when a young volunteer subject responded positively to my suggestion to paint a picture on the wall in front of her and to describe it as she went along. This was one of my first tentative excursions into the realm of the imagination. I venture to say that, had such attempts failed, I might not have further become involved with hypnosis, as I as yet felt no serious commitment. But the attempts succeeded and I continued with many practice inductions and, eventually, investigatory and therapeutic applications of the techniques of hypnosis.

In these latter pursuits it became increasingly clear to me that I was using sensory imagery beyond the standard instructions printed in books and articles on techniques and procedures. I mention this recognition, not at all startling in itself, because I had always thought that I used words as symbols for imageless thought (in the mode of the Wuerzburg School). The ability to create by verbal means visual and other sensory imagery in empathic resonance with the subject or patient therefore came as a surprise. It showed me unequivocally that at a pre- or unconscious level more imagery was present than I had recognized, and that I was tapping into that reservoir. Erika Fromm had always been quite skeptical when I argued for my concept of "imageless thought." I take this opportunity to set the record straight; she was right.

It took some years of working with hypnosis as more or less a "given" before I thought in greater depth about its nature. I had assumed from the beginning that the potential for hypnosis was inherent in the individual and was not created, but only elicited and facilitated, by the operator. Reports and communications regarding the experience itself, when available, gave valuable information about the subjective aspects and revealed a great deal about the personality dynamics of the informant. But were the transferences, the regressions, the literalness of some or the retention of logic by others, and so forth, an integral part of the hypnotic state? Could it be that the whole thing was a hoax, in the manner of a *folie a deux*? After all, most if not all of the so-called hypnotic phenomena were capable of being produced without anything like an induction!

Puzzling questions these, especially in the absence of any acceptable biological markers that would have differentiated hypnosis from ordinary consciousness. The burgeoning research into the presence and function of endogenous opiates in the brain did not lead to the breakthrough I had hoped for. And the development of positron emission tomography (PET) was probably overrated in terms of what was expected from it. Although very useful for delineating cerebral metabolism, PET did not lead to identifying a state of hypnosis as such.

Be that as it may. There were other avenues open to deal with the phenomenon. Descriptions were not lacking, and many workers had systematically explored the phenomena of hypnosis both in normal and in pathological conditions. It seemed that the concept of hypnosis in some form or another could be applied to the whole gamut of the mind–body unit. Any and all organ systems were capable of being influenced, and of influencing in turn the functioning of the organism. It is no wonder then that unwarranted claims and outright quackery at times obscured the very real, solid findings and uses of hypnosis.

How far mutual body–mind influences could go was brought home to me in the context of a research project (Gruenewald & Fromm, 1967). Two young people in particular, one male and one female, were able in response to suggestions to become so immersed in the experience that a psychophysiological state was established that included functional alterations in the central and peripheral nervous system. This was explored by way of an unfortunately, but necessarily, not completely blind neurological examination. Although the neurologist's bias was in a negative direction, it was not possible to overlook or explain away certain changes in these intact subjects on grounds other than "hysterical symptoms, conversion type."

This raised yet other problematic questions in my mind. What do hysteria and hypnosis have in common, and what is *hysteria*? Charcot, Janet, and Freud, to name only a few, had no problem with that term. It was only in the second half of the 20th century that as a category hysteria fell into disrepute. It is now broken down into some of its components, one of the latter being the dissociative disorders.

Dissociative disorders are usually listed under the overall rubric of hysteria—or its successor names. However, as in the case of hysteria itself, it seemed to me to be overly simplistic to reduce them to sexual-genital concerns, as hysteria had largely come to be understood in psychoanalytic parlance. The symptomatology of hysteria tends to be protean, and the word itself allows for the inclusion of traits, symptoms, and personality organization currently assigned to other nosological categories. All of this merely goes to show that neither nomenclature nor diagnostic processes can be pinned down with certainty and exactitude. Furthermore, they tend to change over time.

As for hypnosis, the brilliant Charcot in his time thought it to be a form of hysteria (i.e., a pathological condition). An air of opprobrium clings to hypnosis in some quarters even today. That it has at the same time also been accepted as a manifestation in normal persons is ultimately to be credited to the many serious workers who have painstakingly tried to map out its quantitative and qualitative dimensions and established that the normal person is more likely to be responsive to hypnosis than one with mental or emotional problems.

Hypnotic susceptibility cannot, in my opinion, be pinned down to a cut and dried numerical value, although for statistical purpose it is useful to have a reliable standard measure available. Nevertheless, individuals may not fit into standard measurement as internal or external conditions may impose restrictions or cause facilitation of response (Gruenewald, 1982a). When it comes to therapeutic uses of hypnosis, such aspects as special motivations, transferences, and the like seem to be inextricably interwoven with hypnosis as a condition of the person (Gruenewald, 1982b). It therefore is a most difficult task to tease apart what may or may not in fact be a direct effect of hypnosis per se. Although many clinicians now administer one or another of the extant hypnotic susceptibility scales—for valid enough reasons—and may be guided, at least in some cases, by the obtained values, I would question whether process and outcome of hypnotherapy have much to do with that practice.

I indicated earlier that I became interested in the multiple personality syndrome (MPD). Like my interest in hypnosis, this too was almost accidental in its beginnings. A young woman, previously diagnosed as "borderline psychotic" by competent clinicians, was referred for yet another workup after being hospitalized because of presumptive suicidal tendencies. In the course of meeting with me, she displayed unmistakable evidence of dual personality, previously quite unsuspected (Gruenewald, 1971). Thus began what has over several years resulted in various contributions to the literature (e.g., Gruenewald, 1977, 1978, 1984) and a number of consultations on suspected as well as established cases.

Here too, as with hypnosis, there is a significant element of seduction in the often startling, always fascinating transformations one sees with one's own eyes. It is very tempting to accept the overt evidence as hard fact, without due regard to the potentially self-serving aspects of that evidence and without raising questions of primary and secondary gain in the captivating display. I briefly summarize what I synthesized in my thinking on the basis of such observations as I was able to make. The following aspects and theoretical considerations regarding the etiology and structure of MPD, although based on observation, are of course inferential.

One perhaps superficial but, I believe, important observation has been that MPD persons are highly intelligent people, even if their intelligence does not gain the usual expression. That is, they may show large gaps in knowledge, come across as quite ignorant and inconsistent in many ways, and, of course, "disappear" suddenly. The manner in which the sudden change is carried out seems to depend on what the person knows of the condition. Moaning and groaning, pressing the hands to the temples, complaints of headaches, or a rapid "switch" to another personality are all fairly common mechanisms on display. I use the word "display" advisedly, for such it is. Even if no one else is present, the inner world is peopled by an audience for whose benefit the show can be enacted. This particular characteristic of the MPD has, to my knowledge, not been sufficiently investigated. Altogether it takes considerable mental ability to carry through consistently on the maneuvers that have been identified as belonging to MPD. But let me emphasize that subjectively the person is usually unaware of what is happening and thus is not lying in the proper sense of that term.

Another important element involved in the genesis and maintenance of MPD is that of play and play-acting. It all starts out in a "let's pretend" situation, for very good reasons, to be sure. A history of abuse in various forms and degrees is well enough documented to be accepted, although not necessarily present in each and every case. Thus, the common childhood practice of inventing an imaginary companion becomes solidified, is not relinquished with progressive development, and is gradually expanded into greater and greater complexity. The different "personalities" take on increasing reality as they are fleshed out with the functions they must perform. The upshot is that to the outside observer there are apparently disparate units in one body.

In the realm of memory too there are most interesting processes at work that allow continuty over time among the various apparently discrete elements that make up the "personalities." I have elaborated on the issue of memory elsewhere (Gruenewald, 1984). Suffice it to say that there seems to be no lack of registration in the memory system. There is, however, a profound disturbance of the usual retrieval mechanism, with resulting compartmentalization along unusual dividing lines of the memories that become and remain available to the various segments.

Briefly then, we may assume a basic developmental, or even possibly constitutional, vulnerability of the person suffering from MPD. There is an early inability to coalesce and integrate into a cohesive self along the lines of normal development. The histories of MPD patients almost invariably point to adverse interpersonal experiences, whether factual or subjectively perceived. The young child, in order to survive, has an urgent need to create modes of coping with otherwise intolerable conditions—modes that may later result in the genesis of multiple selves, with different tasks assigned to each. It seemed to me less likely that MPD would originate in a developmentally later, general constellation, as hysteria had been commonly defined in psychoanalytic theory. Rather, its actual roots were more likely to lie in the narcissistic phase of development, even though hysterical mechanisms were significantly involved in its phenomenology and may well have triggered the overt emergence of the disorder.

In their manifestations MPD and hypnosis have much in common and tend to share similar and at times identical pathways for their expression.

Elsewhere (Gruenewald, 1984), I have observed that specific forms of pathology seem tied to prevailing fashions in the culture in which they occur. The same may be said for diagnostic and therapeutic practices. It is easier to make a diagnosis based on the number of certain presenting symptoms than it would be if one took a more comprehensive look at the individual case. For instance, the presence of delusions and/or hallucinations has all too often led to an almost automatic diagnosis of schizophrenia, disregarding the possibility that such symptoms can appear in other conditions as well, including MPD.

Opinions about MPD vary widely, from facile if not overenthusiastic acceptance of the overt signs of the disorder to extreme skepticism regarding its existence. One of the real difficulties in dealing with MPD is to find a balance between the necessary acceptance of the patient's self-presentation and an underlying theoretical orientation that goes beyond outward appearances and seeks meanings. Without the acceptance of what the patient brings to therapy no rapport or working relationship is possible. But to discard one's skepticism altogether at times can lead to reinforcement of the very condition for which one's services were engaged.

The opinions expressed in these pages have evolved over many years. They are a long way from the early days of my work with hypnosis. Erika Fromm always has been an interested listener, contributing ideas whenever she could. She was in many ways an important presence for me. For that I thank her.

Chapter 4

A PERSONAL EXPERIENCE WITH SELF-HYPNOSIS AND CREATIVITY*

ANDREW M. GREELEY
The University of Chicago

"You are going deeper and deeper," Erika Fromm's rich, Middle European voice said reassuringly, "you are climbing back down the ladder of your life and you are feeling very happy, oh, so very happy, deeper and deeper and deeper, you are filled with happiness. Now mentally you open your eyes and look around at this time of your life when you were so very, very happy. Where do you find yourself?"

I was 3 years old and standing on a green, sun-drenched hill, looking at the lawns rolling down to the dull silver platter of a lake. Behind me was a big stately Victorian mansion with turrets and porches, a magic castle perhaps. On either side were wooden buildings painted white with green trim surrounded by screened-in porches. In front of me a bed of thick red flowers surrounded a brilliant reflecting globe, a giant ball bearing; at the side of the lake a dark stone platform covered with a peaked roof and on the lake itself speedboats (Hunter Deluxe Specials!) and sailboats puttered about. Children and adults sat on a quaint wooden pier that jutted into the lake and kids my age were frolicking on a great slide that sloped into the warm, comforting waters. I rushed quickly down the slope of the hill and into the lake to join them.

Dr. Fromm's age regression had brought me back to ecstatically happy experiences at the outer fringe of my conscious memory. Here was where it

*Reprinted from Greeley, A. (1986).Prologue. In *Confessions of a parish priest* (pp. 1–4). New York: Simon & Schuster.

all started. Commodore Barry Knights of Columbus Country Club, a magical place with a vast lake, towering jungle-covered hills, lawns and gravel-covered paths on which to run (and make shambles of one's knees), a dining hall with real mashed potatoes, gleaming corn on the cob, thick gravy, an endless supply of roast beef, crowds spread out on the lawn on a Sunday morning in front of the pergola following the progress of the Mass, a distant drama marked by a tinkling of a bell, barely to be heard over the summer sounds of the lake.

In the dining hall men wore ties although air conditioning was unknown; and at Mass on Sundays, they put on coats and even carried their straw hats in their hands (many of them, my father included, were in "plus four" knickers instead of long trousers and carried caps instead of hats). The priests who said the Mass lived in a secluded wooden house at the fringe of the country club, and enjoyed their quiet vacations, discreetly separated but not completely isolated from the laity.

My reexperienced happiness in Erika Fromm's hypnotic trance was generalized and unspecific. *Everything* about Twin Lakes made me happy. The lake, the jungle-covered hill, the lawns, the boats, the clubhouse (as my magic castle was called) with its slot machines, my friends running down the hill and jumping into the water, the lurking mystery of the pergola at night. The fat man who was in charge of the club and told jokes in the dining hall, the limitless supply of food, chasing my father on the golf course, dreaming about the possibility that we would have a house of our own on the lake, looking through the thick overgrowth on the hill behind the club, excursions to Lake Geneva and the Fox Lake chain during which we actually were permitted to ride in Hunter Deluxe speedboats instead of gazing wistfully at them. There, at Twin Lakes, the early and middle 1930s was the matrix of my childhood and the matrix of my life.

There were some unpleasant memories: the smell of the outdoor toilets; the death during the winter of a dearly loved Twin Lakes friend (tonsil infection, poor radiant little girl); the day that my father, weary, worn and tired, came to Twin Lakes to tell my mother his business had been wiped out by the advancing Great Depression. Somehow Twin Lakes was never quite the same after that.

The images that had surfaced when Erika was teaching me the age-regression technique of self-hypnosis exploded out of my brain for weeks thereafter. First in my own self-hypnotic exercises, then in ordinary waking consciousness, the whole world of Twin Lakes in the 1930s recreated itself, benignly, vividly, overwhelmingly in my imagination. It was not that I was unaware of the Commodore Barry Country Club's role in my life before Erika had taught me (I was helping her design a questionnaire for a study she was doing on techniques of self-hypnosis in psychoanalytic therapy and she offered to teach me the technique). In the fragment of a memoir I wrote for Gregory Baum's book *Journeys*, published in the early 1970s, I mentioned the

Twin Lakes phenomenon. John Kotre in his "intellectual biography" also cited the Twin Lakes experience in my life. The hypnotic interludes, however, revealed to me the critical influence Twin Lakes still is on my imagination.

The sheer raw vividness and power of the memories constrained me to turn to fiction writing. What until then had been a pipe dream became an obligation, a necessity. In most of my novels the experience of summer and summer resorts while growing up is important not merely as background against which the stories unfold, but as integral parts of the novel's structure. . . .

II

THE NATURE OF HYPNOSIS

For the last three decades Erika Fromm has been quite interested in the nature and phenomena of hypnosis. She views hypnosis as an altered state of consciousness, as a stable reorganization of various ego functions. In this section several of her colleagues address the issue of the nature of hypnosis. Helen J. Crawford's chapter, "Cognitive and psychophysiological Correlates of Hypnotic Responsiveness," seeks to identify psychophysiological correlates to the hypnotic state. Previous reviews on this topic, notably those appearing in Fromm's book on modern hypnosis research (Fromm & Shor, 1972a, 1979), were largely inconclusive. Erika Fromm has always believed that there is a physiological basis to hypnosis. This belief traces its roots to Fromm's interest in the interaction of physiological and psychological processes early in her career following her training with Kurt Goldstein. Crawford gives some more definitive findings on the physiological basis of hypnosis. Taking advantage of sophisticated research technology now available, Crawford is able to demonstrate a variety of physiological parameters to hypnosis. High but not low hypnotizable subjects manifest consistent changes in cerebral metabolism, theta EEG, laterality, and integrated power amplitude during certain hypnotic tasks. Crawford believes that these studies lend physiological support for Fromm's ideas about the shift to primary process activity and the problem-solving nature of hypnosis.

Levitt, Baker, and Hulsey (chapter 6) study the extent to which the hypnotic trance is stable and therefore resistant to situational and relational influences. Their cognitive dissonance experiment is designed to ascertain the extent to which situational manipulations can influence both the stability of the trance state and the transference perceptions of the hypnotist. Their largely negative results suggest that hypnotizability and the relational aspects of hypnosis are relatively stable and resistant to external influences. These results lend support to Fromm's belief that hypnosis is the subject's, not the hypnotist's ability. The permissive hypnotist does not try to direct or manipulate the subject's trance experience as much as to provide a supportive context for the subject's own creative exploration of his or her ability.

The last chapter in the section by Stephen Kahn (chapter 7) elaborates on Fromm's view of hypnosis as an example of creative mastery. Kahn summarizes nearly two decades of research conducted by Fromm and her associates on self-hypnosis. He presents the so-called Chicago Paradigm for self-hypnosis research in which highly hypnotizable subjects were asked to initiate their own self-hypnosis experiences daily over a duration of 4 weeks. This research supports Fromm's evolving view of the ego active/ego receptive nature of hypnosis.

Chapter 5

COGNITIVE AND PSYCHOPHYSIOLOGICAL CORRELATES OF HYPNOTIC RESPONSIVENESS AND HYPNOSIS

HELEN J. CRAWFORD
Virginia Polytechnic Institute and State University

As a sensitive and intuitive clinician, Erika Fromm, through her clinical practice, publications (e.g., Brown & Fromm, 1986, 1987; Fromm, 1987b), and many well attended workshops, has contributed immensely to the furthering of hypnotherapy and hypnoanalysis in the United States, Europe, and Australia. She has had an impact on not only fellow clinicians but also experimental psychologists of rather differing theoretical orientations. Although Fromm emphasized clinical aspects of hypnosis, she recognized equally the importance of validating clinical insights and has pursued laboratory studies of adaptive regression (Gruenewald, Fromm, & Oberlander, 1979) and self-hypnosis (e.g., Fromm et al., 1981). As she noted (Fromm, 1987b):

> In order to generalize our intuitive insights and make them valid insights that are worth transmitting to others, however, we need to test our hypotheses on statistically significant samples of patients. Clinical intuition and scientific exploration must walk, and now *do* walk, hand in hand. (p.215)

This chapter highlights some of the cognitive and psychophysiological research findings, particularly from our laboratory, that support some of Fromm's astute clinical observations about hypnosis.

Fromm (1987b) has further hypothesized that hypnosis involves a dramatic shift in cognitive functioning such that a hypnotically responsive individual shows a significant decrease in sequential, analytical thinking and an increase in holistic, imaginal, and nonanalytical thinking. As Fromm (1987b) noted, during hypnosis this imagery

> constitutes a very powerful uncovering technique because it is a symbolic representation of the activity of the patient's internal world, of unconscious feelings, thoughts, and conflict (Reyher, 1963; Shorr, 1972). Imagery reveals these undercurrents more clearly than logical, reality-oriented, rational thinking . . . hypnotic imagery has often been found to represent problem-solving activity. . . . (pp.216-217)

According to Fromm (1987b), the "most important structural components of the hypnotic process are imagery and fantasy, absorption, dissociation, and various ego modes and attention postures" (p. 216).

Her clinical observations are borne out in numerous correlational studies that demonstrate that hypnotically responsive individuals report more vivid imagery and absorptive involvement during their normal activities as well as during their inner-directed, imaginative experiences (e.g., Crawford, 1989; J. R. Hilgard, 1979; Sheehan, 1979; Tellegen & Atkinson, 1974). Hypnotic responsiveness loads positively on a happy, vivid, and positive daydreaming style in both adults (Crawford, 1982) and children aged 8 to 12 (Allen, 1985). The absorptive involvement leads high hypnotizables to report much greater affect intensity than low hypnotizables to a given emotional experience (e.g., sad or happy emotions) in waking states (Crawford & Brown, 1989) and even more so in hypnosis (Crawford, Clarke, Kitner-Triolo, & Olesko, 1989). Emotional intensity is unrelated to frequency of affective experiences (Diener, Larsen, Levine, & Emmons, 1985).

Interestingly, it is these very cognitive skills of imagery, absorption, and intense, focused, and dissociative-like attention that seem to be magnified during hypnosis. Enhanced imaginal processing of information, particularly when the information to be remembered is literal or untransformed representations, has been shown to be enhanced during hypnosis among hypnotically responsive individuals in visual memory studies (Crawford & Allen, 1983; Crawford, Nomura, & Slater, 1983). In addition, a very small percentage of high hypnotizables can produce eidetic-like visual memory for complex Julesz stereograms during hypnosis (Crawford, Wallace, Nomura, & Slater, 1986; Walker, Garrett, & Wallace, 1976; Wallace, 1978). These studies suggest that "this enhanced processing may be accompanied by reports of shifts in cognitive processing modes from a more verbal, detail-oriented style during waking to a more imaginal, holistic style during hypnosis" (Crawford, 1989, p. 156).

With the advent of psychophysiological studies of cognitive functioning that demonstrated differential hemispheric laterality correlates accompanying analytical and nonanalytical tasks (e.g., for review, see Springer & Deutsch, 1989), a commonly espoused hypothesis since the 1970s has been that hypnosis involves greater right-hemisphere involvement, as evidenced by the enhanced imagery and holistic processing just discussed. Many attempts have been made to identify possible electrocortical correlates of hypnosis (for reviews, see Crasilneck & Hall, 1959; Sabourin, 1982; Sabourin, Cutcomb, Crawford, & Pribram, in press; Sarbin & Sable, 1979). It is only recently however, that there has been growing evidence that there are (a) EEG differences between low and highly hypnotizable individuals, and (b) EEG differences between waking and hypnosis conditions as moderated by hypnotic level.

A robust finding of interest here is differences in characteristic patterns of hemispheric arousal associated with hypnotic susceptibility. During waking, high hypnotizables show significantly greater EEG hemispheric specificity in the alpha band or overall total power at several bipolar recording sites. The EEGs of high hypnotizables are more activated in the left hemisphere when doing analytic tasks and more activated in the right hemisphere when doing holistic, visuospatial tasks. Low hypnotizables are more equally activated in the two hemispheres and show less shifting (e.g., DePascalis & Imperiali, 1984; DePascalis & Palumbo, 1986; DePascalis, Silveri, & Palumbo, 1988; Karlin, Goldstein, Cohen, & Morgan, 1980; MacLeod-Morgan, 1979; MacLeod-Morgan & Lack, 1982; Mészáros, Bányai, & Greguss, 1985). Differential bipolar fronto-central and parieto-occipital asymmetries in the low and high alpha bands during waking and hypnosis were found in low and high hypnotizables during rest, math, and imaginal tasks (Crawford, 1989; Mészáros, Crawford, Szabó, Nagy-Kovács, & Révész, 1989). Sabourin et al. (in press) found that highly hypnotizable individuals demonstrated characteristically higher left-hemisphere power in the beta band, across frontal, central, and occipital monopolar recording sites, during waking rest conditions and hypnosis rest and suggestion conditions than low hypnotizables. There was no difference in right-hemisphere power. Crawford et al. (1989) found consistent asymmetries in frontal and parietal monopolar sites during suggested sad and happy emotional states during waking and hypnosis: Highs showed greater right-than left-hemisphere power in both low and high alpha bands, and low to high beta bands, whereas lows were fairly equal in power in both hemispheres and lower than highs in the right hemisphere. Although much more research needs to be done in this area, we believe these hemispheric specificity differences found between low and high hypnotizables support our hypothesis that highs demonstrate greater cognitive and physiological flexibility than do low hypnotizables (e.g., Crawford, 1989; Crawford & Allen, 1983).

Using laterality ratios (left − right/left + right) of integrated amplitude in different EEG frequency ranges, shifts toward greater right-hemisphere relative to left-hemisphere involvement during hypnosis have been reported for bipolar derivations of occipital-parietal alpha (MacLeod-Morgan, 1982), occipital-temporal total power (Karlin, Cohen, & Goldstein, 1982; LaBriola, Karlin, & Goldstein, 1987), and frontal-occipital alpha and beta (Bányai, Mészáros, & Csokay, 1985; Mészáros et al., 1985). LaBriola et al. (1987) reported greater overall total amplitude in the right hemisphere at occipital-vertex bipolar derivations, whereas two other studies (Mészáros & Bányai, 1978; Morgan, Macdonald, & Hilgard, 1974) did not. However, laterality ratio studies can be criticized as the relative contribution of left-and right-hemisphere activity cannot be determined (e.g., Beaumont, Young, & McManus, 1984).

Using spectral power measures rather than laterality ratios, Crawford, Mészáros, and their associates (Crawford, 1989; Mészáros et al., 1989) found enhancements in alpha and beta power in the right parieto-occipital location during hypnosis in rest, math, and imaginal tasks, in high, but not low, hypnotizable subjects. Chen, Dworkin, and Bloomquist (1981) examined EEG activity at frontal-parietal derivations while a patient was going through dental surgery with hypnosis as the sole anesthetic. They found the total energy output of both left and right hemispheres to decrease, with a greater decrease in the left than right hemispheres in theta and alpha bands.

Studies using monopolar recordings during rest and hypnotic suggestions (Sabourin et al., in press) and during induced sad and happy emotional states (Crawford et al., 1989) found no shifts in power at anterior, central, and posterior (parietal or occipital) locations. The greater inhibition of the left hemisphere during hypnosis has been reported in studies of electrodermal shifts (e.g., Gruzelier, 1987; Gruzelier, Brown, Perry, Rhonder, & Thomas, 1984), but no hemispheric shifts were reported in regional cerebral blood flow studies of hypnosis and waking (Crawford, 1989; Crawford, Gur, Skolnick, Gur, & Benson, 1986).

These divergent findings point out the difficulties we presently have in developing a cohesive evaluation of the cognitive psychophysiological studies of hypnosis as moderated by hypnotic responsiveness level. Individuals were often screened for hypnotic susceptibility level in different manners. Waking and hypnosis conditions are often not comparable across studies due to differences in tasks and rest instructions. Studies of the relationships between electroencephalogram, electrodermal, and cerebral region blood flow arousal patterns are only now beginning. Although most of the psychophysiological work on hypnosis has examined electrocortical (EEG) activity, we are even here limited in our comparisons because of major differences across studies in their choices of electrode placements, recording methods (monopolar vs. bipolar), EEG analysis methods, and EEG frequency bands chosen to be examined.

Certain psychophysiological research does support Fromm's (1987b) observation that "hypnotic imagery has often been found to represent problem-solving activity" (p. 217). If there is an enhancement of problem-solving activity during hypnosis, one might find accompanying psychophysiological changes supportive of such activity. Crawford et al. (1986; Crawford, 1989) studied the effects of rest, ischemic pain without suggested analgesia, and ischemic pain with suggested analgesia in conditions of waking and hypnosis on regional cerebral blood flow as measured by the xenon inhalation method. Low hypnotizables had essentially the same regional cerebral blood flow metabolism patterns across frontal, temporal, parietal, and parieto-temporal regions in both waking and hypnosis conditions, regardless of the presence or absence of pain. High hypnotizables showed dramatic increases from 13% to 28% (highest being in the temporal regions) in regional cerebral blood flow, equally in both hemispheres, in hypnotic rest, pain, and suggested analgesia conditions. These unanticipated findings make sense if we think that hypnosis requires absorption and focused attention—it requires effort and work to be in hypnosis. The enhanced cerebral metabolism is reflective of the enhanced cognitive effort and absorption that accompanies hypnosis. This enhanced cognitive effort is in contrast to the often observed external muscle relaxation during hypnosis.

Increments in theta (approximately 3 to 7 Hz) EEG activity has been associated with many problem-solving, perceptual processing, and cognitive tasks as well as with the production of imagery (for review, see Schacter, 1977; Vogel & Broverman, 1964). Vogel, Broverman, and Klaiber (1968) differentiated between two classes of theta. "Class I inhibition" is associated with general inactivity or drowsiness. "Class II inhibition" is associated with more efficient and attentive performance and represents "a selective inactivation of particular responses so that a continuing excitatory state becomes directed or patterned" (p. 172). If hypnosis involves greater attentional involvement in problem solving, when tasks or problems are presented, then one might anticipate an enhancement of theta during hypnosis (Sabourin, 1982). Increased theta during quiescent meditative states in experienced meditators has also been reported (Banquet, 1973; Corby, Roth, Zarcone, & Kopell, 1978; Elson, Hauri, & Cunis, 1977; Hebert & Lehmann, 1979; Kasamatsu & Hirai, 1969; Saletu, 1987; Taneli & Krahne, 1987). Although not consistently found across studies for reasons yet unknown, several early studies (Galbraith, London, Leibovitz, Cooper, & Hart, 1970; Tebecis, Provins, Farnbach, & Pentony, 1975; Ulett, Akpinar, & Itil, 1972) reported high hypnotizables generated more theta activity than low hypnotizables. In a study of stringently screened high and low hypnotizables, Sabourin et al. (in press; also Sabourin, 1982) found that mean theta power was positively related to hypnotic responsiveness. In both waking and hypnosis, highs generated substantially more theta than lows at occipital, central, and frontal locations. Interestingly, both low and high hypnotizables showed a substantial increase in mean theta power after the hypnotic induction and during hypnotic suggestions, although highs continued to have significantly more power than lows. These differences were most prominent in the frontal and central locations.

Further support for the relationship between theta and problem solving comes from a quite recent preliminary study of the EEG correlates of cold pressor pain (Crawford, 1990). Seven low hypnotizables and four high hypnotizables were stringently screened for hypnotizability level on several hypnosis measures and for strong right handedness. Highs had to be able to eliminate completely all perception of pain during a preliminary cold pressor training session before being accepted into the main study. Monopolar recordings at frontal (F3, F4), temporal (T3, T4), parietal (P3, P4), and occipital (01, 02) regions with references to balanced earlobes was done in counterbalanced conditions of waking and hypnosis on the same day. Within waking and hypnosis there were the following conditions: Prerest baseline, pain dip with no analgesia, suggested hypnotic analgesia without pain, suggested hypnotic analgesia with pain dip, and postrest baseline. The left hand was dipped into cold water for 60 seconds; after 10 seconds the EEG recording was started. During prerest, from 13 to 19 Hz (low beta) and 37 to 42 Hz (high beta) there was more integrated power in hypnosis than waking. Given that hypnosis involves focused attention and the 40 Hz band is associated with focused attention (for review, see Sheer, 1984), this may be indicative of the more overall focused state of all subjects.

As anticipated, during hypnosis, high hypnotizables demonstrated significantly greater power than low hypnotizables within the theta range: high theta (5.5 – 7.5 Hz) but not low theta (3.5 – 5.5 Hz). A comparison of hypnotic pain dips with and without suggested analgesia revealed some fascinating interactions that support our previously stated hypotheses. As shown in Fig. 5.1, during pain and suggested analgesia dips, lows show no significant power asymmetries between the left and right hemispheres at the frontal, temporal, parietal, and occipital regions, whereas the highs showed significant asymmetries in some regions. In the temporal and parietal regions, more so the temporal, the highs were significantly more left hemisphere dominant in the pain dip when they were experiencing pain, and then showed a dramatic shift during the pain dip in which they experienced no pain at all: There was a significant decrease in left-hemisphere theta power and a significant increase in right-hemisphere theta power. Temporal theta may be reflective of hippocampal generated theta (Stumpf, 1965). Thus, the shifts in theta laterality may be indicative of laterality shifit in the septal-hippocampal system. The shift to greater right-hemisphere involvement during hypnotic analgesia when the subjects were vividly imagining themselves to be elsewhere and dissociated from the pain is quite supportive of evidence that

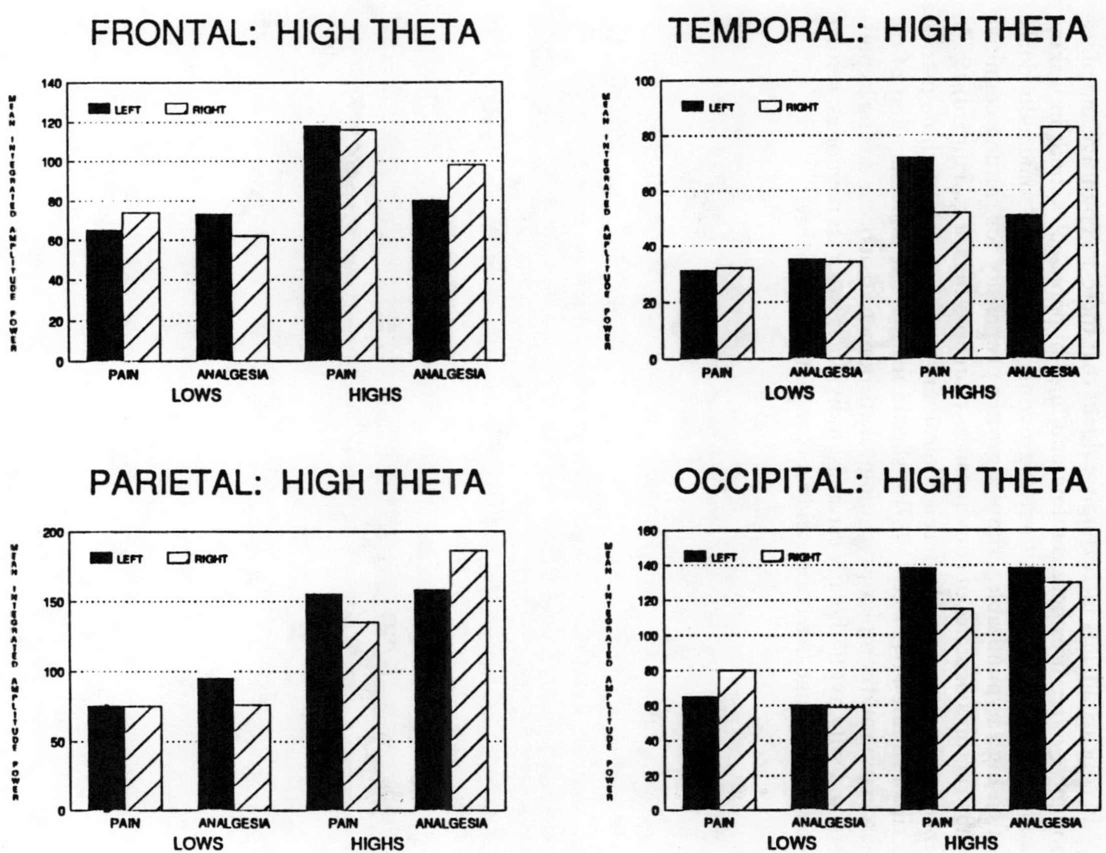
FRONTAL: HIGH THETA
TEMPORAL: HIGH THETA
PARIETAL: HIGH THETA
OCCIPITAL: HIGH THETA
MEAN INTEGRATED AMPLITUDE POWER
LEFT
RIGHT
PAIN
ANALGESIA
LOWS
HIGHS

FIG. 5.1

suggests that the maintenance of vivid imagery is a right hemisphere dominant activity (e.g., Farah, 1988; Springer & Deutsch 1989). Thus, we have evidence for (a) differential hemispheric specificity patterns during painful stimuli in low and high hypnotizables, and (b) shifts in hemispheric dominance during successful hypnotic analgesia in the high hypnotizables.

In conclusion, it is increasingly evident that there are cognitive and physiological differences between low and high hypnotizables, both in waking and hypnosis. In addition, there is growing evidence that some individuals, often high hypnotizables, show a greater propensity for shifting cognitive substructures or states of consciousness than do others (e.g., Hilgard, 1977). Increased cooperation between clinical and experimental psychologists, as Erika Fromm advocated (1987b), should further our understanding of the fascinating and complex psychological phenomena that occur during hypnosis, and why hypnotherapy can assist individuals to access memories, resolve conflicts, change behaviors, and reorganize the personality.

Chapter 6

COGNITIVE DISSONANCE AND THE RESPONSIVENESS OF HIGHLY HYPNOTIZABLE SUBJECTS

EUGENE LEVITT
Institute of Psychiatric Research, Indiana University Medical Centre

ELGAN L. BAKER
Indiana Center for Psychoanalysis and Indiana University School of Medicine

TIMOTHY L. HULSEY
University of Tennessee

The essence of hypnosis has been the focus of a continuing controversy among investigators and theorists since the end of the 19th century. This controversy has spawned a variety of competing constructs for describing and explaining the nature of trance and of hynotic responsiveness. Two significant dimensions along which these theories have varied are the issue of the "involuntariness" of hypnotic behavior and the role of trait versus state variables in determining the specific parameters of responsiveness and experience in trance. Experimental investigation of these core dimensions of hypnosis have been ongoing for at least the past 50 years and have produced a variety of inconclusive or conflicting data, typically interpreted to confirm the pre-existing theoretical bias of the investigators. The current *zeitgeist* of the experimental hypnosis literature has recapitulated these ongoing controversies with the competing views of the contextualists (including Coe, Chaves, Barber, and Spanos) who tend to emphasize situational, social role variables and the neo-dissociationists (including Evans, Fromm, Hilgard, Nash, and Orne) who emphasize the stable centrality of "hypnotizability" with its hypothesized antecedents and phenomenological correlates.

Over the last decade, our laboratory at Indiana University School of Medicine has undertaken a series of empirical studies designed to simultaneously examine the comparative contributions of trait (hypnotizability) versus state (social cues, expectations, motivation, relationship factors) variables to determining hypnotic responsiveness, with a specific focus on the phenomenon of involuntariness as it is perceived by the subject's self-reflection and measured by operationalized behavioral response. Our research has produced a series of publications (Baker & Levitt, 1989; Levitt & Baker, 1983; Levitt, Baker, & Fish, 1990; Levitt et al., in press). The core design of this research has essentially revolved around attempts to induce hypnotized subjects to resist hypnotic suggestions by manipulating a variety of state variables that are "pitted against" the subject's measured level of hypnotizability. Observed responses to hypnotic suggestions have been clarified by examining interview, self-report, and phenomenological inventory data in order to determine the nature of the subject's experience, with special attention to issues of cognitive dissonance, conflict resolution, amnesia, and efforts to give meaning or understanding to the hypnotic experience.

Our results, like those of other researchers who have attempted to examine variables central to the definition of hypnosis, have been somewhat inconsistent and complicated. A summary of our findings to date seems to point to several preliminary conclusions.

First, the experience of hypnosis is heterogeneous. Individuals experience and respond to trance in a variety of ways and likely reflect in their hypnotic responsiveness differing configurations of determining variables. For some subjects, social cues are more potent; for others, relationship factors that may involve transferential projections are more significant determiners of behavioral response. For some subjects, hypnotic experience is primarily motivated by contemporary variables; for others, stable, trait factors appear to be more powerful.

Second, in general, individuals who evidence high levels of hypnotizability seem to be less impacted by contemporary state and contextual variables than subjects with moderate or low hypnotic ability. However, our data suggest that it must be considered highly possible for at least *some* situational variables to alter or to override the influence of at least *some* ordinarily critical trait variables.

Third, interpersonal-relationship factors appear to be powerful variables that may often have a moderating effect in determining hypnotic responsiveness. Further, these variables appear to be even more potent in shaping how individuals process and give meaning to their trance experiences, regardless of their role in producing that experience. These relationship factors often seem to operate in a nonconscious fashion that subjects may not be able to articulate or to rationally explain, suggesting at least some similarity to traditional notions of "transference." In addition, positive perceptions of the hypnotist appear to enhance trance involvement. However, negative perceptions of the hypnotist or other figures attempting to influence hypnotic responsiveness seem to be even more powerful variables in decreasing the subject's behavioral response and post-hypnotic sense of the trance experience.

Finally, external incentives can impact motivational variables and serve to increase hypnotic responsiveness, involuntariness, and the experience of trance, even among high hypnotizables. However, external incentives differ in their ability to impact trait susceptibility. The nature of the difference is probably idiosyncratic to the subject and reflective of his or her dynamics, history, and personality style.

Based on these emerging trends from our data, additional studies have been designed to attempt to further explicate relationships suggested by our earlier work. In particular, efforts have been made to examine the experience of high hypnotizable individuals whose relatively stable capacity for trance involvement and involuntariness has proven the most robust variable across the preceding projects. Further, our data have suggested that high hypnotizable subjects are those most often able to tolerate the inherent conflict or cognitive dissonance produced by the external motivation without alteration of hypnotic responsiveness. The current study was designed to more directly investigate the impact of such dissonance on trance behavior among a group of individuals with measured high hypnotizability.

SUBJECTS AND PROCEDURE

The subjects were 28 volunteers all of whom had scored 8 or higher on the Stanford Hypnotic Susceptibility Scale, Form A (Weitzenhoffer & Hilgard, 1959) and who were able to comply with the time requirements of the project. All subjects were clerical or technical workers, except for three professional persons in the experimental group and one in the control group. They were drawn from a pool of nearly 100 subjects that had been developed for our hypnosis experiments. Subjects were assigned randomly to experimental and control groups with the intent of having 20 in the former and 10 in the latter. Due to failures to report for the experiment, there were actually 19 experimental subjects and 9 control subjects. Of the subjects, 24 were women; there were 2 men in each of the groups. The mean ages for the two groups did not differ (experimental = 36.3; control = 41.0; $t(26) = 1.06$, ns).

The experimental group had a mean score on the SHSS:A of 10.05. The control group mean was 9.11. The difference is not significant [$t(26) = 1.47$, ns].

The experimental group was given the following lecture by one of the experimenters (ELB) in groups of four or five subjects:

> Scientists have been interested in hypnosis for more than 100 years. During that period of time, a great deal of research has been done to try to understand more

> about what hypnosis is and what it can do. Perhaps your experience with being hypnotized has made you curious, too. I would like to tell you some things about hypnosis and some ways that it can be applied in psychology, psychiatry, and medicine. . . . Nearly everyone can be hypnotized. Researchers have determined that hypnosis is an ability that each individual possesses to some degree. Some people have a lot of this ability. Some people don't have very much. That ability, when combined with good motivation in the right situation, can help the individual enter a hypnotic trace. *Some people believe that only people who aren't very bright can be hypnotized. They think that the less intelligent you are, the more you will respond to the hypnotist's suggestion.* It is clear that feeling comfortable with the hypnotist is also an important variable in determining what the experience of hypnosis will be like. . . . Most of the time, hypnosis produces some degree of relaxation.
>
> People who have been hypnotized often describe feeling very comfortable, calm, and quiet. Most people like the experience and feel that it leaves them feeling relaxed and refreshed. Researchers have determined that different people experience trance in different ways. Some people feel like they are floating away; other people feel very, very heavy. Some people can develop very vivid images in trance, much more so than when they are awake. *Some people believe that people will lose all self-control when they are hypnotized and that the hypnotist could make them do anything he wanted, even silly or embarrassing things.* Most people can describe some changes in their experience when they have been hypnotized. Studying these experiences helps us to learn more about the nature of the trance. . . . Hypnosis has been applied in many different clinical situations. It has been used to treat pain problems very effectively. Hypnosis has also been used to help people who have psychological problems like depression or anxiety. Researchers have found that hypnosis can work very well for some people in treating specific kinds of physical problems like high blood pressure, warts, and asthma. *Some people believe that only very dependent, weak-willed, and needy people will respond to suggestions in trance.* Perhaps the most frequent uses of hypnosis in clinical work today are for treating obesity and smoking. Some people are very successful in using hypnosis to work on these problems . . . We hope that your experiences with hypnosis are positive and enjoyable. While I cannot answer any of your questions just now, we would be happy to answer all of your questions and discuss your experiences after this study is complete. . . . Our researchers will now meet you to conduct you to a quiet, private office where you will again have the opportunity to experience hypnosis.

The control group, in two subgroups, heard the identical lecture with the exception of the italicized text. The intent of this misinformation was to implant the notions that susceptible hypnotic subjects tend to be less intelligent, extremely dependent, and out of control under hypnosis compared to less susceptible subjects.

The Stanford Hypnotic Susceptibility Scale, Form B (Weitzenhoffer & Hilgard, 1959) was then administered to each subject individually. Subjects were awakened from the trance immediately after administration of the scale had been completed and the following instruments were employed in an effort to determine possible effects of the pre-trance lecture: an adjective rating form (ARF; Baker & Levitt, 1989) to assess feelings toward the lecturer and the hypnotist; the Archaic Involvement Measure (AIM; Nash & Spinler, 1989) to assess the occurrence of transference-like experience during the trance; and a structured interview in which subjects were asked to tell what they recalled of the lecture. If the three topics were not mentioned spontaneously, experimental group subjects were specifically asked whether they remembered, and what they could recall, about references to intelligence, dependency, and loss of control in the lecture. They were asked how the statements affected them and whether or not they had tried to resist the hypnotist, successfully or unsuccessfully. They were also asked what they thought was the purpose of the experiment.

RESULTS

Exposure to the experimental stimulus had no effect on susceptibility as measured by the SHSS:B [means = 10.16 for the experimental and 8.78 for the control group - $t(26) = 1.47$, ns]; on the perception of the lecturer as measured by the ARF [means = 41.16 for the experimental and 47.44 for the control group, $t(26) = 1.01$, ns]; on the perception of the hypnotist [means = 38.33 for the experimental and 43.78 for the control group, $t(26) = 1.22$, ns]; and on the AIM [means = 73.32 for the experimental and 66.11 for the control group, $t(26) = 0.70$, ns]. Three experimental group subjects and one control group subject reported in the interview that they had attempted to resist the hypnotic induction. This difference is not significant [corrected chi-square (1) = 0.00]. None of the four subjects believed that they had resisted successfully and none had according to SHSS:B scores that were the same as on the SHSS:A, except for one subject who attained a score 1 point higher. A lone control group subject attained a score of 2 after having a pre-experimental score of 10. She did not claim to have resisted and was unable to explain the difference in scores. There were no differences in SHSS:B scores as a function of hypnotists (F 4,23 $= 0.68$, ns).

Recall of the three statements in the experimental lecture was varied but tended to fall into three groups: accurate recall, usually accompanied by an expression of disbelief; inaccurate recall, usually the opposite view or denial attributed to the lecturer; or no recall. Because of the small number of cases, we grouped recalling into accurate and inaccurate, including in the latter absence of recall and the occasional distorted recall ("He said you don't have to be smart to be hypnotized").

For the IQ statement, there were 12 accurate and 7 inaccurate reports; for the dependency statement, 13 accurate and 6 inaccurate; and for the control statement only 4 accurate and 15 inaccurate.

No significant differences were found between the accurate and inaccurate recall groups on any of the dependent variables of the experiment. For example, the SHSS:B means for the accurate and inaccurate recall groups were 10.25 and 10.00 for intelligence, 10.50 and 10.00 for dependency and 10.25 and 10.13 for control. The respective $t(17)$s are 0.51, 1.00, and 0.20, none of which are significant.

Each experimental subject was carefully debriefed by the interviewer after the interview to be certain that the distorted statements were not believed. Despite this customary precaution, no subject in the experimental group, or in the control group as well, correctly identified the purpose of the experiment.

DISCUSSION

On the whole, our results appear to be negative. The lecture failed to produce any behavioral trance effects in the experimental subjects, either in their susceptibility or their perceptions of the experimenters. Failure may be due in part to the simplistic nature of the distortion interventions and to their lack of definiteness. It is probably also partly due to the sophistication of our subjects. For example, 10 of the 12 subjects who correctly recalled the distorted statement linking intelligence and susceptibility indicated that they did not believe the statement. Because this was the first of the three interventions, it may have increased skepticism about the remaining two distorted interventions.

An interesting sidelight of the results is the degree of accurate recall in general. For the intelligence intervention, accurate recall was 63%, about what might be expected with the narrative-interrogatory procedure used by the interviewers (Loftus, 1979). Accurate recall was only 26% for both the dependency and control interventions. The difference between the frequency of accurate recall for the intelligence intervention, and the combined dependency and control interventions is statistically significant [corrected chi-square (1) = 5.88, p .02]. Most of the inaccurate recall for the dependency intervention is due to the 12 subjects who did not recall the intervention at all. However, only one subject failed to recall the control intervention. Two subjects did not recall the intelligence intervention.

Some allusion to repression seems unavoidable. We might speculate that most of our subjects easily brushed aside the distortion concerning susceptibility and intelligence but were forced to adopt stronger measures to avoid the dissonance that would follow from accepting the distortions concerning dependency and control.

Chapter 7

PHENOMENOLOGICAL EXPLORATIONS OF SELF-HYPNOSIS*

STEPHEN KAHN
The University of Chicago

One of the more significant contributions Erika Fromm has made to psychology is in the area of self-hypnosis. Beyond having pioneered the field, she has at the same time advanced the application of phenomenological psychology. Although countless clinicians had utilized self-hypnotic techniques for many years, they have not been systematically explored. Erika Fromm and her colleagues began their research in the early 1970s at the University of Chicago, examining self-hypnosis (SH) by taking an experiential rather than a behavioral approach. By taking this tack, the Chicago group could more completely study aspects of the self that could unfold and come to fruition in the practice of self-hypnosis. A number of questions were posed: What are the contours and boundaries of the SH experience? How does SH compare to traditional, hypnotist-present hypnosis? Can SH be taught by establishing guidelines based on traditional hypnosis? Is there a learning curve involved in the assimilation of SH techniques? What type of individual is more susceptible or skilled in SH?

Research based on these questions, conducted at the University of Chicago by Dr. Fromm and her colleagues since the 1970s, came to be known as the Chicago Paradigm (Johnson, 1981).

---

*Adapted from Fromm E., & Kahn, S. (1990). Summary and thoughts for future research *In Self-hypnosis: The Chicago paradigm* (pp. 219–233). New York: Guilford.

THEORY AND DEFINITIONS

Definitions of hypnosis and self-hypnosis vary according to assumptions that are made about and the perspective that is taken toward them. Expectations of what hypnosis is like define and delimit the parameters of the hypnotic experience, just as expectations, attitudes, and beliefs in general affect and control our perceptions and behavior. Attending to certain aspects of reality enhances one kind of experience, whereas attending to different aspects of the same reality can create a completely different kind of experience. The culture in which one lives provides the basic template of experience and a multitude of options and possibilities with which to frame reality. An individual living within a given culture can "choose" any or all of these possibilities. Usually it is through the consensual validation of other individuals critical to one's physical or emotional survival that specific beliefs are assimilated. Individual beliefs and attitudes thus emerge in the context of the culture.

With respect to hypnosis, a trance or trance-like experience emerges in the context both of the culture and of individual beliefs and attitudes. For instance, although our culture maintains a limited belief in such phenomena as voodoo, a number of Third World cultures validate such activity, considering it to be a crucial part of religious experience. Hypnosis per se, however, is more a Western phenomenon, although it does share some of the same elements, at least for certain individuals. Within our culture, some individuals consider hypnosis to involve a total loss of both control and consciousness, with complete power given to the hypnotist. At the opposite end of the spectrum, hypnosis is conceived of as an active rather than a passive state, with power and will located entirely within the individual.

Hypnotists and subjects alike vary in their views of the hypnotic experience. Hypnotists for many years maintained an authoritarian stance vis-à-vis their subjects; the style, content, and the very wording and intonation utilized reflected this attitude. The hypnotic subject likewise believed that rendering him or herself to hypnosis meant surrendering or even eradicating his or her will. Since World War II, this view has evolved into a more permissive approach. The hypnotist views him or herself as a collaborator or a facilitator of the experience. The capability and the skill for creating and maintaining the trance is seen as residing in the subject. The more sophisticated subject whose contact with hypnosis has gone well beyond that of stage hypnosis or depictions in movies realizes that he or she is the repository of talent for the experience, and that the hypnotist merely provides direction and enhancement for this capability. Thus, as the culture modified general attitudes toward and beliefs about hypnosis, so too has individual experience changed and evolved accordingly.

Rather than reify hypnosis as one specific phenomenon, it is more precise to speak of different kinds of hypnotic experiences. One way of construing hypnosis is to ascertain the relative levels of self (subject) involvement and other (hypnotist) involvement in the experience. At one end of the spectrum, hypnosis is controlled and directed by the hypnotist. At the other end, the phenomenon is qualitatively different; the self initiates and directs the process. (A heuristic representation of this continuum is shown in Fig. 7.1.)

Over the last 17 years, the Chicago group has endeavored to isolate and describe the differences in the hypnotic experience at each end of the spectrum. Hypnosis at Point 5 (other-initiated) was defined by the Chicago group as *hetero-hypnosis* (HH) and the hypnosis at Point 1 (self-initiated) was termed *self hypnosis* (SH).

Both ends of the spectrum do share certain aspects of the hypnotic experience in common. For example, both can be conceived of as an altered state of consciousness in which perception of and interaction with the external environment is changed and absorption in internal experience becomes more profound. Within our culture, certain characteristic changes common to both self-and hypnotist-directed hypnosis are usually involved, including the selective focus of different modes of attention, a more tranquil state of mind and body, perceived involuntarism, incongruous (trance) logic, time distortion, increased memory and imagery, and dissociation.

It should be noted that neither the self (subject) nor the other (hypnotist) can entirely predominate at either end of this continuum. The self cannot solely initiate the experience, because beliefs and expectations have been shaped and colored not only by the culture in which he or she lives, but by exposure to various kinds of hypnosis. Perhaps the purest example of an entirely self-initiated hypnotic trance would be one that spontaneously occurred to someone who had no notion of trance and had never heard of hypnosis before. However, it would be difficult for this individual to comprehend what had occurred, let alone describe it to others.

Similarly, it would be impossible for the self to be entirely eliminated at the opposite end of the spectrum, where the other or hypnotist predominates. No matter how forceful and authoritarian the hypnotist and no matter how much an individual believes his or her will and consciousness will no longer be

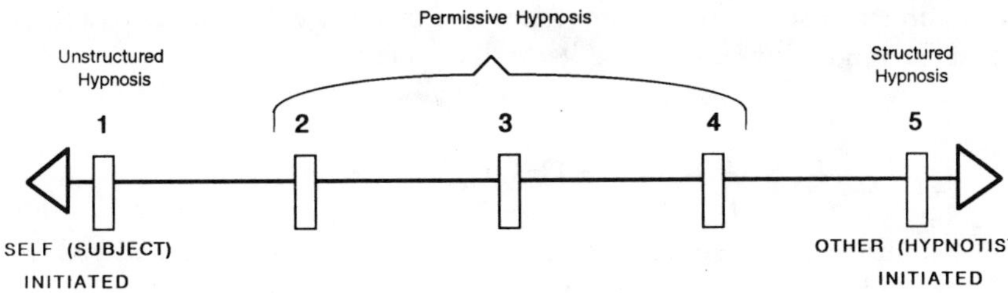

FIG. 7.1 Linear continuum of self (subject) and other (hypnotist) involvement in hypnosis

under his or her control, there still remains a part of the self that is involved. Whether this be called the hidden observer or the idiosyncratic aspects of the fantasies or images suggested by the hypnotist, there is still some aspect of the self that is involved.

At any point during trance, one can locate the kind of experience along the continuum. However, during a particular trance, the relative involvement fluctuates. Although experiences can cluster at one position, they do not remain static. For example, a permissive hypnotist can periodically be silent during trance to allow the subject to pursue more of his or her own private thoughts, fantasies, and suggestions. However, when the hypnotist is giving suggestions and describing them, he or she may move the experience more toward the hypnotist-initiated end of the continuum.

The presence or absence of the hypnotist is irrelevant in determining where on the continuum the subject experiences his or her involvement. An individual can achieve a deep state of hypnosis without any kind of hypnotic aids (e.g., a pendulum) and in the absence of a hypnotist. Moreover, the individual may still find him or herself more toward the "other-initiated" end (Point 5) of the spectrum than toward the "self" end (Point 1). For example, a subject without a hypnotist can vividly imagine his or her presence and create a very rigidly defined and constricted experience based on suggestions and responses enacted "as if" hypnotist and structure were very much present.

Similarly, in the presence of the hypnotist an individual can use the structure provided to create an experience very much attuned to what the hypnotist is suggesting (Point 5). In the absence of structure, an individual can create an experience based on direction provided by the self (Point 1). A subject even in the presence of an authoritarian hypnotist who intrusively attempts to direct and structure as much of the experience as possible may engage in a self-directed experience despite the intrusions. Thus, SH (with the hypnotist absent) is not necessarily to be found at Point 1 and HH (even with the hypnotist present) is not necessarily at Point 5, although this is certainly more likely.

With this clarification of self-versus-other involvement, it is useful to view *all* hypnosis as falling along this continuum of initiation, because who initiates, directs or suggests different aspects of the trance determines to a large extent the kind of hypnotic experience that emerges.

RESEARCH METHOD AND RESULTS

The Fromm group defined SH as hypnotic experiences engendered by self-directed suggestions as well as by self-directed responses. The focus of investigation here involves the experiential rather than behavioral aspects of SH. The subjects in these studies each were given a standard set of "laboratory-defined" hypnotic tasks, but were encouraged to use this only as a point of departure for exploring self-hypnosis. This gave more reign to the self and opened up the possibility for all to experience SH at Point 1 on the spectrum.

The research conducted by Dr. Fromm and her colleagues on SH falls into three distinct phases. Throughout these phases, the clinical implications and applications of SH were being formulated and expressed. Each successive phase explored the phenomena more systematically and fully. The results, however, were comparable.

Phase I, 1972–1975

The first phase involved conceptualization and two preliminary studies. In the first, 36 male and female students at the University of Chicago were given a hypnotic and a self-hypnotic experience, each lasting 90 minutes. All were interviewed extensively afterward in a relatively unstructured manner. In the second study performed about 1 year later, three male and three female subjects were given three standard hypnosis experiences and were asked to induce self-hypnosis each day for 4 weeks. Each subject chronicled his or her SH experiences in a daily journal entry.

From the study it was readily apparent that reality-oriented and primary-process imagery characterized the SH experience more vividly than in the standard hypnotic experience. Also, the role of a directing part of the ego came to light through the pilot studies in SH. In standard hypnosis, researchers have identified a split between the part of the self that watches (observing ego) and the part of the self that undergoes the experience (experiencing ego); an additional directing and suggesting self (ego activity) is prominent in SH. Ego Receptivity—a mode of consciousness in which deliberate control of internal experience, critical judgment, and goal-directed activity are temporarily relinquished, and preconscious material is allowed to emerge—was also a salient feature of successful SH (Deikman, 1971). Further, successful subjects were more able to structure their own SH experience, discovering new features and approaches. This seemed to foster an ability to incorporate SH into their lifestyle. Finally, only highly hypnotizable subjects seemed able to discern differences in the self- versus other-directed hypnotic states. This set of capabilities represented the first glimmerings of a personality type that seemed to flourish in SH.

Phase II, 1976–1981

In the second phase, working hypotheses and other questions about successful SH and SH subjects were formulated in detail. Extensive questionnaires based on ideas that had been gleaned from the results of the pilot studies were created, administered, and analyzed. In these questionnaires, the subjects were asked to retrospectively rate and judge how much or how little of various phenomena they had experienced during SH. This represents a subjective experiential approach (Shor, 1979).

Three extensive surveys were designed to assess the many facets of SH. The first examined these experiences in and of themselves without reference to another mode. The second survey examined SH over time (4 weeks), and the third compared SH to standard hypnosis. The surveys were administered to 58 highly hypnotizable subjects free from psychopathology, that were selected from an original group of 425 volunteers. Highly susceptible individuals were selected for participation because pilot studies indicated that these subjects would be the most capable of making distinctions and discriminations among the various kinds of hypnotic states and because facility in being induced into a standard hypnotic state seemed to aid some subjects in experiencing self-hypnosis. Examining the self-hypnotic state, and charting its boundaries and features at higher levels of hypnotizability could facilitate clarification and discrimination at lower levels.

The subjects were given a number of measures including: HGSHS:A (Weitzenhoffer & Hilgard, 1959); the SHSS:C (Weitzenhoffer & Hilgard, 1962); the SPSHS, forms I and II (Weitzenhoffer & Hilgard's 1967); the Rorschach (1949); the Minnesota Multiphasic Personality Inventory (MMPI) by W. G. Dahlstrom, Welsh, and L. E. Dahlstrom (1972, 1975); Jackson's (1974) Personality Research Form (PRF); and the Personality Orientation Inventory (Shostrom, 1972). Of the 58 highly hypnotizable subjects, 33 volunteers formed the pool of subjects that participated for the next decade. Nearly all were undergraduate or graduate students at the University of Chicago, 17 to 26 years of age. The oldest was 46. The mean age of the sample was 25.18, with a standard deviation of 9.04. These subjects evidenced a strong theoretical orientation, a high level of curiosity, and a disregard for the opinions of others. The men demonstrated "sex-role flexibility," whereas the women tended to be more stereotypically feminine.

Before the experimental sessions began, subjects were given Weitzenhoffer and Hilgard's (1967) SPSHS:I as well as the HGSHS, and the SHSS:C. Thus, subjects had become familiar with standardly defined laboratory hypnosis. The personality measures were administered before the subjects began practicing SH.

During the 4 weeks of the experiment, subjects kept daily journals in which they detailed the contents of their self-hypnotic experiences. Each subject practiced SH alone in a stimulus-free environment, daily, for 1 hour. Subjects were instructed to make entries in their journals every day immediately following their self-hypnotic sessions. The descriptions of the self-hypnotic sessions in these journals served as the raw data from which imagery production, SH Imaginative Involvement, and Ego Receptivity ratings were made.

Subjects were told to monitor their self-hypnotic depth with the slightly revised version of the Extended North Carolina Scale (ENCS; Tart, 1979b) three times per self-hypnotic session, recording these in their journals. The SPSHS:I was given before the experiment began and readministered at the end of the experiment. Form II was given midway through the experiment. At the end of the 4 weeks, each subject completed a series of questionnaires detailing their experiences over the month.

In order to minimize experimenter effects, monitoring of the subjects during the 4 week period was limited to weekly telephone calls and biweekly meetings. No suggestions were given during these meetings as to the content of the journals. Throughout the month-long experiment, the subjects' SH experiences were essentially self-directed.

Results indicated that the fading of the GRO and Absorption provided the structure for both SH and standard hypnosis, whereas Ego Receptivity (ER), free-floating attention, and fluctuations in trance depth characterized self-initiated SH. Ego Activity (EA) was also clearly present in SH, as was a shifting or mixture of ER and EA. Not all attention was expansive; selective concentration provided a backdrop for the experience. In terms of the content, vivid, idiosyncratic imagery again was powerfully salient, with personal memories and adventures emerging with great frequency. Although a number of subjects specifically attempted age regression in SH, most felt that they were more successful with age regression in the structured hypnosis situation. Time distortion was a part of the SH experience as well. Longitudinally, Ego Receptivity, imagery, confidence in the ability to enter and maintain trance, and Trance Depth increased over time, whereas anxiety and doubt decreased. The personality results were mixed, although it was clear that individuals with a seeking, more open, spontaneous stance toward life were more successful in SH.

Phase III, 1982–1990

The third phase of the Chicago group's research focused on the analysis of SH experiences chronicled in daily diary entries. These analyses isolated patterns and themes by examining the process of the immediate experience. This represented a phenomenological approach that enlists the subject as a collaborator in surveying the experience and in delineating its underlying structure and dimensions (Shor, 1979). In this third phase, the constructs delineated in the first two phases were explored in finer detail in the diaries. Through systematic analysis of the subject's experiences, as documented in their own words in the diaries they kept, the results emerged with greater power and clarity, and could be related to personality factors that appeared on the PRF and the POI.

The frequency and function of Ego Activity (EA) and Ego Receptivity (ER) and alternations between them were tabulated and scored. EA occurs more frequently than ER and provides the structure for the unfolding of SH. ER allows facets of the self to emerge by providing the context to allow them to bubble up from the unconscious. Although more EA is actually found in SH, ER seems to be more at the heart of the experience. The rhythm of alternation between EA and ER is dictated by the needs of the individual, who at times needs structure and guidance in the face of overwhelming affect, and who at other times, can work through some of the emotions salient in his or her unconscious and preconscious life. One of the most important findings was that a specific cluster of personality traits influences the experience. An independent person who is at ease with him or herself, is spontaneous and open to experience and to his or her emotions, is able to allow more ER in SH. When EA predominates heavily over ER, the experience becomes dull and constricted. The rigid, nonspontaneous, and externally oriented individual tends to have this torpid type of SH trance.

In terms of SH imagery, both reality-oriented and primary-process imagery were found at the core of SH, particularly for females. ER and imagery go hand in hand, but imagery is the *sine qua non* of self-initiated SH, in that it influences trance depth beyond the influence of ER. Again some striking sex differences emerged, and personality characteristics were found to be influential primarily for the women in the sample. The more available one's impulses, the more outgoing, and the more self-actualized, the more profound and vivid is the imagery.

The assessment of SH trance depth with the ENCS was demonstrated to be quite effective. Although trance depth seems to indicate the overall quality of the experience, it is a less central variable than either ER or imagery production. Personality characteristics are less influential here. The pattern parallels the findings with ER and imagery; the more spontaneous, outgoing and self-actualized individual experiences greater trance depth in SH.

The Fromm group also measured how engrossed and involved the subjects became *during* trance (i.e., an *in vivo* assessment, which was called SH Absorption/Fascination). Although related to the trait of Absorption (Tellegen & Atkinson, 1974), this was a very different measure, in that it occurred less frequently than other aspects of SH and was a specialized feature. Not every SH trance was completely absorbing and filled with wonderment, but when the SH trance was heightened to this extent, the influence of personality characteristics became the most profound. Again, the self-actualized individual and who readily experiences impulses also found him or herself more easily absorbed and fascinated.

Finally, when the SH variables (Ego Receptivity, Depth, Absorption, and Imagery Production) were summarized into one composite measure and the personality variables (Self-actualization, Impulsivity, Outgoingness, and

Susceptibility) into another, a very strong relationship between the two sets emerged.

DISCUSSION

Why did personality style make such a difference when research previously has been hard put to find a relationship between hypnosis variables and personality traits? Understanding the ways in which this research differs from previous studies may shed some light on this question.

As mentioned previously, the Chicago group took an experiential approach to the study of SH. This approach differs markedly from a behavioral line of research in SH, taken by Lynn Johnson (Johnson, Dawson, Clark, & Sikorsky, 1983 ; Johnson & Weight, 1976). Johnson defined SH as hypnotic experiences induced and maintained through self-directed responses. Its exponents hold that the subject is engaging in SH as long as the subject is directing his or her own hypnotic activity, regardless of whether the task is suggested by the hypnotist or even regardless of whether the hypnotist is present or absent. Taking standard hypnosis as its baseline, this definition is operationalized as a specific set of *behaviors* that are readily observed and recorded. Thus, referring back to Fig. 7.1 researchers like Johnson and his collaborators or Ruch (1975), who found little difference between what they call SH and standard hypnosis, may simply have compared two experiences at the same point on the continuum of other versus self-direction depicted.

By contrast, Fromm and her associates assessed via the phenomenological method, thereby tapping its richer and more varied aspects. Specific behavioral aspects of SH were considered less important and therefore occupied a less central focus. Furthermore, the specific type of SH examined was self-*initiated*, rather than simply being the self-directed execution of hypnotist-initiated tasks. This allowed more of the self to emerge, making for more individual differences in the experiences. Consequently, personal style could have more of an impact. Finally, each of the aspects of SH (Ego Receptivity, Imagery, Depth, Absorption/Fascination, etc.) was assessed separately by objective judges and a great number of data points were analyzed. Hypnotizability assessment generally involves much fewer instances of behavior. It is likely that the increased frequency of response over a period of time heightened the accuracy of the measures.

In summary, the Fromm group took a different approach and emerged with new and exciting results. Later phenomenological research confirmed and validated earlier, more exploratory subjective findings through a more painstaking and refined method that tapped a more profound aspect of the phenomenon of self-initiated SH. The level of correspondence with the earlier findings may provide some of the convergent validity (Campbell & Fiske, 1959) that is so essential to scientific endeavor. However, given the exploratory nature of our research, there are a number of caveats and guides for the future taken up in the next section.

FUTURE RESEARCH

The Sample. The small size of our sample, although allowing a wealth of intraindividual (ideographic) analyses, nonetheless limits more general (nomothetic) considerations. It is appropriate for exploratory research. But such a small sample (33 subjects) limits statistical inference and generalizability. Future research should be conducted on larger samples.

These samples should also be randomized to include the full range of hypnotizability and motivation. In order to most clearly discriminate differences between SH and standard hypnosis, only highly hypnotizable subjects were used in the final sample. Future research needs to explore the differences in the population at large to be certain that the effects we found are not simply artifacts due to a rarefied sample.

Gender differences need to be consistently explored as well. These emerged in the two variables at the heart of SH, Ego Receptivity and Imagery. Furthermore, different personality characteristics influence imagery for men and women. Future research on self-hypnosis needs to examine and take into account gender differences.

Motivational and personality characteristics also need to be randomized. An unpaid subject who for 4 weeks spends 1 hour daily in SH is indeed unusual considering that almost half of our original sample dropped out of the experiment at various points. The remainder, our experimental group comprised entirely of volunteer unpaid subjects, must have been very highly motivated. A study of less motivated individuals might yield different results.

One final consideration regarding the sample involves the historical context in which the experiment was conducted. It was a period following the political unrest and social ferment of the 1960s. Those high-minded individuals who were interested in political change also seemed to gravitate toward an interest in expansion of the limits of the mind (and thus to experiments in hypnosis). Would a sample taken at a time less characterized by idealism, interest in social change, and the popular search to understand the inner workings of the mind, react the same way to SH and demonstrate the same results found in our sample?

Standards of Comparison. Throughout the research, the different aspects (e.g., Imagery) of SH were compared to each other and to standard hypnosis.

However, there is no standard of comparison to the waking state. Although certain phenomena occur more frequently in SH than in standard hypnosis, it is not clear how much more frequently. Future studies can remedy this situation by instructing a group of subjects to report daily over consecutive stretches of time on the occurrence of such phenomena in the waking state, in HH, and in SH.

Combination of Approaches. Research with the Chicago Paradigm derives its theoretical research base from the phenomenological perspective (Fromm, Brown, Hurt, Oberlander, Boxer, & Pfeifer, 1981). As Orne and McConkey (1981) suggested, one must utilize behavioral measures along with phenomenological approaches to provide convergent assessment of the phenomenon of SH. Convergent assessment can clarify the boundaries of SH, throw into further relief the distinctions between SH and standard hypnosis, and further specify how personality influences the hypnotic experience. Thus, in addition to administering retrospective questionnaires (the subjective approach) and rating or analyzing ongoing accounts of the subject's experience (the phenomenological approach), observable and operationally defined behaviors need to be developed further and assessed (the behavioral approach).

CONCLUSION

The study of self-initiated SH undertaken at the University of Chicago under the auspices of Erika Fromm has clearly borne fruit. The experiential approach is a viable and productive strategy for highlighting the phenomena of self-initiated SH and clarifying the relationship of personality to this particular altered state of consciousness. Crucial differences between self-initiated SH and standard hypnosis have emerged, primarily in the area of Ego Receptivity. SH seems to be characterized by the relinquishing of active control in favor of allowing the stream of consciousness to dictate the direction of the trance, thereby enhancing the emergence of preconscious material. In addition, the more spontaneous, self-actualized and open to internal impulses an individual is, the more likely it is that a fuller, richer SH experience will unfold. The research has demonstrated that hypnosis and self-hypnosis are not unidimensional phenomena that can only be assessed through behavioral measures. It has clearly shed some light on the varieties of hypnotic experience and the kinds of people who experience them.

III

THE CLINICAL RELEVANCE OF HYPNOSIS

Erika Fromm had a major interest in hypnosis because of its clinical application. In this section a variety of her colleagues discuss the application and efficacy of hypnosis in clinical practice. Germain Lavoie's chapter, "Clinical Hypnosis: A Psychodynamic Approach," is a substantial overview of the field of clinical hypnosis written from an ego-psychoanalytic perspective. The chapter begins with a discussion of hypnosis as an ability of the patient, not of the hypnotist. Lavoie then reviews the main features of the hypnotic trance that are relevant to clinical practice, such as changes in attention, hallucinations, dissociation, dreams, imaginative involvement, access to memories and feelings, age regression, reactivation of self and object representations, transference manifestations and the operations of defenses in trance. He and Erika Fromm share an interest in the psychodynamics and ego activity of trance. Although Fromm puts greater emphasis on the exploration of primary process manifestations and coping resources in hypnoanalysis, Lavoie discusses the interpretation of transference in hypnoanalysis in great detail. The chapter concludes with an overview of the clinical applications of hypnoanalysis in the treatment of psychosomatic conditions, neurotic adjustment and behavioral problems, and in the treatment of severe psychopathology such as psychotic and borderline conditions.

Spinhoven's chapter, "The Clinical Relevance of Hypnotic Susceptibility," reviews the complex issues of assessing hypnotizability in the clinical setting. Standard scales designed to assess hypnotizability have been commonly used in clinical research. However many clinicians have objected to their use in clinical practice. Spinhoven reviews the pros and cons of using such standard instruments in the clinical situation. These scales may be useful in apportioning the relative influence of expectations effects, relaxation, the therapeutic relationship and hypnotizability, to the overall treatment effect. However, standard scales of hypnotizability do not provide adequate information to assess the complex interplay of variables that may affect clinical outcome.

Spinhoven's perspective on the measurement of hypnotizability is reminiscent of Fromm's early work on psychological testing. Fromm did not see intelligence as a unitary and stable trait. She saw it as composed of a variety of complex dynamically relevant variables. Likewise, Spinhoven reminds us that hypnotizability may not be a unitary and stable trait, as has been assumed in research, but a gestalt of numerous dynamic, state, and trait variables that shift according to the clinical situation. The sensitive hypnotherapist is able to appreciate this complexity and accurately assess the relative influence of the many factors which affect the response of the patient to treatment.

Jean Holroyd's chapter, "How Hypnosis May Potentiate Psychotherapy," focuses on the clinical efficacy of hypnosis. She reviews nine characteristics of the hypnotic trance relevant to the effectiveness of hypnotherapy over nonhypnotic psychotherapy. These trance characteristics bear some resemblance to Erika Fromm's discussion of ego parameters in hypnosis and other altered states of consciousness (Fromm, 1981). In fact, both Holroyd and Fromm began writing independently about the clinical efficacy of hypnosis around the same time and later discovered that their views had much in common. In Holroyd's chapter, and also in Fromm's work on the clinical efficacy of hypnosis (Brown & Fromm, 1986), we see a similar view of how the hypnotic trance facilitates greater access to imagery, affects, bodily processes, and archaic self and object representations central to the process of change in hypnotherapy.

The final chapter in this section, by Strauss, addresses the possible negative effects of hypnosis. Strauss reminds us that the incidence of psychological sequelae to hypnosis is low (3%), and that most reported problematic effects are mild. The sources of negative effects in either the clinical or experimental situation may be patient characteristics, therapist characteristics, the nature of the hypnotic intervention, or the way particular suggestions are worded. In her thorough review, Strauss emphasizes that hypnosis is rarely dangerous, but can become an instrusive experience for particular patients treated by some therapists with certain approaches. Erika Fromm might add that such negative effects are less likely to occur when permissive hypnosis is used and open-ended suggestions are given that support the patient's coping ability.

Chapter 8

CLINICAL HYPNOSIS: A PSYCHODYNAMIC APPROACH*

GERMAIN LAVOIE
Hôpital Louis-H. Lafontaine
and
Université de Montréal
Montréal, Canada

HYPNOSIS

Definition

According to Kihlstrom (1985) hypnosis can be defined as:

> a social interaction in which one person, designated the subject, responds to the suggestions offered by another person, designated the hypnotist, for experiences involving alterations in perception, memory and voluntary action. In the classic case, these experiences and their accompanying behavior are associated with subjective conviction bordering on delusion, and involuntariness bordering on compulsion.(p. 386)

Hypnotizability

Contemporary research regards hypnotizability (or the capacity to be hypnotized) as an aptitude of the subject. Using the Stanford scales (Weitzenhoffer & Hilgard, 1959, 1962), subjects undergo a process of hypnotic

*Translated from Lavoie, G. (1988). Hypnose clinique. In P. Lalonde, F. Grunberg et al. (Eds.), *Psychiatrie clinique: Approche bio-psycho-sociale* (pp. 1216—1240). Montreal: Gaëtan Morin.

induction and are then submitted to 12 suggestions. The success rate of young adults according to form C of the Stanford scales is as follows (Hilgard,1965):

- very high hypnotizability (11 out of 12 items): 5% of subjects;
- high hypnotizability (8–10 items): 21% of subjects;
- average hypnotizability (5–7 items): 29% of subjects; and
- low hypnotizability (0–4 items) 45% of subjects.

The Stanford scales serve as the standard against which other scales of hypnotizability are validated (Hilgard, 1979b, Kihlstrom, 1985). The reliability of the Stanford scales (Formula 20 of Kuder-Richardson) is approximately 0.85. The test–retest reliability is in the order of 0.90 with change of hypnotist in the retest situation (Hilgard, 1965). Michaud, Lavoie,Elie, and Amar (1987) obtained a correlation of 0.68 across two measures of hypnotizability at an interval of 10 to 17 years in a group of 27 male schizophrenics. Piccione, Hilgard, and Zimbardo (cited in Hilgard, 1987) reported a test–retest correlation of 0.69 in a group of 24 normal male subjects tested at an interval of 25 years. Such stability over such long periods is close to that of intelligence tests. Some cross-sample studies suggest that hypnotizability decreases with age after having attained a peak around the age of 9 or 10. However, recent longitudinal studies (Hilgard, 1987, Michaud et al., 1987) report no decrease in hypnotizability with age. Finally, the correlation between the "depth" of the hypnotic experience and hypnotizability score is high, being somewhere in the order of 0.85 to 0.88 (Perry & Laurence, 1980).

Hypnotic responsiveness thus appears to be a stable individual ability. Over time most subjects show minor changes of aptitude in the range of one or two points; in a small number of subjects changes of three to four points are observed, and major changes are the exception. These changes can be explained either by an actual change in ability itself, or by situational factors.

Measuring Hypnotizability

The most expedient and certain way to discover the hypnotizability of any subject is to measure it. Any one of Forms A, B, or C of the Stanford scales (Weitzenhoffer & Hilgard, 1959, 1962) requires approximately 45 minutes to administer. Stanford clinical scales, either adult or children's version, require approximately 20 minutes (Morgan & Hilgard, 1979a, 1979b) while the Hypnotic Induction Profile (Spiegel & Spiegel, 1978) takes from 5 to 10 minutes. The longer scales have of course a higher reliability than the shorter forms (E. Hilgard,1982; Kihlstrom, 1985). Weitzenhoffer's (1957, 1989) classical works provide an excellent starting point for the clinician interested in hypnosis, along with that of Crasilneck (1980) concerning the preparation and evaluation of patients. Clinical practicum and supervision and enrollment in training seminars given by professionally recognized scientific associations are normal requirements.

Hypnotic Induction Phase

Given high hypnotizability, strong motivation, a favorable context coupled with an attitude of curiosity and interest on the part of the subject and total clinician–patient rapport, the formal induction phase is reduced to a minimum. A simple gesture, word, or sign may suffice to engage the patient in the hypnotic experience. There are even reports of hypnosis being induced merely upon meeting the clinician by whom the subject wished to be hypnotized, without the least intention on the part of the clinician to engage in hypnosis at that moment. Although the first induction may take from 15 to 45 minutes, subsequently in the clinical setting it may often require no more than 2–3 minutes.

An Example of a First Hypnotic Induction in the Context of Psychotherapy. Above all, the clinician should take his or her time and speak slowly. He or she should ask the patient to sit down comfortably, take a moment to adopt a relaxed position, then keeping the head straight, fix a point placed somewhere in the upper part of the visual field, to put aside all preoccupations, and to do nothing other than listen effortlessly to that which the clinician is about to say, without trying to understand or remember anything. The clinician indicates to the patient that there is nothing to decide, nothing to analyze, nothing to plan for the the moment, and that once again all that is required is that the patient listen freely and effortlessly just as he or she has already been doing. Observing attentively, the clinician reflects as best as possible that which the patient is likely to be feeling, such as tired eyes, blinking of the eyelids "which feel like they want to close," a feeling of ever increasing relaxation, of interest in what is happening and in what is going to happen. The clinician supports the patient in this experience and encourages him or her to let his or her eyelids close when they become too heavy, to let his or her body relax and to observe his or her breathing, which is becoming deeper, more even, and more regular, saying that with each breath the patient is becoming more relaxed, calm, and tranquil. The clinician points out that all this is happening effortlessly. He or she helps the patient to observe the effect of his or her words and how readily they work through him or her encouraging the patient once again to continue listening freely for the moment without trying to understand what is happening.

If the patient feels that what is happening is real to the point that his or her only experience is that of basking in the voice that surrounds him or her, or he or she has already internalized the voice to the extent that it is molding his or her subjective experience, then the patient is well and truly committed to the hypnotic path.

From then on the clinician may point out to the patient how very easy it is for him or her to direct his or her attention to different aspects of the experience, starting for example with the state of total immobility in which the patient now finds him or herself, but of which undoubtedly, he or she had been quite unaware until this moment. He or she may say for example that if the patient is not moving it is not because he or she was unable or because he or she is no longer able to do so, but because in fact the patient has not been asked to move, and that actually the patient really does not feel like moving. The clinician may say, for example: "Obviously you could move if you had to but you are feeling very good now just the way you are. You realize, in fact, how easy and comfortable it is to do just one thing: to listen to my voice and let my words act through you."

The clinician takes care to observe and monitor the patient's reactions in order to construct his or her discourse according to the subjective experience of the patient. Empathy and identification play a most important role at this point. The clinician reflects the patient's own images, giving verbal feedback about what the patient is silently experiencing. The patient should be able to recognize him or herself in the words of the clinician. If, for example, by way to verifying intersubjective rapport, the clinician interjects into his or her speech the simple question: "Isn't that so?", the patient typically responds by nodding the head or an "hm hm" indicating: "You are right, things are happening in me just as you say " (Erickson, Rossi, & Rossi, 1976).

The clinician may also add: "You are doing very well. This is your own experience and you may let it deepen as much as you wish, easily, effortlessly, whether you speak or you remain silent, whether I speak to you or I remain silent. In hypnosis you don't have to attend to time or space. In fact you can readily and without effort transport yourself anywhere you wish. You may remain in this state until I let you know clearly, in time and place, the hypnosis is terminated."

Involuntary Resistance to Induction

Situational Resistances. The clinician should be especially attentive to the various situational resistances that may occur during induction and that may manifest themselves through such indications as frowning or facial tension, body rigidity, perspiration, or a worried expression. Sometimes the patient simply opens his or her eyes and announces: "It's not working." After having invited the patient to talk about what is bothering him or her and to say if he or she wishes to continue the trance but is afraid that he or she won't succeed, the clinician then ascertains that there is no contraindication, transference, or countertransference obstacle in the way, and simply reminds the patient of the basic rule, which is to do nothing and suspend all critical judgment for time being. The clinician reminds the patient that he or she does not need to ask him or herself if he or she is able or not, if things are going well or not. The patient may be advised, that if distractions or questions arise in his or her mind, all that is required is that the patient do his or her best not to pay attention to them, in order to attend as best as he or she can to the words of the clinician. All that the patient has to do is to let him or herself be carried away by the voice and the words of the hypnotist, if that is what the patient really wants. One may go so far as to assure the patient that he or she can always interrupt the process and resume communication in the usual way if he or she wishes. The apprehension that may be experienced during the first hypnotic induction requires the utmost attention. It is usually tied to fantasies of danger related to the emergence of memories of traumatic experiences. The difficulty is often related to anxious and nonverbalized memories of anesthesia related to childhood operations. This kind of resistance also reveals the way in which the patient is experiencing the immediate relationship with the clinician (J.R. Hilgard, 1979).

Techniques of Utilizing the Resistance. Milton H. Erickson refined the technique of utilizing resistance to advantage in hypnosis (Erickson et al., 1976). One of the essential elements in this approach consists of the use of paradox and double bind during the induction process. Also every response of the patient, no matter what, may be interpreted as being adequate:

"Do you wish to sleep now or wait a few minutes ?"

"Let's wait and see if your eyes will stay open or if they will close, and if later on you will feel heavy or light, or just simply normal."

"Let's see if your mind will be clearer or confused, or if it will see some things clearer than others."

"Perhaps your right hand will feel lighter than your left, unless the opposite occurs. Or maybe both will feel the same, equally light . . . or heavy."

"If your unconscious is ready to experience the trance your right hand will rise by itself . . . if not, it will be your left hand."

Each of these statements implies that the response of the subject, whatever it may be, will in fact be the right one, and moreover will serve to indicate the progress of the induction process.

To imagine that all resistance can be overthrown and the subject thus "tamed" by the masterful use of paradoxical communication would be a distortion of Erickson's thinking. Above all, it would place the clinician in an attitude of manipulation contrary to his or her own best interests and those of the patient. Likewise, it would promote the consolidation of an illusion and dominance–submission in the area of the intersubjective relationship exactly where in fact the task is to discover, with the help of another, that it is possible to free oneself from needless pressures. One of the best analyses of Erickson's clinical attitude in this respect is that of Haley (1967a). Elsewhere, Hilgard (1984) and Weitzenhoffer (1989) published thoughtful scientific evaluations of Erickson's thinking. Unfortunately, the current vogue in Ericksonian practice goes far beyond its scientific foundation (Baker, 1987; Fromm, 1987b).

The Hypnotic State (Trance)

The concepts of hypnotic state or trance are far from being clear (Hilgard, 1987), especially when we take into consideration the distribution of hypnotizability and the variations in hypnotic "depth." It is not a state of limited consciousness complete with exact boundaries and specific physiological characteristics. The clinician will be attentive for the following processes likely to support his or her endeavours, and that are defined more or less by what is referred to in the literature as the "hypnotic state" (Gill & Brenman, 1959; Hilgard, 1965,1977):

1. an exclusive relationship between patient and clinician that strikes the observer, as patient and clinician alike seem to be set apart from the surrounding world; it is the "hypnotic rapport" of the ancients, the hypnotic transference, ancestor of the psychoanalytic transference (Lagache,1952).
2. the selective, voluntary relinquishing by the patient of
   - critical judgment,
   - reality testing,
   - planning and executive functions, which are placed at the disposal of the development and maintenance of the trance;
3. a feeling of effortless experiencing on the part of the patient;
4. a particular attentional mobility that readily cathects representations that are more difficult to access in the awake state;
5. an intense capacity for absorption and focusing on certain emotions and representations;
6. a strong imaginative involvement where the word takes on the significance of the thing and where what is ordinarily experienced as imaginary becomes real;
7. the possibility of producing temporary modification of ego functions (see section on "Phenomenology of Hypnosis")

8. the possibility of establishing dialogue and intersubjective communication analogous to that of the waking state (see "Choice of approach")

9. an increase in suggestibility evoking a flexibility in which the patient has the tendency to appropriate the words of the clinician and genuinely live that which is expressed only in a complex play of introjection, projection, and identification (see "Object Relations").

Termination of Hypnosis

The termination should be clear, clean, precise, and verified to avoid the risk that the patient remain in a state of confusion or dissociation. The clinician may say, for instance, "in a few moments, I will wake you up by counting from 1 to 5." although one may use any signal whatsoever. "On the count of 5, you will find yourself in your normal waking state."

Unless there is some reason to favor the establishment of a partial or total amnesia, which in any event is always reversible, the clinician may then say to the patient: "You will remember clearly everything that we have done since the beginning, and if you want to, you may talk freely about anything you may wish. Are you ready?"

The patient will then indicate yes, or utter a "hm hm" or a "yes." If the patient is engaged in a deep personal experience, he or she may feel skeptical: "How does he expect me to come back from so far so quickly?" However, on the count of five the patient will find him or herself wide awake, in a normal state and will remember progressively all that he or she has experienced; the patient will be ready to talk about the experience while at the same time remaining free not to do so.

It could happen that the patient does not awaken on the given signal. It may simply be that what we have just described has happened; that the patient prefers to pursue his or her own personal experience and lets you know this without actually saying so. However, the patient will accept a suggestion, somewhat reluctantly, that all good things must come to an end, that time is passing, and that he or she could readily return to the experience in the next trance should he or she wish.

PHENOMENOLOGY OF HYPNOSIS

Laboratory studies have examined a whole gamut of psychological and psychophysiological functions under the effect of hypnosis. Clinical hypnosis is supported not only by the findings in experimental hypnosis, but also by an adequate theoretical background, clinical training, and practice in diagnosis and psychotherapy. Taking these prerequisites for granted, the mastery of hypnotic phenomena offers the clinician more treatment options.

Sensation, Perception, and Ideomotor Phenomena

Visual, auditory, olfactory, cutaneous, and kinesthetic delusions and hallucinations are common in capable hypnotic subjects. Under hypnotic analgesia, the patient may feel something such as pressure as a reaction to a painful stimulus, without feeling pain, or the patient may totally ignore any sensation (E. Hilgard & J.Hilgard, 1975). Classical effects of hypnosis on the motor system are included in modern inductions and measurement scales (E. Hilgard,1965; Weitzenhoffer, 1957).

Splitting of Consciousness and Dissociation

Splitting, spontaneous or suggested, may take several forms (E. Hilgard, 1977, 1987; Laurence & Perry, 1981). For example, an aphonic patient of mine was made able to speak in hypnosis, on condition that "it was not *she* who spoke" but rather an hallucinated double, she herself remaining unable to speak. This other "me" was led to testify out loud to the reality of the awakening process. In the awakening process the task of the double was to say "yes" at each count as I went from 1 to 5. The double complied with this except for the last "yes" (the fifth one) when the patient herself replied yes because presumably she was awake. She then remarked excitedly that she had obviously recovered her speech.

Attention

According to the nature of the instructions, attention may be focused on predetermined or suggested representations, or it may float freely following the pattern of primary processes (Gill & Brenman, 1959; Karlin, 1979).

Association

In hypnosis the patient may be more capable of free association (with the exclusion of thoughts that may have a disruptive effect on hypnosis), or the patient may follow restricted streams of association related to a theme, for example, father or mother, which would appear in the waking state in a somewhat more stereotyped form (Wolberg,1964, 1967).

Memory

Amnesia, paramnesia, and hypermnesia all play a part in the process of reconstruction of personal history, whereas imagination confounds reality. Such ambiguity poses serious problems, especially in the realms of legal evidence and testimony. Moreover, the process of restoration of memories remains central to psychotherapy, with or without hypnosis. Hypnosis may facilitate the production of memories, but it does not necessarily aid interpretation (American Medical Association, 1985; Kihlstrom & Evans, 1979; Orne, 1979b; Orne, Whitehouse, Dinges, & Orne, 1988; Laurence & Perry, 1988; Pettinati, 1988).

Age Regression

Age regression is a term used more or less to describe the capacity of the patient to relive in an extremely convincing subjective manner "forgotten" events or childhood episodes and to behave in a way compatible with the child the patient believes him or herself to have been (Fromm, 1970). Some subjects experience a duality in experimental age regression, simultaneously feeling like a child and like an adult observer. These subjects experience Hilgard's hidden observer effect (Laurence & Perry, 1981).

Affect and Representation

Hypnosis is an excellent laboratory for the study of the relationship between affect and inner representations. Affect may be blocked, displaced, amplified, or minimized. Left to itself, affect becomes omnipresent and strongly invests images and memories, the contents of which appear different in the waking state. Thus, one patient who distinctly detested her mother in the waking state, felt a deep love for her in hypnosis. Another patient who insisted in the waking state "to have nothing to say today" proceeded to have a strong abreaction in hypnosis concerning a childhood drama. It is notable that the therapeutic effect of abreaction is not directly related to dramatic intensity, but rather to the manner in which the ego succeeds in integrating the affect (Gill & Brenman, 1959).

Dreams

Hypnosis has an effect on dream activity (hypnotic and nocturnal) and on the associative capacity of the patient with regard to his or her dreams. With guidance, the patient may learn to recognize the symbolic value of his or her dreams and to integrate them into his or her life. Hypnosis itself may to some extent have the same value as dreams (Gill & Brenman, 1959; Lavoie, 1985b; Moss, 1967; Sacerdote, 1967; Wolberg, 1967).

Defense Mechanisms

Hypnosis is characterized by a temporary rearrangement of defense mechanims and ego investment. Reality testing and critical judgment are partially suspended to facilitate trance maintenance. The patient may have less tendency to deny certain wishes or conflicts that he or she refused to admit or especially to feel in the waking state, but the patient will hide others, willingly or not. It is important to know in legal settings especially that the subject is perfectly capable of simulating or lying in hypnosis. Furthermore, hypnosis may camouflage certain resistances, especially those that make the hypnotic transference itself possible (Gill & Brenman, 1959; Lavoie 1985b)

Thought and Language

The hypnotizable patient has access to the process of concrete thinking, where the word evokes the thing. This is where the realms of ideomotor phenomena and direct suggestion come into play. You say to the patient that he or she is sleeping and the patient will tell you he or she is sleeping; you state that the patient is awake and he or she will reply that he or she is awake; you suggest to the patient that he or she is angry and you will see him or her blush; you assure the patient that he or she feels good; she or he smiles. Symptom abolition may be achieved through simple instructions of this kind; this is an example of the classical use of direct suggestion. The patient may adhere literally verbatim to instructions, and simultaneously maintain a deep sensitivity for metaphorical thinking and symbolism. Exploration of this potential is the foundation of Milton Erickson's work (Haley, 1967a; Rossi, 1980).

Imaginative Involvement

In hypnosis, what is ordinarily perceived as imaginary is often felt as being real. The capacity for absorption that characterizes the hypnotic subject has been well documented in contemporary research (J.R. Hilgard, 1979).

It can be seen, therefore, that clinical hypnosis is fertile terrain for the development of delusion, enthusiasm, deceit, and disappointment. The articulation of imaginative involvement within reality and the uncovering of the symbolic significance of this experience in the overall life of the patient constitute the most delicate shared task of patient and clinician.

Regression in the Service of the Ego

In adaptive regression the patient is able to allow representations normally repressed to come into consciousness, and provide a glimpse of the derivatives of the unconscious. Above all, the patient is able to master this process and to use it as an aid to adaptation. This experience, which is facilitated by hypnosis, can lead to the emergence of new configurations and in turn lead the patient to new ways of seeing and feeling. The role of adaptive regression in hypnosis constitutes the basis of Gill and Brenman's (1959) theory of hypnosis. The validity of this theory has been supported by studies with normal subjects (Gruenewald, Fromm, & Oberlander, 1972) and with schizophrenics (Lavoie & Elie, 1985; Lavoie, Sabourin, Ally, & Langlois, 1976).

Ego Autonomy

Hypnosis underscores the fact that the autonomy of the ego is relative to the interdependence of external reality with the unconscious, the id (desire and the erotic or aggressive drives), superego (unconscious prohibitions), and ideals (ego ideal and ideal ego). By modifying the conditions pertaining to the external world through hypnotic induction, one provokes, ipso facto, a modification of the usual relations between conscious, preconscious, and unconscious (Gill & Brenman, 1959).

Synthetic Function

Hypnosis implies a modification in the customary hierarchy of control systems (Hilgard, 1977). It is agreed that in hypnosis a "waking ego" (Gill & Brenman, 1959), an "executive ego" (Hilgard, 1977), or a "watching part of the self" (Freud,1900) continues to function. In this respect:

1. hypnosis may provide the subject with the opportunity for a better synthesis of conflictual or dissociated elements;
2. integration by the ego of contradictory hypnotic experience requires a process of interpretation and assistance;
3. there are patients who are capable of living flamboyant hypnotic experiences without these having much impact on their daily lives; and
4. certain patients may experience substantial difficulty in recovering from a badly directed hypnotic trance (see section on "Dangers")

One should not propose to a patient in hypnosis even more than in the waking state an undertaking too difficult for him or her to accomplish.

Object Relations

Without doubt, hypnotizability relies on a certain object relations structure. Freud (1921) recognized in the subject an unconscious desire to submit to an all powerful figure, and for identification with this figure from which the ego draws its own sense of omnipotence. Gill and Brenman (1959) have insisted on the reciprocal character of the process; the hypnotist also identifies with the subject and participates in his or her experience. Accordingly, there is a significant risk of lover-like idealization by the hypnotist of the hypnotic subject (do we not speak of the subject as "remarkable," a "virtuoso," "exceptional" and of the hypnotic interaction itself as "the ripe couple," "the unique experience in which both protagonists participate"?) By contrast, hypnosis is also exposed to the risk of devaluation when real therapeutic gains fail to measure up to the reflected promises.

The Kleinian therapist will appreciate the fact that hypnosis intrinsically reactivates a repetition of primitive modes of being and relating, including fantasies and mechanisms of the schizoparanoid position, and confronts the patient and therapist with a choice between avoidance, or confrontation and working through the depressive position.

Posthypnotic Suggestion

This is a technique by which the experimenter seeks to lead the subject to accomplish certain predetermined acts outside of the hypnotic state, with or without the subjects knowledge of the hypnotic source of his or her actions. In clinical practice, one may make use of posthypnotic suggestion in the hope of seeing the patient accomplish a certain psychological task in the waking state, or deal better with personal handicaps of all kinds, with or without recourse to self-hypnosis. Most frequently, these handicaps refer to inhibitions, or unhealthy attitudes or habits or fall under the heading of what the psychoanalysts term *motives of defenses* (e.g., anxiety, shame, guilt, and disgust).

We should not underestimate possible problems with posthypnotic suggestions (Orne & Hammer, 1974), even if they seem to be fully acceptable to the patient. They may readily become a source of conflict in so far as the patient may experience them as ego-alien. In all cases, this delicate and uncertain technique requires solid clinical experience.

With regard to hypnoanalysis related to psychoanalytic technique, or to a focused hypnotic intervention in the course of analytic therapy, it may be difficult to reconcile posthypnotic suggestion itself with the theory, techniques, and objectives of such therapies, unless the suggestion is related to further spontaneous and undirected associations the patient may have.

Self-Hypnosis

Hypnotizable patients are often surprised to find, on coming out of hypnosis, that they can learn to initiate and terminate the hypnotic state themselves, using the same instructions. This exercise in itself implies a mechanism of dissociation. If heterohypnosis can be considered to be an interpersonal endeavour, then self-hypnosis can be considered to be a private one. These two undertakings have neither the same meaning or impact in the life of the patient. Once the initial anxiety has been assuaged, attention, imagery, and even dreams can be utilized in a remarkable fashion (Fromm et al., 1981). In certain cases, self hypnosis seems to increase mastery over anxiety. The correlation between the behavioral effects of hetero- and self-hypnosis are only modest, in the range of 0.33 to 0.62 (Johnson et al., 1983; Kihlstrom, 1985).

Some therapists include practice in self-hypnosis in their overall treatment plan (Clarke & Jackson, 1983). Others reserve the technique for specific purposes such as sensory control (pain), or problems of self-control in patients who underestimate their capacities in this regard. In either case the function of self-hypnosis remains subordinate to the therapeutic relationship.

Although there is a solidly established body of research on hypnosis, self-hypnosis research is still in the early stages (Orne & McConkey, 1981). Caution is the rule, especially because the problem of adverse side effects has been practically ignored to date. Outside of the appropriate therapeutic context, many patients fall victim to the commercialization of self-hypnosis (the cassette market) where one is led to believe that interpersonal difficulties can be solved by a "do it yourself kit," without seriously examining underlying dynamics.

Neuropsychology and Psychophysiology

Several recent studies suggest that hypnosis and hypnotizability are related to a preference for right hemispheric processing. Hypnotic induction itself is accompanied by a displacement of cortical activity from the left to the right hemisphere (Kihlstrom, 1985). Hilgard, (1977) noted that division of consciousness cannot be explained without invoking both hemispheric differences and a relative balance between the cortex and the limbic system. Hebb (1975) suggested that there could be a connection between the kind of splitting that underlies hypnotic pain control and his own concept of cell assemblies, which he considered to be the physiological substratum of cognitive structures (see also Hebb, 1980).

Relative Difficulty of Hypnotic Experiences

None of the existing hypnotic phenomena can adequately account for the hypnotic experience, even though they contribute to its understanding (Hilgard, 1965). What is more, the degree of difficulty varies among items. For example, the simple sensorimotor experiments (postural sway, heaviness, and involuntary movement) are easy to accomplish; they are experienced by 70% to 80% of subjects. Hypnotic dream and time regression are experienced by 45% of subjects. Negative visual hallucinations and auditory hallucinations are achieved by only 9% of subjects.

CRITERIA FOR CLINICAL APPLICATIONS

The clinician will have recognized by now that it is precisely those functions that are observed and evaluated in the course of a normal clinical examination that undergo alteration during hypnosis. The concept of ego functions (Bellak, Hurvich, & Gediman, 1973) affords a psychodynamic reading of the phenomena observed and offers an understanding of how and why the general principles of psychotherapy take precedence over any decision as to whether to utilize hypnosis, especially in crisis situations (Bellak, Faithorn, & Plishka, 1981). Criteria include:

1. *Diagnosis*: Functional, affective, and interpersonal aspects of the symptom or syndrome as evident contraindications are ruled out.
2. *Hypnotizability*: Sufficiently high for the ends currently pursued. The fastest and surest way to know is to measure it.
3. *Motivation*: Present but not based on blind faith. Skepticism regarding hypnosis often conceals a strong interest and in itself is not a contraindication.
4. *Free consent*: The patient should feel absolutely free to accept or decline hypnosis, free also to withdraw and discover for him or herself that the method, or the particular clinician or context, does not suit him or her.
5. *Transference*: The clinician should have sufficient knowledge and control of the desires and fantasies that hypnosis may awaken in both the clinician and the patient.
6. *Ego activity*: The clinician should allow the patient to participate as actively as possible on the psychic level.

7. *Nature of the request*: The request of the patient should be reasonable, that is to say, reconcilable with the limits of hypnosis.

Recognition of Transference and Countertransference

From both an historical and epistemological point of view hypnosis precedes psychoanalysis. [1]Hypnosis represents a kind of expanded "no man's land" ; an area where it is possible for both protagonists to make certain moves in the hope of sparing oneself the fray of battle. This is the best metaphor that Freud could have found when he explained why he gave up hypnosis, in practice if not in fact in his theories (Freud, 1910a).

The price paid for the enormous freedom of movement in hypnosis between conscious and preconscious, foreground and background, the mind and the back of the mind (those very phenomena that so interested Erickson), are prohibitions that reinforce repression at the frontier of the unconscious. We know from Freud (1910a, 1917) that what is hidden behind the "insurmountable walls" of hypnosis is the entire transference scene whose discovery gave birth to psychoanalysis (Lavoie 1985a, 1985b).

In fact, the ambivalent mixture of latent loving and aggressive impulses are evident even in the questions patients ask if given the opportunity: "Will I remember what I have said and done while under hypnosis?" "Can someone be made to do or say something in hypnosis that they would not do or say normally?" "What will happen if I don't waken up?" "Is it possible to hypnotize someone against their will ?" "Can someone be forced to commit a crime under hypnosis?"

These questions must be understood in their true sense: "If I abandon myself to you, will you promise not to take advantage of the power I invest in you?" Or, "Is it not possible that my desire puts you in a delicate or intenable position?"

These questions suggest that the mere mention of hypnosis may bring to consciousness fantasies and conflicts about rape, abuse of power, seduction, domination, submission, sadism and masochism, exhibitionism and voyeurism, dependence and passivity, which touch on questions of truth and deceit,

[1]Space precludes a summary of the history of hypnosis. Accordingly, we have but scratched the surface of the vast body of experimental literature on the subject. Suffice to say only that the French at the end of the 19th century had already enunciated several problems with which contemporary researchers still wrestle (see Barrucand, 1967; Chertok, 1983; Chertok & De Saussure, 1973; Ellenberger, 1970; Laurence & Perry, 1988). Those readers interested in source material would be well directed to an article by M. Gravitz (1987). Concerning the connection between hypnosis and psychoanalysis, recently a most stimulating book has been published in French by Chertok and Borch-Jacobsen (1987). Here several collaborators react to a text by Borch-Jacobsen. To mention just one fundamental point raised by Merton M. Gill in that book "hypnotizability in its deepest form is not universal while transference is" (p.87).

fraud and simulation, and the possible plundering of liberty and reason. Before even submitting to hypnosis the patient is testing the hypnotist's fantasies with his or her questions. The dynamics or projection and introjection, which are going to play such a fundamental role in hypnosis are immediately evident. "Are these my own wishes or those of the other?"

The testimony of a psychoanalyst reported by Gill and Brenman (1959) illustrates perfectly the fact that this instinctual infrastructure can pervade the hypnotic undertaking:

> I gave up hypnosis as a regular procedure very early in my career because I am aware of the fact that for me personally, it was an unhygienic situation. Without elaboration of details, I may now say that my decision to hypnotize a man was motivated ultimately, with almost immediate awareness, by some sadistic impulse to dominate him. With a female, the comparable situation manifested itself in the form of an erotic impulse. In my emotional economy therefore I have to look upon hypnosis as an acting-out with implications ramifying beyond even the conscious phenomena which I have stated. (p. 93)

Other fantasies include regression to early stages of childhood in the hope of retrieving the joy merging with the all powerful mother, or of clarifying the ambiguity that governs this strange union. In this regard, Ferenczi (1909/1950) made a distinction between paternal and maternal hypnosis. It is an acknowledged fact that by their very nature, the dependance and totally obedient behavior of some highly hypnotizable subjects nourish the hypnotist's narcissism and sense of omnipotence.

As long as the hypnotist is unable to recognize these dynamics within him or herself and the subtle way in which the patient stirs them up, recourse to clinical hypnosis is hazardous.

Keeping in mind these fundamental ingredients of hypnosis that perhaps constitute the essence of its power and limitations, the clinician will find that the patient will usually be satisfied by a literal response to his or her questions. "In so far as you wish to remember everything you will be able to remember everything. You will do and say under hypnosis what you wish to do and to say. In so far as you are a hypnotizable person you will awaken just as you will have gone into trance. And even if you are a highly hypnotizable person you will be hypnotized only if you really want to be." These utterances amount to saying: "I respect and affirm your freedom as a subject. Your best interests are what interests me. I am here to work with you in a different sort of way which may help you to change your condition in a significant and enduring fashion."

In fact, in hypnosis the patient becomes extremely sensitive to the fundamental attitudes of empathy, respect, kindness, and authenticity, perhaps precisely because he or she senses that hypnosis can evoke less desirable and respectable motives or desires (Fromm, 1968b).

Activity and Passivity

At this point one can imagine, if one has not already had the experience, that the natural position of the hypnotized subject is one of waiting, expectation, receptivity, and open mindedness with regard to the experience. The subject has, shall we say, a yearning desire to be passive, and he or she could spend hours and days in a sort of "sleep" akin to a drugged state (Gill & Brenman, 1959).

However, the patient retains his or her capacity to choose. The patient can take initiative, even in the absence of any indication from the hypnotist (Sheehan & McConkey, 1982), especially if he or she is made aware of this potential. We see him or her also weaving the very fabric of every hypnotic experience with Ego Activity and Ego Passivity (Frankel, 1976; Fromm, 1972a; Fromm & Hurt, 1980).

To work effectively in hypnosis the ego should be active and should be a fairly good mediator. It should be capable of renunciation that, as we see here, may go so far as to renounce hypnosis itself. It should be able, if necessary, to confront and metabolize the conflict without resorting to excessive dependence, denial, or splitting; or to stubborn idealization and devaluation. One of the fundamental challenges in hypnosis is to safeguard the mediating activity of the ego in a situation where the call to passivity is extremely strong.

The Nature of the Request

One final criteria rests with the more or less reasonable character of the subject's request and the looked-for results. In the realm of psychopathology, successful hypnotic treatment is not necessarily tied to levels of hypnotizability. For example, chronically depressed, hallucinating schizophrenics, those suffering from severe obsessional neuroses, men and women otherwise well established in life but who carry with them old interpersonal conflicts, or deep feelings of guilt, inferiority, doubt or uncertainty, delude themselves if they come to hypnosis expecting it will easily alleviate their conflicts. In these cases, hypnosis may eventually contribute to a therapeutic process but will in no way take the place of therapy. Once again the hypnotist must be certain that recourse to hypnosis does not constitute an avoidance or diversion. Were it so, untimely failure is to be expected, even in the presence of some short-term gain.

All the same, the perspective will be different depending on the task; to resolve a long-term psychopathological problem, clarify a current situational problem, or alleviate the sequelae of physical illness or some acute neurotic or psychotic episode.

Sickness is accompanied by feelings of anxiety, suffering, and often by strong feelings of helplessness. Many hypnotizable patients, regardless of the nature of their illness may recover their sense of control, reduce their anxiety, and attenuate their suffering through hypnosis. The work of Hilgard (1980) and Hilgard and LeBaron (1984) with pediatric cancer patients is an eloquent demonstration of the optimal use of individual hypnotic potential, and is based solidly on laboratory research.

Choice of Approach

The tone of the hypnotic relationship will depend on the nature of the demands of the situation (Orne, 1980); that is, according to what the patient and the clinician recognize as the latent or manifest specific requirements of the situation.

At one extreme, there are hypnotic inductions in which the therapist talks continually with a pacifying tempo, using a profusion of metaphor and evocation, while the subject allows him or herself to be molded by everything that the monologue evokes in him or her (Erickson et al., 1976). At the other extreme, the hypnotist may remain silent after having given a word or two to the patient, and intervenes only to help the patient to overcome blocking of associations. Under this condition the patient has the feeling of a vast opening of the preconscious and of his or her past history, and a great flow of associations. Affect is ever present and may break out in sporadic bursts of abreaction. This phenomenon represented in fact the turning point in the evolution of psychoanalytic technique (Freud, 1900).

If hypnoanalysis is used, over time the usual resistances are sure to make themselves felt (e.g., transference and superego resistances, repetition compulsion, and secondary gain). To this list must be added another resistance specifically related to dependence and secondary gain with regard to hypnosis itself.

In the transference neurosis, for example, the patient may reproach the therapist for not helping enough and let him or her know rather vigorously, that he or she could, if desired, make things easier for the patient with the help of hypnosis. On his or her part, the therapist will have to deal with this additional dimension of therapy. Clarification, confrontation,interpretation, construction,and the possible renunciation of hypnosis when it serves only as an alibi may be necessary here. On the other hand, there are persons (see the section on "Personality and Borderline Disorders"), even with transference issues, who benefit if they are able to put hypnosis at the service of adaptation rather than defense.

Between these two polarities there exists a gamut of possible dialogues where suggestion plays a more or less prominent role, according to patient's and clinician's personal and theoretical preference, the nature of the objective problem at hand and the hypnotic phenomena on which we rely.

Hypnosis may also be included adjunctively within the framework of psychoanalysis, psychoanalytic psychotherapy phenomenological and existential psychotherapies, behavior therapy, and psychosomatic medicine (Baker 1987; Bourgeois, 1981; Brown & Fromm, 1986, 1987; Frankel, 1987; Fromm, 1987b; Spinhoven, 1987; Watkins & Watkins, 1979; Weitzenhoffer, 1989).

Thus, at the present time, the term *hypnotherapy* can only indicate a heterogeneous group of techniques. The titles *hypnotherapist* or *hypnotist* lend confusion, especially because they are often adopted by persons without sufficient medical or psychological training. These terms may give the impression that the practice of hypnosis is based on a unified body of knowledge distinct from those of the medical and psychological disciplines. This is not the case. Nonetheless, the term *hypnotherapy* seems to be passing into current usage to the degree that clinicians and researchers define its boundaries.

What is important to remember is that for clinical purposes, hypnosis is a way of relating, and not a general system of therapy, and that the clinician may use hypnosis as an adjunct in the practice of his or her normal therapeutic activity.

The Interpretation of the Hypnotic Transference

In all therapies that do not require systematic interpretation of the transference, hypnosis can be integrated into the therapy relatively easily. Lasting results can be obtained by optimal utilization, as opposed to interpretation of the hypnotic transference. In more severe cases, however, and when there are indications for analytic therapy, hypnosis is subordinate to analytic technique (free association, free floating attention, and interpretation).

According to Wolberg (1967), hypnosis may be used advantageously in psychoanalytic psychotherapy when the patient presents one or more of the following conditions:

- the patient lacks motivation for psychoanalytic therapy; refuses to begin therapy unless he or she is assured of immediate symptom relief;
- has a negative transference or depressive characterological detachment that obstructs the development of a working relationship;
- is unable to verbalize freely;
- is unable to engage in free association;
- is unable to dream or remember his or her dreams;
- seems blocked in bringing up transference material;
- has certain repressed traumatic memories, elucidation of which may help the therapeutic process;

- seems to "dry up" productively and is unable to produce any further significant material;
- is unable to deal with forces that inhibit a translation of insight into action; and
- has problems in terminating therapy.

However useful these guidelines may be, the clinician, may quickly find him or herself confronted with a problem. In fact, what distinguishes the psychoanalytic method from all other methods of psychotherapy, is the deepening interpretation of transference. Therefore, it is necessary to examine the impact of hypnosis on the analytic technique, and above all to determine how the interpretation of the transference may be applied to the hypnotic transference itself.

One way of dealing with the problem consists in looking at hypnosis as a particular aspect of the containing function of the therapist. The therapist contains hypnosis, which in turn partially contains the emotional experience of the patient. In this respect hypnosis becomes an envelope within an envelope sealed by a double seal such that if you ask the patient what has taken place or what he or she has experienced during the session the patient may respond "In which session, hypnosis or the other one?"

Hypnosis thus introduces a splitting of the transference and the countertransference within the session. This splitting will be more evident to the degree that the therapist differentiates between hypnosis and the rest of the relationship. The splitting will be less evident to the degree that the therapist emphasizes the similarity and continuity of the hypnotic experience with the rest of therapy. Nevertheless, introducing hypnosis even in the most continuous and natural way possible still introduces splitting.

This splitting facilitates the repetition of conflicts and of the unconscious primitive mechanisms of projection, introjection, incorporation, and projective identification, as well as attitudes of triumph and contempt, idealization and devaluation that characterize the manic defenses. These processes are especially clear in the hypnotic transference, and it therefore becomes easier to point them out to the patient. This is not possible, however, unless the analytic *distance* is preserved and the therapist does not allow him or herself to become engulfed in uncontrolled projective identification. If the therapist has a fairly clear perception of the split generated by hypnosis he or she may interpret and use it to analyze the other splits that this situation evokes, in particular splits of the first object relations and later ones concerning the Oedipal complex.

The imperviousness of the wall that separates that which the patient can experience *in* hypnosis and that which the patient can experience *outside* of hypnosis gives the measure of importance of the split that separates these two populations of emotions and feelings and thoughts.

For example, one of my borderline patients with long-standing depressive tendencies and acute episodes of depression, successively visualized this wall as a wall of ice, a wall of concrete, and a prison-like wall before discovering that it was in fact an interpersonal barrier that he had first erected between himself and his parents, intent on revenge and punishment and between himself and others in general. Thus he realized that for years while in therapy with others and now with me, he had erected and maintained the same barrier out of fear and shame. The interpretation of the hypnotic transference, that is to say, of the defensive function of hypnotizability and of hypnosis for him, reestablished, to a large extent, circulation between these two parts of himself; that hidden revengeful part that he showed only in hypnosis, and the other sick part, suffering and "cut-off," that he readily showed to the therapist outside of hypnosis. In the beginning, his subjective experience in hypnosis was dramatically different from his experience outside of hypnosis. In the end, there was a great deal of continuity between the two realms and he could explore in free association as many aspects of himself without hypnosis as with hypnosis. Love did not shift so violently to hatred, and a feeling of freedom, unity, and emotional stability developed.

This interpretative process, long and arduous, presupposes the working through of the schizoparanoid position with its threats, envy, fits of rage, hateful projections, despair, and feelings of isolation and rejection. It presupposes also the renunciation of the sadistic control and omnipotence by which the infant dreams of overcoming his or her suffering and handicap once and for all. A great deal of time is spent in the process of mourning as the patient has to give up manic repair and forceful control of objects in order to reach true reparation, that which is grounded in love.

Over the years I have adopted an attitude that I believe maximizes the possibilities of integrating the interpretation of the hypnotic transference into the mainstream of the analytic process. When I see an indication for hypnosis in the course of analytic psychotherapy, especially with severe cases, I proceed as follows:

1. Present hypnosis as a possible means to overcome whatever difficulty we are presently confronting;
2. Use hypnosis solely as a transference envelope and as support in confrontation, clarification, and interpretation. Basically, I capitalize on the exploratory potential of hypnosis, interpreting and analyzing catharsis wherever it occurs.
3. Exclude, as much as possible, all forms of suggestion except to encourage the patient to follow the same analytic rules in hypnosis as outside of hypnosis.
4. Wherever possible interpret the difference between subjective experience *in* hypnosis and *out* of hypnosis as a manifestation of transference

resistance, involving the use of splitting as a defense against anxiety, shame, or guilt.

5. Also interpret the fear, fantasies, and mechanisms that prevent the patient from expressing outside of hypnosis what he or she can experience in such a dramatic way in hypnosis.
6. In so far as the defensive and protective functions of hypnosis are uncovered, the thoughts and feelings that were previously maintained through the yoke of hypnosis can find a way out and break into ordinary conscious experience. This coincides with substantial reinforcement of the mediating function of the ego and ego mastery over primary processes.
7. This experience is felt by the patient as a deep change in his or her subjective and interpersonal relationships, and typically results in an attenuation of primitive defense mechanisms.
8. To summarize, that which is experienced in hypnosis but cannot be translated into the relationship outside of hypnosis is interpreted as transference. The consequent uncovering of the transference resistance contributes to freeing the patient from unconscious conflicts, liberating feelings that previously could be experienced only in hypnosis.

Hypnosis may thus help the hypnotizable patient to work through, in vivo, fantasies and mechanisms by which he or she actively prevents certain vital rich and creative parts of him or herself from being fully manifest in his or her everyday life.

CLINICAL INDICATIONS

Various Medical and Psychosomatic Conditions

By typically leading the subject to imagine a physiological effect, or to strongly imagine that he or she is in a position to produce the sought after effect, experimental research has elucidated the benefits of hypnosis on cardiac, vasomotor, respiratory, genitourinary, and gastrointestinal systems. Hypnosis can modulate oral temperature, superficial skin temperature, electrodermal response, and perspiration. Induction is often accompanied by temporary alterations of body image, which the clinician can explore in the trance state. Paralyses, contractures, catalepsies, and various spasms are classical phenomena of hypnosis.

Sometimes a change in attitude can make a huge difference. A neuropsychologist colleague requested consultation for a young man suffering from Wilson's Disease. The patient had the greatest difficulty walking, sitting, getting up, or making himself heard. One hypnotic session brought about substantial improvement in motor control and made his daily life less arduous.

Controlled studies have shown the usefulness of hypnosis as an adjunct in the treatment of migraines, asthma, and acute and chronic pain, especially when the pain has a well-defined organic basis. Clinical literature shows that in all medical specialties (psychosomatics, anesthesiology, cardiology, gastroenterology, urology, obstetrics, gynecology, dermatology, oncology, pediatrics, and dental medicine) some portion of the patient population is likely to benefit from hypnosis (Bowers, 1976; Brown & Fromm, 1987; Burrows & Dennerstein, 1980; Clarke & Jackson, 1983; Crasilneck & Hall, 1985; Frankel, 1976; Gardner & Olness, 1981; Kroger, 1963; Kroger & Fezler, 1976; Turk, Meichenbaum, & Genest, 1983). However, claims that hypnosis can act on the immune system and thereby modify the course of cancer currently lack scientific validation (Frankel, 1987).

Neurotic Adjustment and Behavior Problems: Brief Hypnotic Intervention

In this category there are patients for whom the hypnotic context serves to remove the symptom in just a few sessions, even in a solitary trance experience. These patients are neither naive nor gullible. They often are sophisticated with regard to intersubjective relations and sensitive to transactions other than words. They are persons who are capable of undertaking an introspective and reconstructive approach, but do not have the means or the interest at the time to invest in such an undertaking. They are willing to use any means available to rid themselves of the symptom. Such persons often have a subtle intuition about the unconscious significance of the symptom: It is as if they would like to satisfy themselves with regards to this intuition, at the same time making it very clear that it is sufficient just to obtain symptom relief. The psychopathological blow, although acute, is not serious; the ego is active and relatively strong; the request rational, and there is hope for a substantial improvement or even total remission through hypnosis.

Symptoms of simple phobia (300.29)[2] or conversion (300.11) such as aphonia, paralysis, and spasms of the esophagus may occur following surgery for a hiatal hernia. Cases of conversion I have seen were the consequence of recent stress: marriage, loss of employment, spouse's illness, and surgery. Follow-up visits 4 years later in the cases of phobia, and 8 to 14 years later in the cases of conversion syndromes, revealed total remission without any

[2]The numbers in parentheses refer to DSM-3 categories.

symptom substitution. All but one patient had been treated in one session varying from 25 minutes to 2 hours.

Although certain phobias may readily give way under hypnosis, others are more resistant. One should carefully examine the function that the symptom serves, the structure of the personality, and the possible consequences of removing the symptom through hypnosis to the overall clinical picture (Frankel, 1976).

The literature reports numerous examples of brief treatment in cases of various extreme sexual and other inhibitions, work or eating habits, certain substance abuses (e.g., the 20%–25% of smokers who remain abstinent after a single hypnotic trance), and situational problems demanding ego control in otherwise well adjusted individuals.

Neurotic Adjustment and Behavior Problems: Hypnosis as an Adjunct to Psychotherapy

The difference between these patients and those just described is that for this group, hypnosis controls the symptom sufficiently, but does not eradicate it completely. In general the symptoms serve a more complex function than those in the first category, and hypnotic resolution leads to a new formulation of the latent aspects of the initial demand. This "new" request, which translates into words what the symptom was expressing on the psychophysiological level, relates specifically to the subject's conflicts in the areas of work and love.

Examples include cases of: (a) vaginismus (306.51); (b) inhibited female orgasm (302.73); (c) anxiety neuroses without phobic structure and with work inhibition (300.01, 309.23); (d) anxiety neuroses with psychosomatic elements and loss of sexual appetite (300.01, 300.81, 302.710); (e) problems of adjustment to married life, accompanied by depression and anxiety (309.00, 309.24); and (f) speech disorders and difficulties in public speaking (307.21, 300.23).

In most of these patients the presenting symptom was resolved after 2 to 10 sessions of hypnosis, but the change in the symptom picture provoked an immediate request for psychotherapy, which lasted from 3 months to 3 years. Follow-up visits ranged over a period of 10 to 16 years, and there is no doubt that hypnosis was the pivotal point for major personal changes.

One young woman originally presented with a somatoform disorder (300.7). Hypnotic therapy, which centered on control of her anxiety, nausea, and distaste for certain food items, produced satisfactory results. She returned 8 years later with panic, major depression, and suicidal ruminations requiring psychiatric intervention. The patient engaged in analytic therapy with me, improved for 2 years, and then worsened. After two hospitalizations with a diagnosis of major affective disorder (265.5) she received antidepressants and then lithium therapy without significant improvement. A Rorschach at that time strongly indicated an Axis 2 diagnosis of borderline personality (302.83). I explained to the patient what that meant to me in a way that she found strikingly close to her own inner feelings. I then reintroduced hypnosis as an adjunct to analytic psychotherapy in the manner described earlier. She gained dramatic insights into the roots of her problem, improved rapidly, got rid of medication, suspended hypnosis,although not therapy, went back to work, and is now feeling stronger than at any previous time in her life. In the course of the psychotherapy of hysterical neurosis of the dissociative type (300.12–14) similar delayed reactions and complications may occur.

Personality and Borderline Disorders

The attempt to bring about any substantial change in state of ego functioning when dealing with personality disorders (301.00–301.89) is fraught with difficulties. It is a major undertaking for the clinician for several reasons. Patient traits such as deep emotional wounds; splitting of the ego; denial; idealization and devaluation with difficulty in reality testing; repetition compulsion; depressive tendencies; and exhaustion; and major problems with object relations and internalization that compound lasting dependency needs often lead to major problems in therapy. Although the patient may need lifelong therapy, as noted by Kernberg (1977) and by Bergeret (1974), often the patient is not able to remain in and tolerate the austerity of the classical analytic framework.

For some borderline patients the hypnotic induction allows access to a state of mind that seems unavailable otherwise, unless by the use of certain drugs. Through hypnosis emotional experiences, memories, associations, and introspection are facilitated in such a way that the patient feels a growing internal unity of control and authenticity.

Both the literature and personal experience confirms the fact that characterologically impaired patients often seek hypnosis after having tried everything else; Gestalt therapy, Jungian therapy, personal development groups, one or two attempts at psychoanalysis, analytical therapy. The hypnoanalytic method described earlier is well suited to a number of these patients, furnishing both the protective and reassuring atmosphere which they need and the possibility of effective reconstruction and reparation (Baker, 1983c; Copeland, 1986; Scagnelli, 1980).

I have used hypnosis in long-term analytic psychotherapy with several borderline patients for periods ranging from 5 to 15 years. Interpretation of the transference itself is a powerful way to access some of the most deeply repudiated pockets of conflicts in such patients. Typically, patients would measure their progress through lowered anxiety, increased capacity for free association, more comfort exploring areas of the self and life previously avoided, if not ignored. They achieved increased capacity and new freedom to give and receive love and to make choices in that area and in others that they never had before. Hostility decreased with fewer attacks on oneself and others. They developed sharper ego boundaries and improved body ego with attenuation or disappearance of psychosomatic disorders, clear reduction of pharmacological needs, or even total freedom from drug treatment. Patients enjoyed renewed capacity for work, fewer feelings of persecution coupled with increased hope, confidence, and compassion, along with keener reality testing. These gains stemmed out of their growing insight into their own particular unconscious structure, repetitions, and fantasies as revealed in part through the interpretation of the hypnotic transference.

Severe Neuroses, Pre-Psychotic Patients, and Pseudoneurotic Psychosis

In these instances also, the subject may obtain certain gains from hypnosis but in other ways may be unable to eliminate or control the symptoms. Moreover, the patient may not be able to effectively utilize the symbolic realm. In the majority of these cases, the patient is fixed in an attitude of expiation common in neuroses with irreconcilable submission of the ego to the imperatives of the superego. In the domain of psychosis we find egosplitting which produces denial on one hand of what is observed on the other.

Examples of such cases include: (a) paranoid delusions (297.90), camouflaged by strong phobic elements; (b) extreme agoraphobia (300.21) with highly systematized counterphobic rituals and deep mistrust; (c) panic with many changing phobias, witness to a poorly affirmed ego; (d) depersonalization with feelings of possession (300.60, 300.15) and with fixed delusions of influence which resist all attempts to dissolve them; (e) cases of apparent conversion (300.11) well compensated by public funds and who would consult only to keep their neurologist quiet, being firmly convinced of a permanent neurophysiological injury despite the negative results of all medical and neurological experts; and (f) cases of obsessive neuroses (300.30) highly ritualized, with substantial alterations in reality testing. In all of these cases the contribution of hypnosis to the treatment was extremely limited or nonexistent.

Florid Psychoses, Schizophrenia

For a long time it was believed that psychotics, and in particular schizophrenics could not be hypnotized due to their attentional deficits. Modern research, however, demonstrates the opposite. Among these patients the distribution of hypnotizability is close to that of normal subjects (Lavoie & Elie, 1985; Pettinati, 1982). Nevertheless, within clinical cross sample studies, hypnotizability rises as formal thought disorder is less manifest (Lavoie et al., 1976; Spiegel & Spiegel, 1978).

Hypnotizability also has a prognostic value in longitudinal studies. In a blind study of schizophrenics followed over a period of 10–17 years we observed an inverse relationship between hypnotizability and formal thought disorder (Lavoie, Michaud, Elie, & Amar, 1987). Finally, in schizophrenia, high hypnotizability significantly increased the probability that the patient would obtain his or her release from the hospital in the 10 to 17 years that followed (Michaud et al., 1987). The prognostic value of hypnotizability can be observed in other less severe psychopathological conditions, whether or not hypnosis is actually used in treatment.

Among the classical studies on hypnotherapy with patients suffering from schizophrenia are those of Wolberg (1964) and Biddle (1967). Hypnosis can also be used adjunctively with psychotherapy with certain schizophrenics. Clinical and experimental data on hypnosis and schizophrenia have been reviewed by Lavoie and Sabourin (1980).

In the course of a 6-year psychotherapy with a hospitalized schizophrenic (295.3) we used hypnosis with age regression to explore the mother child relationship. What was discovered was much more subtle than the stereotype on which the patient had remained fixated. The effect of this breakthrough, inspired by Wolberg (1967), was far reaching on the development of therapy and the actual reparation of this patient's relationship with his mother.

Affective Disorders

Although there are findings on the use of hypnosis in the treatment of neurotic depressions, they are sparse with regard to severe depression and even more sparse with regard to manic-depressive states. Hypnosis is often contraindicated in major depressions where there may be a serious risk of suicide, except perhaps when the intervention is undertaken in a hospital setting (Burrows & Dennerstein, 1980; Crasilneck, 1980).

In every case of severe depression the risk of acting out must be explored in overtly, which is the reason why hypnosis should be used only with the greatest of care. In cases of depression where the patient is aware of and accepts his or her illness and where suicidal compulsion capitulates under interpretation, hypnosis can provide a special source of hope and trust. In particular, hypnosis allows the patient to see that the bonds between affects and representations are neither lawless nor immutable. Such a case was presented earlier.

DANGERS OF HYPNOSIS

When one is simply obtaining measures of hypnotizability in a laboratory setting, using freely volunteering subjects, and standardized methods of induction and measurement, we see only minor side effects in 2%–3% of subjects. These include slight numbness, slowing down, slight dizziness, or a brief headache. The advantage for the beginning therapist in studying the standardized scales (apart from their predictive value) is that they serve to contain, almost perfectly, the unforeseen effects of transference even in neurotic and psychotic patients. They are strongly recommended as an initial learning tool, and as a measure of current hypnotizability, but particularly as a way to predict and avoid pitfalls in treatment situations.

Once we engage in further diagnostic and/or therapeutic activities, the transference or countertransference may contain surprises. To deny that hypnosis thus presents a certain danger is to deny the existence of aggressivity and the regulating function of the symptom.

Dangers to the patient

Cases have been reported of dissociative reactions, hysterical conversion, homosexual panic, and acute psychotic reactions following hypnosis. The recognized treatments for suicidal depression and latent psychosis have absolute priority over the use of hypnosis that is contraindicated at certain points in treatment.

Even hypnotic pain suppression, when it is possible, can engender complications or compromise the course of treatment. In general all intervention associated with a physical illness must be absolutely subordinate to the medical diagnosis in order not to obscure the clinical picture.

A young male schizophrenic who acted as an experimental subject experienced homosexual panic. He received help from the staff on his ward. After a session conducted by a trainee, a young lady developed partial paralysis of the legs. Fortunately, the paralysis disappeared after a few days when, after supervision, the psychologist in training interpreted the phenomenon to the satisfaction of the subject, who then asked for psychotherapy at the University Clinic. She found in fact that the experience had presented her with an opportunity to confront long lasting personal problems.

Dangers for the Professional

The professional (doctor, psychologist, dentist), before even wondering what he or she could do with hypnosis, should ask him or herself what can be done without hypnosis. The clinician who engages in hypnosis without sufficient prior training in psychopathology, dynamic psychology, and psychotherapy, would be exposed to a series of blind risks and blunders. The therapist risks thinking that hypnosis confers him or her with a special power; that hypnosis may compensate for his or her lack of experience; that hypnosis can give him or her direct access to the unconscious; worse yet that hypnosis will allow the professional to tame the unconscious; that everything that happens in hypnosis is more real than that which happens in the waking state; that the diagnosis has but relative importance; and finally that the request for hypnosis coming from the patient is sufficient reason to go ahead with it. This last pitfall, if ignored, implies a fatal blind spot with regard to the essential process of evaluation of the dynamics that underlie the request. The professional risks also promising to the patient infinitely more than he or she is, in reality, capable of delivering. Above all the hypnotist may slip unknowingly into domination, manipulation, seduction, overprotection, and activism; he or she may consolidate the ego of the patient in a passive attitude of self-alienation and above all, deprive the patient of a more appropriate therapeutic approach.

By contrast, when used with care by a competent professional who limits its use to the field of his or her proper expertise, hypnosis presents neither more nor less danger than those medical, psychiatric, psychological or psychotherapeutic contexts in which it is used.

ACKNOWLEDGMENTS

I thank my colleague and former student, Maureen Glynn,M. Sc. ,who with her usual competence and *bonne humeur,* completed the English translation of this chapter. I also thank the Direction of Hôpital Louis–H. Lafontaine for supporting the preparation of both the English and French texts.

Chapter 9

THE CLINICAL RELEVANCE OF HYPNOTIC SUSCEPTIBILITY

PHILIP SPINHOVEN
State University of Leiden, Leiden, The Netherlands

Although hypnosis is one of the oldest therapeutic techniques, research on the clinical application of hypnosis is still in its infancy. Since the 1950s, many researchers have tried to dispel old myths about hypnosis by introducing a scientifically careful and critical approach to the field. In line with experimental research on hypnosis, clinical research currently focuses to a great extent on the importance of individual differences in hypnotizability.

This chapter is a survey of the research done on the therapeutic relevance of the degree of hypnotizability. The first part reviews the development of hypnotizability scales for experimental research and the second part for clinical research. Objections of hypnotherapists to the measuring of hypnotizability are discussed in the third section. The ways in which hypnotizability scales can be used in a clinical situation are dealt with in the fourth part. Finally, some conclusions and recommendations are presented on the use of hypnotizability scales.

EXPERIMENTAL HYPNOTIZABILITY SCALES

How does one measure hypnotizability? As early as the 19th century, a number of authors such as Bernheim pointed out that some persons are more capable of responding to hypnotic suggestions than others (Hilgard, 1978). The first scales invented to measure differences in hypnotizability (e.g., the

Davis and Husband Scale in 1931) were unreliable, because a standardized procedure to induce hypnosis and to give suggestions was not available. There also were no clear criteria on the basis of which one could decide whether a specific hypnotic phenomenon had occurred or not. Although these early scales may have offered some guidance to the hypnotherapist, as an instrument for the investigator they were useless.

From 1957 on, Weitzenhoffer and Hilgard started to develop a series of laboratory scales, the so-called Stanford Hypnotic Susceptibility Scales (Forms A, B, and C) and the Stanford Profile Scales (Forms I and II). In all five scales, standardized methods of administering inductions and presenting suggestions are used, and there are strict criteria for scoring whether a suggestion is or is not followed. The scales include a series of phenomena, associated historically with hypnosis, such as ideomotor responses, challenges, hallucinations, amnesia, and posthypnotic suggestions (Weitzenhoffer, 1980). Besides the Stanford Scales, a few other laboratory scales have been developed since the 1960s. A short description of the Stanford and two other widely used scales can be found in Table 9.1.

Laboratory measurements of students' hypnotizability taken with hypnotizability scales have over and over shown that hypnotic reponsivity is approximately normally distributed, and that it is a relatively stable attribute. Ten percent of all subjects are capable of responding to almost all suggestions, 10%–15% are not or are poorly hypnotizable, whereas the remaining majority (75%–80%) is able to carry out suggestions to a greater or lesser degree (Hilgard, 1965). In addition, when a hypnotizability scale is administered to assess a subject's hypnotizability on two different occasions, the subject will score practically the same both times. Hypnotizability not only remains stable for a short time, it also changes little over a period of some 10 years (Gwynn, Spanos, Gabora, & Jarrett, 1988; Morgan, Johnson, & Hilgard, 1974) or even 15–25 years (Hilgard, 1987).

CLINICAL HYPNOTIZABILITY SCALES

Scales designed for laboratory research are not always appropriate to assess individual differences in hypnotizability in a clinical setting. Some objections to their clinical use include the fact that the scales are long and fatiguing; a sleep metaphor is frequently used in the induction; the scientific rather than the therapeutic aim of the test situation is stressed; the style is rather authoritative; difficult items are included that one would not routinely use in hypnotherapy (e.g., hallucinations), as are therapeutically contraindicated items (e.g., challenges).

In order to partially meet these objections, a number of clinical scales have been developed, the adminstration of which is relatively easy and shorter than that of laboratory scales (see Table 9.2). In particular, the more permissive

Table 9.1. Survey of Hypnotizability Scales for Experimental Research on Hypnosis

(a) Stanford Hypnotic Susceptibility Scale, Forms A and B (SHSS: A and B) (Weitzenhoffer & Hilgard, 1959).
These two 12-item scales were the first instruments to be thoroughly standardized. The scales are relatively easy, and consist mainly of motor items (such as: "Your hand will become heavy and drop"). The observable behavior of the subject is scored. Each item passed is scored "plus," in accordance with clean-cut criteria, and scores 1 point. The total score of the SHSS:A and SHSS:B ranges from 0 to 12. The administration of either scale requires about 50 minutes, and the correlation between them is .83.

(b) Stanford Hypnotic Susceptibility Scale, Form C (SHSS:C) (Weitzenhoffer & Hilgard, 1962).
It is considerably more difficult to score high on this individual 12-item scale than it is on the SHSS:A and B, as the Form C contains more items related to perception and cognition (such as not being able to smell ammonia, or to have a dream). This scale is often used to determine the limits of a person's hypnotizability. The items of the scale are arranged in ascending order to difficulty (a so-called Gutman scale). As the sequence is based on group data, the items of this scale, when it is administered to a particular individual, may not be experienced by some subjects as falling into an exact pattern of increasing difficulty. The score, ranging from 0 to 12, relates to objective aspects of the response to suggestions. The correlation between the SHSS:A and SHSS:C is .85.

(c) Stanford Profile Scales, I and II (SPS: I and II) (Weitzenhoffer & Hilgard, 1967).
These individual scales are very difficult to pass, with items relating to those phenomena that are historically related to hypnosis (hallucinations, age regression, etc.). The main object of this test is not so much to measure a person's hypnotizability score as to map out his or her profile (i.e., the specific areas of strength in his or her hypnotic capacities). Both scales consist of nine items. Each item can be scored from 0 to 3, so that the total score ranges from 0 to 27.

(d) Harvard Group Scale of Hypnotic Susceptibility, Form A (HGSHS:A) (Shor & Orne, 1962).
This scale is an adaption of SHSS:A for group administration. It enables quick identification of high and low responders. The subjects themselves score their—observable—responses to the suggestions presented to them. The total score ranges from 0 to 12. It takes about 50 minutes to complete the scale. A direct assessment of subjective involvement might enhance the predictive validity of the HGSHS:A, especially when the more dissociative aspects of hypnosis are under scrutiny (Register & Kihlstrom, 1986).

(e) Barber Suggestibility Scale (BSS) (T.X. Barber, 1969).
The specific structure of this individually administered 8-item scale allows administration with or without preliminary hypnosis induction. Barber believes that hypnotic phenomena can occur whether or not trance was induced previously. The scoring is not only based on objective responses to suggestions, but also on the individual's subjective experiences. In the objective scoring, each item scores 0 or 1, so the total score ranges from 0 to 8. In the subjective scoring, the subject chooses from four categories of answers (a Likert scale). Here, the total score ranges from 0 to 24.

style of the Creative Imagination Scale, developed by Wilson and Barber (1978) for experimental and clinical purposes, reflects the changes that are taking place in hypnotherapy. The emphasis is put on the capacities of the patient and not on the alleged power of the hypnotist. However, as pointed out by Gruenewald (1982a), assessment of hypnotic susceptibility is more complex in the clinical situation than in the laboratory. In hypnotherapy,

Table 9.2 Survey of Hypnotizability Scales for Clinical Research on Hypnotherapy

(a) Diagnostic Rating Scale (DRS) (O'Connell, Orne, & Shor, 1966).
Prior to the diagnostic testing for hypnotizability, ample contact is established with the patient. This is achieved, depending on the individual and the situation, either by making him or her feel comfortable by talking about neutral things, or by spending considerable time in removing his or her misconceptions and doubts about hypnosis. When the test is completed, an experienced therapist assesses the patient's hypnotizability, in accordance with the following five categories:
1. absence of response
2. ideomotor response
3. challenge response with subjective involvement
4. hallucination
5. amnesia + posthypnotic response.
Induction and suggestions are adapted to each individual. The score covers both subjective and objective aspects of the response to hypnotic suggestions. The time needed for administration is 1 hour.

(b) Hypnotic Induction Profile (HIP) (Spiegel & Spiegel, 1978).
This rather authoritative individual scale includes two parts: the "eye-roll" (ER), and an induction procedure based on arm levitation (LEV). Irrespective of the "eye-roll" score (ER), an induction score (IND) is assessed on five objective and subjective aspects of the arm levitation, the total score ranging from 0 to 5. This 2-item scale requires an administration time of approximately 10 minutes.

(c) Stanford Hypnotic Clinical Scale: Adult (SHCS:Adult) (Hilgard & Hilgard, 1975; Morgan & Hilgard, 1979b).
This individual scale is an adaptation of the SHSS:C for the use of clinical practitioners and clinical investigators. The scale consists of five items: a motor item (moving hands), age regression, a dream, posthypnotic amnesia, and a posthypnotic suggestion. The score includes both subjective and objective aspects of the response to the suggestions presented. Each item scores 0 or 1, the total score ranging from 0 to 5. The scale takes some 20 minutes to be administered.

(d) Stanford Hypnotic Clinical Scale: Child (SHCS:Child) (Morgan & Hilgard, 1979).
This scale is also an adaptation of the SHSS:C. There are several modifications, particularly when the scale is used with children under the age of 6. It has been found that very young children resist eye closure and the scale is so designed that it can be administered with eyes open.

(e) Stanford Hypnotic Arm Levitation Induction and Test (SHALIT) (Hilgard, Crawford & Wert, 1979).
This single-item scale, in 6 minutes, yields a score predictive of the total SHSS:A or SHSS:C. The eyes are closed from the start. Standardized suggestions for arm levitation follow, with the height of the hand noted at stated intervals. The subject is also questioned about the degree of involuntariness (5-point scale) and the feeling of being hypnotized (10-point scale).

(f) Creative Imagination Scale (CIS) (Barber & Wilson, 1978; Wilson & Barber, 1978).
This permissively worded scale, which can be administered both to individuals and to groups, requests subjects to think of, or to imagine that an arm becomes heavy, a finger numb, etc. The test can be taken with or without formal trance induction in approximately 18 minutes. It is a 10-item scale; scoring relates solely to the subjective experience of the subject. After completing the scale, the subject answers questions about each item choosing from five categories of answers (a Likert scale). The total score ranges from 0 to 40.

hypnotizability scores may become contaminated by variables thought extraneous to the prevailing operational definition of hypnosis, such as the nature of the therapeutic relationship. A short description of the most important clinical scales of hypnotic susceptibility follows.

Given their low correlations with laboratory scales, the HIP and the CIS are hardly appropriate to measure hypnotizability in clinical research. What the HIP actually measures is still being discussed (Frischholz, Spiegel, & Spiegel, 1980; 1981; Frischholz, Tryon et al.; 1980; Hilgard, 1978, 1981a, 1981b; Orne et al., 1979; Sheehan, Latta, Regina, & Smith, 1979; H. Spiegel, 1977; Stern, Spiegel, & Nee, 1979). However, the CIS appears to be a valid and reliable scale to determine a person's capacity for imaginative involvement (Hilgard, Sheehan, Monteiro, & MacDonald, 1981; McConkey & Sheehan, 1982; McConkey, Sheehan, & White, 1979).

The correlation between the DRS and the SHSS: A and B ranges from .75 to .93 (Hilgard, 1978; O'Connell, Orne, & Shor, 1966; Orne & O'Connell, 1967). Given the individual character of the DRS and the lack of norms for unselected populations, the Stanford-type clinical scales are to be preferred as the most valid and easily administered clinical hypnotizability scales. The correlation between SHCS: adult and SHSS:C is .72 (Morgan & Hilgard, 1978-79a). The correlation between SHCS: child and SHSS:A is .67 (Morgan & Hilgard, 1978-1979b). The correlation between SHALIT and SHSS:A is .63 and SHALIT and SHSS:C is .52 (E. Hilgard, Crawford, & Wert, 1979).

OBJECTIONS TO THE MEASUREMENT OF HYPNOTIZABILITY

Many clinicians believe that individual differences in hypnotizability are irrelevant in therapy (Gill & Brenman, 1959; J.Jackson & Merrington, 1980; Sacerdote, 1982a, 1982b; Sheehan & Orne, 1968; Van der Hart, 1982). Some clinicians even believe that the assessment of hypnotizability is harmful to hypnotherapy. More specifically, it is argued that (J. Hilgard & E.Hilgard, 1979):

1. anyone can develop a sufficient level of hypnotic responsivity given a proper individualized approach and style of hypnotic communication;
2. compared with other factors, hypnotizability is of secondary importance to successful hypnotherapy;
3. hypnotizability ratings do not provide clinically useful information;
4. even if persons are not sufficiently hypnotizable at first, they can be trained to acquire the degree of hypnotic responsivity needed to benefit from hypnotherapy; and

5. measuring a person's hypnotizability in therapy may have adverse consequences.

Each of these objections are dealt with separately.

The Importance of Style of Hypnotic Suggestion

Many clinicians are convinced that everybody is capable of developing a clinically suitable hypnotic condition. Joseph Barber's (1980a) main criticism of investigations in which a relation is found between hypnotizability and therapeutic results is that hypnotizability is measured with standardized scales, in which authoritative and direct suggestions are given without taking into account the patient's special capabilities. In addition, standardized and direct suggestions are usually also given in the therapies that were investigated. In short, the clinical relevance of a person's hypnotizability is, according to Joseph Barber, an artifact that results from the high degree of similarity between the measuring and treatment situation (Fourie & Lifschitz, 1988).

Another study by Barber (1977) on the superior effects of a Rapid Induction Analgesia procedure (RIA) raised a lot of excited attention. In this study, Barber described how by using the RIA (a permissive and indirect hypnotic procedure aimed at posthypnotic analgesia), 99 out of 100 patients were able to undergo dental treatment without chemical anesthesia. On the basis of this very high success rate, Barber concluded that individual differences in hypnotic susceptibility are not important in the clinical application of hypnosis, although he failed to measure the level of hypnotizability in his patient sample (Frischholz et al., 1981).

Recent experimental research on the efficacy of the RIA gives some indications that the RIA indeed raises a subject's pain threshold independent of level of hypnotic susceptiblility (Fricton & Roth, 1985). However, a higher pain tolerance (especially for more intense pain) occurs in higher hypnotizable subjects, especially when an experimenter trains subjects in using the RIA, and helps them in maintaining and reinforcing the posthypnotically suggested analgesia (Price & Barber, 1987; Van Gorp, Meyer, & Dunbar, 1985).

Results of clinical research on the RIA are consistent with this interpretation. In the control of very intense pain occurring during hyperthermia treatment of cancer, personal training in using the RIA results in pain reduction in high hypnotizables only (Reeves, Redd, Strom, & Minagawa, 1983). When the RIA is presented on tape, however, almost no pain reduction is achieved during very discomforting dental treatment. In dental procedures with a low level of discomfort, the RIA does result in a successful hypnotic analgesia, irrespective of hypnotic susceptibility level (Gillett & Coe, 1984).

Further, it is interesting to mention in this context a personal communication of Barber that indicates that in his 1977 study he failed to report some important treatment parameters (cited in Gillett & Coe, 1984). Barber himself remained present during the dental treatment and he or the dentist tested and reinforced the posthypnotic analgesia during dental treatment. Moreover, he reported that when a patient requested chemical anesthesia during dental treatment, he or the dentist applied the posthypnotic cue again to reinforce the hypnotic analgesia. This occurred with 7 out of 10 patients.

Besides research on the effectiveness of the RIA the influence of differences in style of hypnotic communication has been investigated in experimental settings, especially during the last decade. One aspect of this research relates to the degree in which hypnotic suggestions are individualized and geared to the subject's capacities and limitations. Van der Does, Van Dyck, Spinhoven and Kloosman (1988) observed no differences in hypnotic response between subjects who received individualized or standardized suggestions for hypnotic phenomena such as ideomotor reactions, age regression, or amnesia.

No firm conclusions can be drawn from studies of the efficacy of permissively/indirectly versus authoritatively/directly worded suggestions because of procedural differences across studies and methodological shortcomings. In most studies no differences in objective responding have been found (Barber & Calverley, 1966; Lynn, Neufeld, & Matyi, 1987; Lynn, Weekes, Matyi, & Newfeld, 1988; Matthews, Bennett, Bean, & Gallagher, 1985; Matthews, Kirsch, & Mosher, 1985; Matthews & Mosher, 1988; Spinhoven, Baak, Van Dyck, & Vermeulen, 1988; Thorne & Hall, 1963; Woolson, 1986). The data with respect to differences in the subjective experience of the suggestions, however, are conflicting.

Alman and Carney (1980) observed that permissive/indirect suggestions for a posthypnotic reaction were superior to direct suggestions, independent of level of hypnotizability. Moreover, Stone and Lundy (1985) found that indirect wording enhanced involuntary behavioral responses, although the effects of both permissive/indirect and authoritative/direct suggestions were related to level of hypnotic susceptibility.

Overall, available research does not indicate that by using a more individualized approach and permissively/indirectly worded suggestions, a more valid measure of subject's level of hypnotic susceptibility can be obtained than by using standardized and authoritatively/directly worded hypnotizability scales. In fact, controlled clinical research along these lines with patients who are perhaps more resistent to hypnosis than volunteer subjects is still lacking.

Hypnotizability Is Not Important

Clinical experience has shown that more patients respond to hypnotherapy than can be expected from laboratory research on individual differences in hypnotic responsivity. Several authors have pointed out that in a clinical situation therapeutic success also depends on factors other than a person's hypnotizability. Sheehan and Orne (1968) claimed that in a clinical situation the intense relationship between the therapist and the patient, and the factor of secondary gain can make hypnotizability an insignificant variable. Lazarus (1973) concluded from a clinical study that the patient's attitude and expectations toward hypnosis contribute more to successful hypnotherapy than his degree of hypnotizability. Perry, Gelfand and Marcovitch (1979), when treating smokers, found hypnotizability to be an irrelevant variable compared to motivation to quit smoking. De Moor (1987) also stated that the complexity of the hypnotherapeutic situation transcends the situational and intrapersonal variables that have been found to influence hypnotic responsiveness in an experimental situation. Especially, the dynamics of the communication system and metacommunicative qualifications of information exchanged are different when clinical hypnosis is involved.

The findings of clinicians and laboratory researchers, however, are not incompatible if one acknowledges that a therapeutic response to a hypnotic induction and hypnotic suggestions is possible even when hypnosis does not occur. The efficacy of any treatment procedure is determined in varying degrees by factors, which although associated with therapy, are nevertheless extraneous to a given method. From a therapeutic point of view, it may seem unimportant to disentangle effects of the treatment procedure used from other nonspecific effects. From a scientific standpoint, however, it is worthwhile to analyze whether therapy results can be ascribed to a specific procedure and to what extent. The specification, identification, and verification of therapeutic factors unique to a special treatment procedure are essential for understanding the mechanisms through which therapeutic change is produced (Kazdin, 1986).

Besides assessing the individual's level of hypnotizability, hypnotizability scales are also expected to aid in distinguishing hypnotic responses from responses associated with other factors such as expectancy, relaxation, or a trusting relationship (Frankel, 1978a,1978b). However, there is no guarantee that high susceptibles in a therapy situation defined as hypnosis will actually enter a hypnotic condition, nor that they will respond to hypnotically conveyed therapeutic suggestions (Gruenewald, 1982a). On the other hand, low susceptibles can respond to hypnotic suggestions without necessarily experiencing their reactions as convincing or involuntary (Sheehan & McConkey, 1982).

Patients come for help and their motives differ substantially from those of research volunteers. These often covert motives may influence their hypnotic responses in ways difficult to control. Responding to a hypnotic induction and hypnotic suggestions is the end-product of numerous overlapping attentional/cognitive, motivational processes interacting with aptitudinal and relational factors probably not totally unique to hypnosis (Sheehan & McConkey, 1982). Measuring hypnotizability may not be entirely successful in teasing apart the extent to which the outcome of psychotherapy is a function of hypnosis.

Scores for hypnotic susceptibility may be helpful in differentiating hypnotic from nonhypnotic therapy responses. However, given the complexity and interactive nature of hypnotic responding, especially in a therapeutic situation, it does not seem that standardized hypnotic susceptibility scales alone can separate the effects of hypnosis per se from nonspecific effects. Further discussion of the use of susceptibility scales is given later in this chapter.

Scales Do Not Give Clinically Useful Information

Sacerdote (1982a, 1982b) has argued that the existing laboratory and clinical hypnotizability scales are not very helpful in formulating treatment plans. More specifically, he asserted that the generally accepted scales give disproportionate weight to some categories of hypnotic responses, but that they are not comprehensive enough to tap all the possible capabilities of individual patients. The scales are blind to some of the qualitative differences in the experience of hypnosis, and are insensitive to some of the dissociative abilities of the patient and to the subtler aspects of the relationship between therapist and patient. Standardized scales rely almost entirely on written or spoken instructions and therefore miss the opportunities of nonverbal communication. In addition they do not give enough emphasis to time as a crucial variable for a positive hypnotic response.

Frankel (1982), in his reply, stated that the purpose of the standardized scales is primarily investigative. However, he did point out ways that performance on the standardized scales can be used to guide treatment strategies. As he said, however, the scales in no way provide rules regarding whether or how hypnosis is to be used clinically.

For clinicians, the clinical scales mark an advance over the earlier laboratory scales, because they are relatively easy to administer and they do not include difficult items (hallucinations) or therapeutically irrelevant or possibly adverse items (e.g., challenges). Still, they present too many deficiencies to be used yet as practical instruments by the hypnotherapist. Their main value is that they can rather easily be integrated into the clinical context in order to assess hypnotizability in a standardized way for scientific purposes.

Hypnotizability Can Be Trained

Hypnosis theorists are sharply divided on the question of whether hypnotizability can best be conceptualized as a relatively stable trait of the individual

(Hilgard, 1975, 1982; Perry, 1977) or whether it can be thought of as a set of potentially modifiable social–cognitive skills and attitudes (Diamond, 1974; Spanos, 1982).

In numerous experimental studies, attempts have been made to raise the level of hypnotic responsiveness by interventions such as personal growth training, sensory deprivation, psychotomimetic drugs (e.g., LSD or Mescaline), biofeedback, and hypnosis training. The initial level of hypnotic responsiveness proves to be highly predictive of the eventual level reached. The assumption that hypnotizability is a relatively stable attribute of the person was not fundamentally challenged by this line of research on the modification of hypnotizability (Bowers, 1976).

In recent years, however, several studies based on a social–cognitive skills model of hypnotic responding have documented appreciable increases on behavioral and subjective measures of hypnotic susceptibility following hypnosis modification training (Gfeller, Lynn, & Pribble, 1987; Gorassini & Spanos, 1986; Spanos, Cross, Menary, & Smith 1988; Spanos, Robertson, Menary, & Brett, 1986). These studies show a much higher degree of methodological rigor than previous studies that also found a positive effect of hypnosis training (Diamond, 1972; Kinney & Sachs, 1974; Sachs & Anderson, 1967; Springer, Sachs, & Morrow, 1977). In these studies a considerable and enduring increase in hypnotic responsiveness has been observed after a training package that includes the following elements: (a) information aimed at enhancing positive attitudes and motivations, (b) the provision of imagery-based strategies for experiencing the subjective effects called for by the given suggestions, and (c) increasing interpersonal and rapport factors between the hypnotist and the subject. After undergoing such training, a great majority of initially moderately hypnotizable subjects achieved a high hypnotizability score. However, it cannot be excluded that demand characteristics influence the achieved suggestibility gains (Bates, Miller, Cross, & Brigham, 1988).

The main value of these investigations seems to be that they provide a growing understanding of the different factors that determine person's hypnotizability score. According to a multifactorial model of hypnotic responsiveness, hypnotizability scores result from a complex set of interacting factors, such as attitudes concerning hypnosis (Cronin, Spanos, & Barber, 1971), involvement in imagery (J. R. Hilgard, 1979), compliance (Van Dyck, 1986), rapport with the hypnotist (Sheehan, 1980), dissociative capacity (Hilgard, 1979a), degree of cognitive distortion (Register & Kihlstrom, 1986), and the fading away of the generalized reality orientation (Shor, 1959). Possibly, some of these factors have to be conceptualized as relatively stable traits, whereas others constitute potentially modifiable cognitive skills.

Generalizing these experimental findings to a clinical context, a substantial number of initially low to medium hypnotizable patients may prove to acquire and develop a sufficient degree of hypnotic responsiveness after hypnosis training. Up until now clinical research of which inter- and intrapersonal factors inhibit or facilitate hypnotic responsiveness in hypnotherapy is lacking.

Measuring Hypnotizability May Be Harmful

Many clinicians believe that one of the prerequisites in a clinical situation is to evoke in a patient positive expectations about his or her capabilities to respond to hypnosis and the hypnotic suggestions. Suggestions that are liable to go beyond the capacity of a patient are therefore not given. The therapist thus avoids disappointment or doubt about the efficacy of hypnosis or of the therapist's abilities to deal with the patient's problem. In this context, measuring hypnotizability is seen as harmful to the process of hypnotherapy, because almost no patient will be able to follow all the suggestions of a scale.

Perry, Gelfand, and Marcovitch (1979) pointed out that these objections result from the tacit presupposition that hypnosis is a means of manipulating a patient's behavior and steering it in a therapeutically desirable direction. In recent years, however, there have been a number of clinicians who agree with experimental researchers that hypnotizability is a skill or a set of skills, which, when understood by the therapist, can be used to alter a patient's experience. With this in mind, Frankel and Orne (1976) stress, in a preparatory session, that the scale is used to give the patient the opportunity to experience hypnosis and to react to different suggestions. In a nonperformance-oriented situation, a hypnotizability test is presented as an instrument that can give indications as to the areas of a person's hypnotic capabilities. Based on this knowledge, the hypnotic procedures can be modified in order to meet the individual needs of the patient.

Frankel et al. (1979), who administered standardized scales to more than 300 patients in 6 years, reported that a vast majority of the patients found exposure to the scales to be of a positive nature, in spite of their own initial hesitation to expose their patients to the probability of not being able to respond to certain items. Sporadic disappointing experiences occurred with the rather authoritative HGSHS:A, which was not administered individually. The fear that failure on a hypnotizability scale interferes with therapy also was not born out by the findings of Stern, Spiegel, and Nee (1979), who administered the HIP to more than 4,000 patients.

Precautions to reassure patients that these scores will not necessarily affect therapeutic outcome can partly prevent pretherapy measurements of patient's hypnotizability from inducing negative attitudes and expectancies concerning hypnosis and hypnotic responding. However, such assurances cannot be given in clinical research settings, where at least single blind conditions have to be met, and the hypnotist is not aware of the patient's hypnotizability score.

Hypnotic susceptibility and extent of pain reduction were significantly correlated in some clinical experimental studies. However, the correlation between these variables was nonsignificant when the assessment of hypnotic susceptibility followed pain testing (Spanos, Hodgins, Stam, & Gwynn, 1984; Spanos, Kennedy, & Gwynn, 1984; Spanos, McNeil, Gwynn, & Stam 1984). These findings indicate that the usual superiority of high susceptibles in suggested analgesia may possibly occur because expectations from the hypnotic susceptibility testing situation are carried over to the pain-testing situation.

In conclusion, clinical experience indicates that the administration of hypnotizability scales only sporadically leads to disappointing experiences, when hypnotists take precautions to counteract negative attitudes and expectancies in low hypnotizable subjects. In a clinical research setting investigation is still necessary to determine to what extent the overlap between the pretreatment susceptibility test situation and the subsequent hypnotherapy leads high susceptibles to approach hypnotherapy with positive attitudes and expectancies. This is especially true when a hypnotist cannot proceed with a more personalized procedure based on the patient's pretreatment assessment of hypnotizability.

CLINICAL APPLICATION OF HYPNOTIZABILITY SCALES

In the previous section it was suggested that hypnotizability scales may be helpful in planning treatment strategy and in familiarizing a patient with hypnosis. It is further argued that these scales may be helpful in differentiating hypnotic from nonhypnotic therapy responses,although outcome as related to hypnosis per se, versus nonspecific effects of the hypnotic interaction, is hard to disentangle. Probably the most useful clinical application of hypnotizability scales is in investigating the relationship between hypnotizability and psychopathology and in problem solving, for example, in overcoming phobias, pain, and various habits and somatic complaints (Frankel, 1978a; Mott, 1979).

Hypnotizability and Psychopathology

In the 19th century, disagreement existed about the relationship between hypnosis and psychopathology. Charcot argued that the hypnotic state demonstrated neurological and mental dysfunctions, whereas Bernheim maintained that hypnosis was a normal psychological phenomenon (Spiegel, Detrick, & Frischholz , 1982). The development of hypnotizability scales has rendered the question subject to empirical assessment. On the average, "normal" subjects prove to be better hypnotic subjects and achieve higher hypnotizability scores than patients (Frankel & Orne, 1976). In some diagnostic categories there appears to exist a nonrandom relationship between hypnotizability and relative mental health.

Coincident with the renewed experimental and therapeutic interest in the concept of dissociation as originally developed by Janet (E. Hilgard, 1977, 1979a; Van der Hart, 1986), several reports have been published in which the level of hypnotic susceptibility was assessed in patients who manifested symptomswith dissociative aspects. In most studies of phobic patients, the level of hypnotic susceptibility appears to be higher than in a normal reference group (Frankel & Orne, 1976; Gerschman, Burrows, Reade, & Foenander, 1979; John, Hollander, & Perry, 1983; Kelly 1984; Spiegel, Frischholz, Maruffi, & Spiegel, 1981). The same holds true for patients with nightmares (Belicki & Belicki, 1982, 1984), sleepwalking (Perrault & Montplaisir, 1984), conversion disorder (Bliss, 1983,1984), posttraumatic stress disorder (Stutman & Bliss , 1985; Spiegel, Hunt, & Dondershine, 1988), or hyperemesis gravidarum (Apfel, Kelly, & Frankel, 1986). Elevated hypnotizability scores have also been reported for patients with bulimia or anorexia nervosa with vomiting (Pettinati & Wade, 1986) and patients with a multiple personality disorder (Bliss & Jeppsen, 1985; Bliss & Larson, 1985). Nash, Lynn, and Givens (1984), who observed that adults who had been physically abused before the age of ten were more hypnotizable then nonabused adults, interpreted hypnotizability from a developmental perspective as a coping mechanism to attenuate traumatic experiences (J. R. Hilgard, 1974a, 1979).

On the other hand, studies on the relationship between hypnotizability and psychopathology did not find differences in hypnotizability scores between normative groups and the following patient samples:

- non-schizophrenic psychotic (Scagnelli-Jobsis, 1982, 1983; Pettinati, 1982; Spiegel, 1983).
- chronic pain patients (Frischholz, Spiegel, Spiegel, Balma, & Markell, 1982),
- patients with a nicotine addiction (Frischholz et al., 1982; Perry, Gelfand, & Marcovitch, 1979; Perry & Mullen, 1975), and
- panic disorder with agoraphobia (Van Dyck, 1986)

A significantly lower level of hypnotizability has been reported in patients with the following diagnoses:

- schizophrenia,
- affective disorder (such as a bipolar disorder),
- generalized anxiety (Spiegel, Detrick, & Frischholz, 1982),

- alexithymia (Frankel, Apfel-Savitz, Nemiah, & Sifneos, 1977), and
- obsessive–compulsive neurosis (Hoogduin & De Jong, 1984, 1986)

It is evident that research on the relationship between hypnotizability and psychopathology is relatively recent and replication studies that better control for possible confounding variables such as unclear diagnostic criteria, age, use of medication, and context effects (Council, Kirsch, & Hafner, 1986) are essential. Also, the possible role of hypnotizability in the pathogenesis of different forms of psychopathology should be investigated in greater detail. Hypnotic susceptibility may constitute a vulnerability factor in the development of psychopathology, and/or the development of hypnotizability may be conceptualized as a coping mechanism to attenuate the impact of traumatic experiences and stress.

Although dissociative capacity is often mentioned as a pivotal concept linking hypnotic susceptibility with certain forms of psychopathology, the boundaries of the concept of dissociation are rather vague and the concept needs to be clarified to a greater extent in order to establish its empirical validity. If this could be accomplished, hypnotherapy may prove to be especially indicated for patients with dissociative characteristics. Hypnosis may help patients to acquire control over these dissociative processes (Frankel, 1976). On the other hand, severe psychopathology may inhibit the development of a hypnotic state and interfere with the concentration of attention and the flexible handling of reality and fantasy, necessary for a successful hypnotic response (Spiegel, Detrick, & Frischholz, 1982).

Hypnotizability and Problem Solving

Mott (1979); Perry, Gelfand, and Marcovitch (1979); Bowers and Kelly (1979); Wadden and Anderton (1982); and Spinhoven (1982) have reviewed the relationship between level of hypnotic susceptibility and the effectiveness of hypnotherapy as investigated in more than 30 outcome studies. The most important results of this line of research are summarized here. Most of these studies relate to the treatment of phobic complaints, chronic pain syndromes, asthma, warts, smoking, and obesity. Irrespective of treatment strategy, in most studies a significant or at least positive relationship between hypnotizability and therapeutic results has been found. Also in the investigations by Lang, Lazovik, and Reynolds (1965) and Marks, Gelder, and Edwards (1968) this relationship was found to exist, even though their therapy was in fact a pseudotherapy, and the hypnotic experience was not aimed at a specific treatment goal (Spiegel, Frischholz, Maruffi, & Spiegel, 1981).

In many investigations, hypnotherapy is seen to produce better results in the group of moderate to high susceptibles. No reliable norms on patient populations being available, we can only assume that as in an unselected student population, 15% of the patients are not or are only low hypnotizable (Hilgard, 1965). The fact that in 15% of the cases, hypnotherapy may not be the most efficient treatment, would make a person's hypnotizability a crucial variable for hypnotherapy. In the light of what clinicians traditionally think about the importance of hypnotizability, this is a striking conclusion.

The conclusion concerning the therapeutic relevance of hypnotizability needs some qualification, however. As mentioned earlier in studies hypnotizability proved to be clinically irrelevant. Most of these studies dealt with smoking and obesity. The relevance of hypnotizability may not only depend on the person's hypnotic ability, but also on the nature of the problem as well (Bowers, 1981; Perry, Gelfand, & Marcovitch, 1979; Wadden & Anderton, 1982).

Direct hypnotic suggestions seem to be particularly effective in the treatment of somatic and psychosomatic symptoms in patients with a moderate to high responsivity to hypnosis. The irrelevance of hypnotizability in the hypnotherapy of obesity and smoking can be understood in various ways. Problems such as pain, warts, asthma and so on are involuntary phenomena. Problems such as obesity and smoking have a stronger voluntary component of self-initiated behavior (Bowers, 1981; Perry, Gelfand, & Marcovitch, 1979). In the treatment of somatic and psychosomatic problems such as pain and asthma, an alteration of subjective experience will suffice to reduce or eliminate the problem to a considerable extent. In the case of habits such as obesity and smoking, subjective alteration does not guarantee therapeutic success. These behaviors can be seen as over-learned responses under tight social and physiologic control (Perry, Gelfand, & Marcovitch, 1979; Wadden & Anderton, 1982). In addition, pain and anxiety, for example, usually create aversion in the short and in the long run, thus motivating the patient to accept therapeutic suggestions. Smoking and eating, however, are quickly rewarding, and have aversive effects only in the long run. This possible conflict between long-and short-term reinforcement may evoke tension and anxiety during hypnotherapy and interfere with responsiveness to suggestions (Perry, Gelfand, & Marcovitch, 1979; Wadden & Anderton, 1982).

Moreover, the therapeutic relevance of hypnotizability many also be related to the kinds of suggestions that are typically used in many hypnotherapeutic approaches for smoking and obesity. Suggestions for relaxation, ego enhancement, or positive future-oriented imagery typically used for smoking and obesity are relatively "easy" suggestions that most patients can pass and that do not require major cognitive/affective/perceptual alterations more characteristic of hypnosis for pain, asthma, and anxiety. The therapeutic relevance may be contextually dependent and require a therapeutic approach in which voluntary control is less prominent and suggestions for more difficult to pass involuntary hypnotic experiences are given (Andersen, 1985; Bowers, 1982; Spinhoven, 1987).

Not all the research available is of equally good quality: Patient populations are sometimes quite heterogeneous (Cedercreutz, 1978; Spiegel et al., 1981); the patient's or the therapist's assessment of the therapeutic results are often subjective ones (Glick, 1970; Stern, Spiegel, & Nee, 1979); and frequently follow-up data are lacking (Lang, Lazovik, & Reynolds, 1965; Sullivan, Johnson, & Bratkovitch, 1974).

Further, the treatment procedure in most of the studies is not described in sufficient detail (Cohen & Alpert, 1978; Deyoub, 1979a, 1979b). One gets the impression that in many investigative studies standardized and direct suggestions are given in an authoritative manner, and that the number of sessions is rather limited. More research is needed on prolonged hypnotherapies (where the therapeutic approach is more in line with clinical practice). Possibly, the therapeutic relevance of hypnotizability will be reduced in studies where hypnosis is used as an adjunct in the context of a more comprehensive treatment. A negative relationship between "width" of therapy and the importance of "depth" of hypnosis may exist. Especially in short-term symptomatic treatments in which suggestions for hypnotic phenomena constitute the main therapy ingredients (such as hypnotic analgesia in pain reduction), hypnotizability may prove to be related to therapy success (Spanos, Hodgins, Stam & Gwynn, 1984; Spanos, Kennedy & Gwynn, 1984).

A positive development is the more frequent use of hypnotizability scales in research on hypnotherapy. However, it seems that double blind conditions were rarely if ever used. Only Perry and Mullen (1975) presented pseudohypnotic items when measuring hypnotizability in order to try and give all the patients the experience of having the necessary capacities to be able to benefit from hypnosis. In most of the studies it is not explicitly stated that the therapist was unaware of the results of the hypnotizability ratings. Such methodological flaws are surprising in the light of the ample literature on "demand characteristic" in hypnotic responding (Orne, 1979a; Sheehan & Perry, 1976).

CONCLUSIONS AND RECOMMENDATIONS

Hypnotizability Scales and Clinical Research

Clinical researchers and therapists interested in research and in the replicability of their findings are advised to assess their patients' hypnotizability with a standardized scale (Frankel, 1981). The effects of hypnotherapy seem to be related to the level of hypnotic susceptibility, the disorder under treatment, and the nature of the therapeutic context and hypnotic suggestions given. It therefore seems warranted to assess the therapeutic value of hypnosis by comparing in high and low hypnotizable patients a nonhypnotic treatment with a hypnotic treatment by the same therapist, including specific hypnotic suggestions relevant for the disorder under treatment (Spinhoven, 1987).

Hypnotizability assessment may also be relevant for case reports. Case reports can contribute to a better understanding of hypnotherapy, if the problem, the treatment and the results are described in some detail. In any therapy situation it is hard to appreciate the relative influence of such factors as expectation, relaxation, the therapeutic relationship and so on; it is therefore important to measure objectively whatever we can. In this context, the assessment of hypnotizability with a standardized scale is a highly useful and easy measure. However a hypnotizability scale can only measure a person's hypnotic capacity; it can not be used to assess whether hypnotic processes actually occurred during therapy. If from a hypnotizability measurement it is concluded that hypnosis has been present, it is taken for granted that a person in a therapy situation defined as hypnosis will actually use his or her hypnotic capabilities after the induction of hypnosis. Even if this is a reasonable assumption, it is nevertheless, an assumption. To assess the presence of hypnosis during therapy, clients could be asked to give a subjective report of their experience of hypnosis in that setting (Shor, 1979; Tart, 1979b). Such methods for the evaluation of hypnotic experience can give important information supplementary to the data gathered by hypnotizability measurements (Laurence & Nadon, 1986; Sheehan & McConkey, 1982).

Hypnotizability Scales and Clinical Practice

Given the results of the research available, it is questionable whether hypnotherapists who are interested mainly in the practical application of hypnosis should be advised to use hypnotizability scales. Although the scales suit the purpose of research on hypnotherapy, they are too narrow to serve as a practical instrument in hypnotherapy (Sacerdote, 1982a, 1982b). Although the degree of hypnotizability in patients with psychosomatic and anxiety problems contributes to the success of hypnotherapy and in at least some studies low hypnotizables treated with a nonhypnotic treatment responded better than low hypnotizables treated with hypnosis (Van Dyck, 1986), the amount of variance in therapy results accounted for is so small that it does not permit reliable individual predictions indiscriminately. There is no justification to withhold hypnotherapy from a patient with such problems solely because he or she has a low hypnotizability score. Such a decision should also depend on other factors, such as the patient's motivation and expectations, the availability of effective alternative treatments, etc . On the other hand, the hypnotherapist who administers a scale will find some guidance that will help him or her to plan the treatment strategy. A hypnotizability scale can give the therapist some indications of a person's hypnotic skills, which will guide him or her to decide what procedure will be appropriate and what therapeutic suggestions can be successfully presented (Frankel, 1982).

But a therapist should not rely blindly on the hypnotizability score of a patient (Tellegen, 1978). The incomplete information from a standardized test must be augmented by an evaluation of the patient's motivation, expectations and attitude toward hypnosis (Gruenewald, 1982a; Frankel, 1982; Udolf, 1981). Furthermore, it is useful to discuss with the patient the phenomena he or she experienced during the test and his of her reactions to it; and to make use of this information by exploring through an alternative approach whether the patient responds better to suggestions different from those used in the hypnotizability scales (Hart, 1985).

The Multifactorial Nature of Hypnotizability

A last remark is related to the question of whether the therapeutic relevance of hypnotizability is fact or fiction. Although some speak of hypnotizability as a concrete entity, one must not lose sight of the fact that hypnotic susceptibility is a theoretical construct used to explain individual differences in hypnotic responding. The actual score on a standardized hypnotizability scale only forms an operational definition for this hypothetical construct.

Few advocates of the clinical use of hypnotizability scales will argue that a person's hypnotizability score can be equated with his or her level of hypnotic susceptibility. Just this ambiguous meaning of the concept of hypnotizability has generated a lot of research. Research into the relationship between hypnotizability and related factors, like the development of the concept of intelligence, has led to a greater specification and differentiation of the concept of hypnotizability. We can no longer assume that hypnotizability is a homogeneous and consistent ability. Rather we find that it is the sum of various dynamic, trait, and state factors. Thus, it may be expected that clinically more relevant predictions can be formulated about the association of dimensions of hypnotizability with different forms of psychopathology and for various problems presented for solution through hypnotherapy. This line of research promises to be a fruitful area for bridging the gap between research and clinical practice.

Chapter 10

HOW HYPNOSIS MAY POTENTIATE PSYCHOTHERAPY*

JEAN HOLROYD
University of California, Los Angeles

What accounts for the effectiveness of hypnotherapy and occasional dramatic results? A noticeable gap between clinical observations and experimental research gives rise to the question, "*How* does hypnosis affect clinical outcome?" Psychotherapists lack a conceptual framework that considers both psychotherapy processes and trance characteristics. This chapter is an attempt to focus our thinking on trance phenomena as they affect therapy, and is directed at the thoughtful clinician. The discussion is limited to the hypnotic *state*, which I take to be equivalent to hypnotic trance. I do not include other dimensions of treatment such as hypnotic context and waking suggestions (Mott, 1982).

The trance-related phenomena I have identified involve changes in attention and awareness, imagery, dissociation, reality orientation, suggestibility, mind–body interactions, initiative or volition, availability of affect, and relationship. Elsewhere I have presented research evidence for many of these trance effects (Holroyd, 1986). This chapter proposes that hypnotherapy exploits hypnotic phenomena—takes advantage of them—in the service of standard therapy endeavors. Hopefully, future papers will provide more detailed examples of exploitation of trance phenomena in connection with specific cases.

---

*Reprinted from Holroyd, J. (1987). How hypnosis may potentiate psychotherapy. *American Journal of Clinical Hypnosis*, 194–200.

In discussing the effects of hypnotic trance on therapy, it is important to distinguish changes attributable to the hypnotic state from differences attributable to personality variability. Research investigating the cognitive, emotional, and motivational changes associated with hypnosis frequently has not made this distinction. Nevertheless, clinically it seems useful to pay attention to the putative effects of hypnosis until the experimental data clarify whether effects are due to person, situation, or their interaction.

TRANCE EFFECTS

Attention

Attention changes in two ways during hypnosis, to become either more focused or more free-floating (Fromm et al., 1981). Both types of changes can facilitate psychotherapy. Attending to awareness is central to Gestalt therapy as well as psychoanalysis. As Fromm (1979) noted:

> Attention cathexis is withdrawn from the normal average range of its distribution *in order* to concentrate it with full intensity on one single spot. If this spot is a piece of reality, better knowledge about it can be gained in hypnosis than in the waking state where it has to share attention cathexis with a much wider range of objects. (p.101)

In fact, Gendlin (1978) postulated that "focusing," is the quintessential therapy process. In contrast, the deautomatized free-floating attention sometimes associated with hypnosis facilitates free association in psychoanalysis.

Imagery

Imagery appears to be reliably vivid for highly hypnotizable subjects, more vivid following hypnosis (Coe, St. Jean, & Burger, 1980), and is an important aspect of many types of therapy (Sheikh & Jordon, 1983). (Whether it is actually more vivid under hypnosis is somewhat controversial, but five out of six controlled studies located in the literature support that position; see Holroyd, 1986.) It is likely that visualization promotes awareness of emotional and symbolic or primary-process material (Reyher & Smeltzer, 1968) and facilitates creative problem solving (Dave, 1979). Furthermore, imagery involving senses other than vision seems useful in psychodynamic explorations. Unfortunately, controlled research on the relationship between imagery vividness and therapy effectiveness has been limited to visual imagery and to behavior therapy and has yielded mixed results (e.g., Dyckman & Cowan, 1978; McLemore, 1972). Furthermore, Kazdin (1979) found that it was the elaboration of scenes in imagination rather than vivid imagery per se that leads to better therapy outcomes. The question is not just whether hypnosis reliably improves imagery, but what that improvement may contribute to imagery therapies.

Dissociation

Dissociation, which is said by some to be fundamental to hypnosis (E.Hilgard, 1977), is also central to the psychotherapeutically germaine concept of an unconscious (Shevrin & Dickman, 1980). Unlike imagery, however, promoting dissociation is not integral to many therapies. Gestalt therapists, more than others, have fostered temporary dissociation to facilitate emergence of previously unconscious attitudes. The patient is encouraged to "talk to" the split-off parts of the self. Watkins' (1978) hypnosis-facilitated ego-state therapy also relies on dissociation in order to discover unconscious attitudes or roles.

Other applications of dissociation in therapy tend to rely on hypnosis to establish the dissociative set. A patient may "view" traumatic memories on a TV screen or recall unhappy childhood memories protected with hypnotically suggested amnesia. A phobic patient may be taught to block awareness of the feared situation, and an obsessional patient may be taught to have a blank mind. The smoker may ameliorate physical withdrawal symptoms by considering the body as separate from the self. In summary, dissociation capabilities that are overlooked in most traditional psychotherapies are particularly salient for hypnotherapy. Like imagery, the mechanism of action for dissociation in psychotherapy is not well understood.

Reality Orientation

Reality orientation decreases during hypnosis; the usual interpretive framework of cognitive understanding is abandoned (Shor, 1959). Correspondingly, there is a preoccupation with internal processes (P. Bowers & K. Bowers, 1979), increased primary process thinking (Fromm, Oberlander, & Gruenewald, 1970), and a higher frequency of dream recall (Stross & Shevrin, 1967). Loss of reality orientation and the accompanying florescence of internal processes may benefit seemingly disparate therapies. The fantasies and primary-process material available during hypnosis provide rich lodes for psychoanalytic exploration. On the other hand, cognitive interventions such as reframing (Watzlawick, Weakland, & Fisch, 1974) also may be facilitated by the absence of continuous reality checking.

Suggestion

Suggestions are the hallmark of hypnosis (Weitzenhoffer, 1980), but well-controlled therapy research in which only experimentally altered suggestibility is varied is scant. Indeed, studies of hypnotherapy that measure suggestibility generally have been limited to populations with physical problems or easily measured behavioral problems. Although positive suggestibility/outcome relationships have been demonstrated for psychosomatic disorders and pain, the relationship seems weaker for more psychological problems (K. Bowers & Kelly, 1979; Mott, 1979; Perry, Gelfand, & Marcovitch, 1979). Research design problems suggest caution in accepting these results at face value, however.

It is unclear how such suggestion operates in nonhypnotic therapies. Because highly hypnotizable people tend to respond to suggestion in the unhypnotized state (Weitzenhoffer & Sjoberg, 1961), they probably internalize remarks of a trusted therapist more readily than their less responsive brethren. In fact they do seem to respond faster to inpatient treatment (paradoxically with subsequently higher rate of rehospitalization; Horne, 1985). It seems logical that increasing suggestibility with hypnosis would improve at least initial response to any "talking cure."

Mind–Body Interface

Hypnosis reveals the *mind-body interface* in an unparalleled manner (Black, 1969), sometimes resulting in motor paralyses, automatic movements, altered sensation or perception, changed physiology, or shifted cerebral lateralization. How the potential for intensifying mind–body communication may influence therapy is not well understood. Our dual nature receives only incidental attention in traditional therapy, which focuses on intrapsychic and interpersonal events even when the presenting problem is psychosomatic. (Bioenergetics and Reichian therapists use physical contact, but like traditionalists they are primarily concerned with characterological impairment.) Of course, behavior therapy and biofeedback have paid more attention to physiology, particularly in training relaxation.

Hypnosis extends treatment of physical disease farther than training for relaxation however, and relaxation is not essential to the hypnotic state (Banyai & Hilgard, 1976). Evidence of the biological effects of hypnosis is particularly strong for skin problems, psychosomatic problems, and pain problems (Barber, 1978; Di Piano & Salzberg, 1979; Hilgard & Hilgard, 1975; Mott, 1979; Perry et al., 1979). The mechanisms of cure are not known, although vascular and endocrinological systems are suspected (Black, 1969; K. Bowers & Kelly, 1979).

Feeling of Compulsion

The seventh attribute, a *feeling of compulsion* or of necessity to do what the hypnotist suggests, is closely related to increased suggestibility (P. Bowers,

1982) and implicates processes of rapport (Sheehan & McConkey, 1982). Commonly subjects say they are simply waiting for the hypnotist to tell them what to do. In psychodynamic terms, the ego has shifted into a receptive mode (Fromm, 1977) and executive functions have been turned over to the hypnotist (Hilgard, 1977).

In nonhypnotic therapies practitioners attempt to deflect patients' desires to comply with therapists' (covert) expectations. Psychoanalysts and client-centered therapists attempt not to give even a clue about the therapist's preferences, although behavior therapists may prescribe treatment activities. Whereas traditional therapists attempt to avoid undue influence in order to support autonomy and self-initiated activity, hypnotherapists use patients' inclinations to fulfill the therapist's expectations as leverage for accomplishing therapy goals (risking the accusation of being considered manipulative). It is paradoxical that encouraging a patient to abandon executive functions can be therapeutic, given the high value we place on patient initiative and self-responsibility in therapy. Exploration of this paradox may provide further clues to psychotherapy change processes in general.

Affect

Affect becomes more available with hypnosis, as evidenced by the spontaneous occurrence of emotion as well as the easy arousal of emotion with hypnotic suggestions (Blum, 1979). Hypnotized people tend to laugh more at jokes (Maslach, Zimbardo, & Marshall, 1979), as well as exhibit a higher heart rate following fear stimulation (Hepps & Brady, 1967).

Why emotional expression is important in psychotherapy is not clear, despite the fact that affect stimulation is a prime function of therapists across orientations. Perhaps it is not just catharsis that is important, but also the emergence of associated memories and conflicts. Childhood memories associated with a hypnotically induced mood are recalled more readily than other childhood memories (Bower, 1981). It follows that therapists who can manipulate moods and enhance experienced affect using hypnosis have better access to psychodynamically important early memories. Watkins (1971) applied this principle as an "affect bridge" in hypnosis to move patients experientially from present feelings to past events. There is an obvious need for controlled research on the effects of the per se expression of affect in therapy, as well as affect-mediated recall.

Archaic Involvement

The relationship between hypnotist and patient entails a *fusional or archaic* element that differs from the psychoanalytic concept of transference (Chertok, 1982; Diamond, 1987; Shor, 1962). Until recently, scientists have not attempted to study archaic involvement, perhaps because it is less likely to be observed during experimental hypnosis than during treatment (Weitzenhoffer, 1980). Also, hypnotic rapport is not experienced by everyone who is hypnotized and is not predicted by standard tests of hypnotizability (Sheehan, 1971; Sheehan & Dolby, 1979). Recent research suggests that the hypnotist–subject relationship is reflected even at the neurophysiological level (Banyai, 1985). The implications of intense mutual involvement between therapist and patient for treatment process and outcome point to areas of unmined gold in hypnotherapy research.

Despite the paucity of experimental studies of fusional and archaic processes, concepts of rapport and transference have been important to dynamic psychotherapy, and central to some theories of hypnosis (Gruenewald, 1982b). Archaic involvement may facilitate treatment by permitting the development of a therapeutic alliance; by neutralizing resistance in selected situations; and by permitting regression with primordial fantasies and child-like transference. On the other hand, there may be instances when these effects are not desired (e.g., when a therapist wishes to work with a full-blown negative transference, minimize a patient's dependent feelings, or observe an adult-to-adult relationship; Diamond, 1987). Freud (1966) stopped using hypnosis in part because he valued interpreting the resistance rather than attenuating it.

CONCLUSION

I have tried to clarify how some psychological phenomena attributable to hypnosis may contribute to the effectiveness of hypnotherapy. In addition, hypnotic responsivity of patients probably improves their responsiveness to nonhypnotic psychotherapy. The concept of a three-way interaction between individual responsivity, changes attributable to hypnosis, and psychotherapy processes such as uncovering, imagery exploration, and so on, may provide a focus for more definitive clinical interventions as well as stimulate research that will lead to more effective hypnotherapy.

The nine trance characteristics noted here are not sacrosanct; they are neither purely theoretical nor empirical. They could be reduced as well as expanded by others who interpret the literature differently. I derived nine characteristics from experimental research and clinical observations of differences in experiencing under hypnosis, and progressed to a discussion of how those capabilities developed in hypnosis can potentiate psychotherapy. This quasi-empirical approach is rather shaky in areas not well researched, but hopefully clinical usefulness and a heuristic function for scientific exploration may compensate for this failing.

Chapter 11

SEQUELAE TO CLINICAL AND EXPERIMENTAL HYPNOSIS

BILLIE S. STRAUSS
Michael Reese Hospital and Medical Center, University of Illinois at Chicago

Although clinicians and researchers trained in and experienced with the use of hypnosis view it as a reasonably safe technique, difficulties have been reported in the literature. These difficulties have been characterized in several ways. The problem may be in the hypnotic experience itself (e.g., a subject does not awaken from hypnosis when suggestions are given) or in the larger therapeutic or experimental context (e.g., substitute symptoms are produced). The complication may range from minimal discomfort to actual harm to patients or subjects. Problematic effects following or during hypnotherapy and hypnosis experiments have been conceptualized as sequelae to hypnosis (J. Hilgard, 1974b; J. Hilgard, & Hilgard , & Newman, 1961), dangers of hypnosis (Conn, 1972; Meares, 1961; West & Deckert, 1965), undesirable effects of hypnosis (Orne, 1965), transient experiences following hypnosis (Crawford, Hilgard, & MacDonald, 1982), deleterious effects of hypnosis (Kleinhauz & Eli, 1987), complications of hypnosis (MacHovec, 1988), and adverse reactions in the use of hypnosis (Mott, 1987). Examination of these problems is useful in order to minimize them in the future and to handle them more effectively should they occur.

Orne (1965) noted that most of the problematic effects of hypnosis occur in the therapeutic situation rather than in the experimental setting because the former creates expectations of change that may threaten a patient's coping mechanisms. The literature reports negative sequelae following experimental, therapeutic, and teaching/demonstration uses of hypnosis (Lazar & Dempster, 1981). Problems sometimes do arise during or following hypnosis experiments as well as during or following hypnotherapy sessions that must be handled and understood in light of the interaction between the subject's characteristics and the nature of the experimental or clinical context.

This chapter considers some of the variables that may contribute to negative effects of hypnosis that occur when hypnosis is used by trained professionals who follow accepted standards of practice, rather than by nonprofessionals or stage hypnotists. Factors related to sequelae of clinical uses of hypnosis, and problems that arose during and after a group hypnosis experiment are presented. Whether and the extent to which hypnosis, or the hypnotic context is related to the unpleasant effects is addressed.

SEQUELAE TO CLINICAL HYPNOSIS

Surveys of clinicians who use hypnosis suggested that in the United States approximately 25% (Levitt & Hershman, 1963) and in Australia 45% (25% in the year preceding the survey. Judd, Burrows, & Dennerstein, 1986) reported complications and/or unusual, or adverse reactions. Negative sequelae of hypnotherapy appear to stem from the interaction between patient variables and therapeutic intervention, including therapeutic strategy, therapist variables, and hypnotic technique.

Patient variables, including anticipation of the reduction of symptoms, transference reactions, and other psychodynamic mechanisms, sometimes contribute to problems attributed to hypnotherapy. For example, a patient whose psychogenic headaches were alleviated with hypnotherapy suddenly awoke from hypnosis, vomited, and refused further treatment (Lazer & Dempster, 1981). This patient had a variety of psychogenic complaints. She spent considerable time seeing her 10 doctors, and made luncheon appointments with their other patients. Other social relationships were limited. She was of borderline normal intelligence and held a job because a relative was an officer in the firm. This patient used her headaches (and other symptoms) as a means of fostering interpersonal relationships and as a way of giving meaning to her somewhat limited and marginal lifestyle. Hypnosis, because it successfully removed her symptom, threatened the coping mechanisms she had developed. Whether symptom removal without the use of hypnosis (e.g., use of cognitive–behavioral techniques) would have held the same threat, or indeed, even have been successful, is unclear.

Specific hypnotic techniques sometimes contribute to negative reactions. Use of relaxation techniques with some patients results in increased anxiety. Some patients experience techniques that foster increased dissociation and nonvoluntariness as similar to the symptoms for which they seek treatment. For example, a patient with a flying phobia, which he related to loss of control, experienced relaxation techniques as "going under," similar to how he felt when in an airplane or otherwise out of control (Strauss, 1986). This patient responded positively to supportive suggestions that emphasized control rather than effortless functioning.

Treatment strategy in conjunction with hypnotherapy may result in negative sequelae. Dramatic examples involve removal of seemingly circumscribed symptoms (one patient's smoking, a second patient's fear of flying, and a third patient's psychogenic abdominal pain) with hypnosis that resulted in personality decompensation and hospitalization (Kleinhauz & Eli, 1987; Meldman, 1960; Oberlander, 1978). Further examination of these cases revealed pre-existing psychopathology, intrapsychic meaning of the symptoms unknown to the therapist, and in one case, coincidental circumstances unknown to the therapist. A more detailed history and a more cautious approach may have prevented these difficulties, although whether another event, independent of hypnosis or therapy, would have precipitated decompensation is unknown.

In these cases, hypnosis did not cause the personality decompensation. Rather, these effects appear to have been the result of the removal of symptoms that were necessary for the patients' intrapsychic economy. The contribution of hypnosis was its effectiveness in removing symptoms by circumventing the patient's weak ego defenses. Healthier patients might have retained their symptoms, substituted another symptom, or become unhypnotizable.

In some cases, the treatment strategy of direct symptom removal may result in symptom substitution. For example, Cedercreutz (1972) presented a case where symptom removal resulted in multiple symptom substitution and even surgeries that could have been avoided by taking an adequate history. Symptoms remitted as the result of an analysis. The cultural meaning of hypnosis and expectations generated may contribute to the "success" of hypnosis in symptom removal, even when patients need the symptoms.

The interaction between patient variables and intervention in producing negative reactions is illustrated in the following case. A professional woman sought hypnosis for relaxation to control back pain, which was attributed to tension. The patient had been treated by her physician for the pain for over 10 years, and no medical reason was found. She was completing an advanced graduate degree that would assure her of a promotion in her field. She sought hypnotherapy at this time because she had to write several papers to complete her degree, and experienced considerable pain when she sat for long periods of time. No psychodynamic function for the pain was evident from the history she provided. She had seen another therapist for hypnotherapy several years earlier and was told she was not hypnotizable. Evaluation suggested that she was a highly intelligent and capable woman with low self-esteem. She also had difficulty with mutuality in relationships.

The patient was hypnotized easily using an eye fixation technique. She reported that she felt as if she was floating and was not quite in control of what she was doing, but that this loss of control was fun. The clenched fist technique (Stein, 1963) was used to promote relaxation and reduce tension. This technique involves having the patient imagine water flowing into a pitcher, and in an analogous way, imagine the excess tension in her body flow into her fist, and soon her fist would open. After a moment, the patient said her fingers could not open, and expressed concern that she was unable to move them. I gently told her that her fingers soon would move just a bit, that they had in fact moved a bit, and she would be rid only of any excess tension she did not need. Within a short time the patient opened her fist.

After the termination of hypnosis, the patient explained that her job and school responsibilities demanded considerable concentration and discipline, and she enjoyed the feeling of not having to be in control. She attributed the failure of her fingers to open to her having to write her papers; she somehow felt that if her fingers remained closed, she could remain in trance and avoid the hard work of writing the papers. Several weeks later, as we continued to explore her feelings about and reaction to hypnosis, the patient talked about her feelings of competition with me because I was an experienced professional woman, and she viewed me as more successful than she viewed herself. She noted that her fingers had not opened because she did not want me to help her, so she would not allow my techniques to work. The patient was able to discuss her competitive feelings toward me, and relate these to her difficulty with mutuality with her friends. A second issue that emerged was her ambivalence about completing her degree, and how the papers that she had to write were a source of conflict.

In this case, a history was obtained, a permissive approach was used, and an attempt was made to allow the patient to relinquish only as much tension as was comfortable. However, the patient still had the uncomfortable experience of not being able to open or move her fingers. Several variables contributed to this negative effect. The specific hypnotic technique certainly was a factor in her catalepsy, although whether an untoward reaction to a different relaxation technique would have occurred is unclear. One can speculate about whether the clenched fist had symbolic meaning, such as anger, for this patient, although this technique has been used with many other patients without incident. The context of hypnosis was a second factor. She previously was told that she was not hypnotizable, and having hypnosis "work" was important to her. Being "unable" to open her fingers was an indication to her that she was hypnotized. Dynamic factors that contributed to the patient's reaction were her competitive transference reaction to the therapist and her ambivalence toward completing the papers and hence, her degree. The strategy of symptom removal in conjunction with some dynamic exploration seemed to be an appropriate one, in that the use of other relaxation techniques resulted in some pain reduction with no further incident.

Discussion

Negative reactions during or following hypnotherapy sometimes are multidetermined. Patient dynamics, transference reactions to the therapist, and pre-existing psychopathology often play a major role in what ensues. The specific hypnotic techniques used and the treatment strategy may result in problematic effects if they do not match patient's needs. The context of "hypnotherapy" may create expectations of change and symptom removal, which in some patients may result in anxiety and problematic reactions. Sequelae to hypnotherapy probably could be minimized through adequate history taking and understanding of the patient's pathology, attempting to fit techniques and treatment strategies to specific patients, and responding empathically and sensitively to patients. However, sometimes, regardless of the precautions, problems may arise that must be handled and understood.

SEQUELAE TO THE HYPNOSIS EXPERIMENT

Previous studies that looked at sequelae of hypnosis experiments (Coe & Ryken, 1979; Crawford, Hilgard, & MacDonald, 1982; Faw, Sellers, & Wilcox, 1968;, J. Hilgard, 1974b; Hilgard, Hilgard, & Newman, 1961) found relatively few and mainly benign negative effects. For example, following the administration of the Stanford Hypnotic Susceptibility Scale, Form C (SHSS:C) (Weitzenhoffer & Hilgard, 1962), studies have found that 29% (Crawford, Hilgard, & MacDonald, 1982), 31% (J. Hilgard, 1974b), and 49% (Coe & Ryken, 1979) of subjects experienced negative sequelae such as headaches, confusion, or anxiety. After administration of the less cognitive but more ideomotor Harvard Group Scale of Hypnotic Susceptibility, Form A (HGSHS:A) (Shor & Orne, 1962), only 5% of subjects experienced negative sequelae (Crawford, Hilgard, & MacDonald, 1982).

The author conducted a hypnosis study in a group setting in which as an incidental finding three subjects manifested negative reactions ranging from strained arms to frank psychosis. Using case material, this chapter looks at facets of this hypnosis group study that may have resulted in these unexpected and unpleasant experiences. In reviewing this material, several questions are considered. First, do subject variables, such as psychopathology, contribute to sequelae? Second, does hypnosis contribute to the problematic experience? If so, are sequelae due to the fact that this is a hypnosis experiment or to the experience of hypnosis per se? Third, with the hindsight of the cases presented, could these negative effects have been prevented?

The Study

This study examined self-perception, perception of others,social interaction, and hypnotizability. Because of the interest in social interaction, the experimenter made carefuly notes of comments made by subjects, beyond what normally would be recorded.

The subjects were 91 college students, ranging in age from 17 to 36 years (*M* = 20.3 year). Mean Wechsler Adult Intelligence Scale Revised (WAIS-R) Digit Symbol SS (Wechsler, 1981) (corrected for age) ranged from 4 to 18 (*M* = 11.6, *SD* = 3.0). Of the subjects, 58 were females; 59% were White, 8% were Hispanic, 13% were Black, and 20% were Asian-American. This was an upwardly mobile sample, in that all subjects planned to graduate from college, and 75% planned to pursue some graduate work; 62% of their fathers had not graduated from college, and only 22% had pursued some form of graduate work. 15% of the sample reported high school grades of A, and 58% reported high school grades of B. Seven of the subjects had prior experience with hypnosis, and 2 reported being in psychotherapy. Psychological adjustment was measured by the Psychiatric Symptom Index (PSI) (Ilfeld, 1976), which gives retrospective self-reports of frequency of 29 symptoms. Scores were consistent with those obtained for a sample that had a hypnosis group and a nonhypnosis control group at the same university (Devens & Strauss, 1989), but suggested more symptomatology than subjects in the stratified normative sample (Ilfeld, 1976). Scores on the HGSHS:A ranged from 0 to 12 (*M* = 6.0, *SD* = 2.9).

The Subjects were recruited from the psychology subject pool by posting a notice on a bulletin board inviting students to participate in an experiment called "Experience with Hypnosis." Subjects received class credit in exchange for participating in the study.

Subjects were seen in 12 groups, each of which had 4 to 10 people. Following administration of various questionnaires and psychometric tests, subjects engaged in a semi-structured discussion about hypnosis. The discussion included why subjects signed up for this experiment on hypnosis, whether they previously were hypnotized or knew somebody who was hypnotized and what were the circumstances and experience of the hypnosis, what they thought hypnosis would be like, and what they would like and not like to experience with hypnosis. Hypnosis was described as involving concentration and imagination, and subjects talked about their experience and ability in these areas. The discussion was structured so each subject was called on at least once if he or she did not speak spontaneously. Following this discussion, sociograms (Moreno, 1934), based on interaction during the session, were completed. Subjects were asked if they had additional questions, and the HGSHS:A was administered. After the administration of the HGSHS:A, subjects were debriefed, discussed their experience during the HGSHS:A, and were told that if they had questions about the experiment or wished to discuss it further, they could call the experimenter. Of the subjects, 36 were seen for additional investigation one to several weeks after the initial session, and were asked about their thoughts or reaction to the first session.

Case Reports

Problems arose with three subjects in this study during the group session.

Subject 3. This subject is a White male, probably between the ages of 18 and 22 who was seen in a group with three other subjects. He attracted no particular attention while completing pencil-and-paper tests. During the prehypnotic discussion, he did not respond when the group was asked about previous experience with hypnosis. When asked what hypnosis would be like, this subject replied "Try to put your mind at ease, reveal thoughts, break down barriers. I came to see if I can be hypnotized. I don't think so without being willing." When the group discussed imagination, he said his imagination was above average, and that he gets involved in things. Following the completion of the sociogram, when I asked the group for any further questions before beginning the HGSHS:A, he asked, "Is this information [acquired during the experiment] available to the public?" I asked what he meant. He said, " If someone wanted—what if the KGB or CIA. I'm a spy for God. If asked if I had psychiatric help, what do I say?" (An item on a questionnaire asked if subjects presently are in psychotherapy.)

I spoke with the subject in private and excused him from further participation in the study. He expressed great concern that someone would find out his responses; we tore up test data that he had completed. The incident was reported to the subject pool coordinator so that mental health services could be obtained for this subject. No further follow-up was available to me. On the sociogram, his frequency of being selected to share various activities was about average for those in his group. No other data are available for this subject because protocols were destroyed.

This subject manifested a psychotic episode during this experiment. During the prehypnotic interview this subject did not stand out until he asked "if this was available to the public." His viewing hypnosis as revealing thoughts and breaking down barriers may raise questions about concern with intrusion, but in and of itself would not predict his delusional behavior. The paranoid episode clearly was not related to the hypnotic condition (Orne,

1977) because it emerged before hypnosis was used. We can speculate about whether the episode is related to the fact that this was a hypnosis experiment; the subject may have become paranoid as a means of avoiding the hypnotic experience perhaps because he fantasied that in hypnosis he would reveal too much. On the other hand, the episode may have been provoked by other factors, such as the subject saying too much during the prehypnotic interview, revealing too much on the questionnaires, or evaluating and being evaluated by other students on the sociogram.

Subject 25. This is an 18-year-old White male college freshman who was seen in a group with nine other subjects. WAIS-R Digit Symbol Scale Score (corrected for age) is 10, and HGSHS:A score is 8. He reported being a B student in high school and hopes to get a masters degree. His father is a high school graduate. He views his health as good and is not currently in psychotherapy. On the questionnaire, he reported he has no previous experience with hypnosis. While completing the subject information form, he raised his hand and said he was not sure how to complete an item that asked about birth order, as he had been in two families. During the prehypnotic interview, he did not respond when the group was asked about previous experience with hypnosis. When asked about what would happen in hypnosis, this subject said "someone takes control." He did not participate further in the discussion.

On the sociogram, his frequency of being selected to share various activities was about average for those in his group. Results of the PSI were within one standard deviation of scores for this sample, although depression scores were in the range that may suggest mild depression for the normative sample.

Following debriefing and dismissal of the group, he remained in the room and said he had a headache, which he attributed to this study. He said the headache began when I told people they would touch their ankles [posthypnotic suggestion on the HGSHS:A], and he resisted. I rehypnotized him and suggested that he comply with the posthypnotic suggestion, which he did. He said the headache was better, but he felt tension in his neck. I suggested he relax his neck muscles. He awoke from hypnosis, said he felt better,and left. A few minutes later he returned and said he felt "weird and uncomfortable." He told the following story.

The subject's parents died when he was 3, and 2 years later, his younger brother died of diabetes; the subject blames himself for not making sure that his brother received his medication. Subsequently, the subject was adopted into a family, and acquired an older brother. The family thought the subject was autistic because he did not talk and they took him to a therapist who tried to use hypnosis with him; the subject is not sure if he was hypnotized and thinks he may have resisted. The subject indicated that after a time, he did begin to talk, and now feels that he functions normally.

The subject discussed with the experimenter his feelings evoked by this study. When the questionnaire asked about birth order, the conflict and guilt around his brother's death was re-evoked, and the subject became confused. He is both the oldest of two siblings (in his original family) and the youngest of two siblings (in his adopted family).

Although the subject indicated on the questionnaire that he was not previously hypnotized, he acknowledged that a therapist had attempted to hypnotize him when he was a child. He viewed his response to the questionnaire as a lie and experienced much tension because he sees himself as very moral and ethical person,and feels that his word is very important. The initial resistance to the posthypnotic suggestion likely evoked his childhood experience in that he perceives himself as having resisted the therapist's attempts to hypnotize him.

The questions about birth order and previous hypnotic experience, the hypnotic experience itself, and his resistance to the posthypnotic suggestion contributed to re-evoking a very painful time in his life. The subject felt that the questionnaires were particularly conflictual, and said he felt better and was glad to talk about his experience and his background. We discussed psychotherapy as a vehicle for him to talk further about his background.

The subject was seen 3 weeks later for follow-up. He experienced no further discomfort, and was not sure if he wished to pursue psychotherapy.

Subject 68. This is a 19-year-old White female college student who was seen in group with nine other subjects. WAIS-R Digit Symbol Scale Score (corrected for age) is 8, more than one standard deviation below the mean for this sample. She reported being a B student in high school and hopes to get a doctorate. Her father has a masters degree. She views her health as fair and is not currently in psychotherapy. While the group completed questionnaires and psychometric tests, she raised her hand and said she wanted to ask questions about hypnosis. She looked ahead to other instruments in the test packet, although she was told not to do so.

During the group discussion, she reported having a positive experience when she previously was hypnotized by her mother's friend, who was a psychiatrist; she was aware of what was going on but was not in control of her body. She noted that other people in her family also were interested in hypnosis. When the group was asked if they had seen other people hypnotized, she said, "at camp, people were getting hypnotized by campers, but I was never put into a trance there." Her expectations of hypnosis included "I feel I'm going to say things in my subconscious, they will be drawn out." She would like to be hypnotized and feel hypnotized, but does not want to have a "scary" experience. Following the sociogram and just prior to administration of the HGSHS:A, when the group was asked if they had any questions, she asked "Are we going to sit here? The chair is uncomfortable."

During the debriefing following the administration of the HGSHS:A, she described the experience as feeling different, but better. She scored 12 on the HGSHS:A (and 10 on the SHSS:C several weeks later). Results of the sociograms suggested that this subject was less well liked than the other nine subjects in her group. The PSI suggested moderate depression (frequency of symptoms more than one standard deviation above the mean for this sample) and anxiety (frequency of symptoms more than two standard deviations above the mean for this sample).

The day following the group session, she telephoned to say her arms felt like she had been exercising. Her biceps hurt when she straightened her arm, and she felt sluggish. She attributed straining her arms to hypnosis. Discussion over the phone revealed that in the past, she had similar feelings after doing exercises such as push-ups or swimming, but would feel better quickly. The subject was told that as in the past, the pain was likely to remit quickly, but if not, she would have to go the Student Health Service, and that she should keep me posted. The subject called 4 weeks later to say that her arm was fine 2 days after she spoke with me, and was calling because I told her to keep me posted. Follow-up several weeks later revealed no further problems, and this subject appeared less anxious than she had during the group session. Subsequent administration of the SHSS:C revealed no problems that were called to the experimenter's attention.

This subject may have strained her arm during one of the ideomotor items on the HGSHS:A while attempting to resist a paradoxical suggestion. Why she strained her arm might be considered in light of the meaning of participating in the hypnosis study. She seemed to be fascinated by hypnosis, and expressed considerable interest in and fear of it. She felt that her family was interested in hypnosis and apparently had their support for its use, but also manifested anxiety around hypnosis, both while filling out the questionnaires and during the prehypnotic interview. She was a very suggestible subject and may have taken my comment to call if there was anything subjects wanted to discuss very literally.

Discussion

The incidence of reported negative effects in this group hypnosis study (3%) is comparable to those reported by Crawford, Hilgard, and MacDonald (1982). Although subjects were not asked specifically about effects of the group session as was done by Crawford, Hilgard, and MacDonald (1982), the three subjects were identified without direct questioning or follow-up. In addition, 36 of the subjects were seen in subsequent sessions where they were asked for thoughts about or reactions to the first group session, and reported no additional negative reactions.

Subjects bring their experiences, character structure, motivations, and affects to the hypnosis experiment. Psychopathology contributed to some of the negative effects described in this study, but not to all. Many subjects express concern about hypnosis and intrusion but do not become paranoid, as did Subject 3. Although fantasies about hypnosis as well as responses to questionnaires, sociograms, and discussion may result in anxiety or behavior that delays or prevents the hypnotic induction, they do not cause psychosis in people who are not so predisposed. Previous studies with normal college students (Coe & Ryken, 1979; Crawford, Hilgard, & MacDonald, 1982; Faw, Sellers, & Wilcox, 1968; J.Hilgard, 1974b; J. Hilgard, E.Hilgard, & Newman, 1961) found that when negative effects occur, they tend to be mild, such as headache, confusion, or tension. For example, Subject 25, whose level of adjustment was about average for this sample, experienced headache and a "weird feeling" when his traumatic childhood was re-evoked by the study.

Some college students experience mild symptomatology following usual college activities such as taking an exam, attending a lecture, and participating in a nonhypnosis experiment as well as following participation in a hypnosis experiment (Coe & Ryken, 1979). Sequelae of hypnosis experiments may not always be due to hypnosis. For example, although the hypnotic experience appears to be related to Subject 68's arm pain and Subject 25's discomfort following failure to execute the posthypnotic suggestion, it is clearly unrelated to Subject 3's paranoid presentation and Subject 25's confusion while filling out the questionnaire because these occurred prior to the use of hypnosis. Had Subject 3 become psychotic following administration of the HGSHS:A, this episode very likely would have been attributed to hypnosis. Thus, one must be cautious in attributing apparent sequelae of hypnosis experiments to the hypnotic condition.

The label of *hypnosis experiment* may contribute to the subject's reaction. Whether Subject 3 would have become paranoid during a nonhypnosis experiment is unknown. The episode occurred just before hypnosis was to begin, which suggests that his anticipation of a hypnotic experience may have played some role. On the other hand, it occurred just after completing sociograms, and concern about evaluating and being evaluated by other students may have played an equally plausible role. For Subject 25, the question about birth order seemed to evoke memories of his brother's death; whether this was potentiated by the hypnotic setting is unclear. The question about previous hypnosis experience evoked memories of his childhood hypnosis experience, and further revivified his childhood trauma.

Sequelae to hypnosis experiments are the result of interaction among subject variables including history and psychopathology, the hypnotic condition and particular suggestions given, the labeled *hypnosis experiment* and its meaning, and other facets of the experimental setting. Which of these contribute to particular reactions during or following experiments must be evaluated on an individual basis.

Crawford, Hilgard, and MacDonald (1982) made some recommendations for avoiding negative sequelae to hypnosis experiments, including developing rapport with subjects, assessing their reactions, and discussing their experiences. In the present study, where a group hypnotic induction was conducted during the initial session, and clinical instruments and individual interview were not used for screening, these recommended procedures did not prevent the development of negative effects for three subjects. The group prehypnotic discussion did exclude Subject 3 from the hypnosis portion of the experiment. Because Subject 25 appeared about average in adjustment for this sample, his background probably would not have been revealed without an in-depth individual clinical interview, which is not realistic for research purposes. Screening with the PSI would have identified Subject 68 as exhibiting symptoms of anxiety and depression, although the relationship between symptomatology and negative reactions to hypnosis is unknown.

In conducting group hypnosis experiments, as in conducting nonhypnosis experiments and other activities of life (Coe & Ryken, 1979), some negative sequelae probably cannot be prevented. However, understanding the contributions of experimental and subject variables to the production of sequelae as well as adhering to the recommendations of Crawford, Hilgard, MacDonald (1982) may help to minimize these negative effects.

CONCLUSION

Although clinical and research uses of hypnosis differ in purpose, expectations and type of subject seen, negative sequelae may result in both contexts. Hypnosis, per se, is neither a dangerous tool nor a risky procedure, although it is an intrusion into the patient or subject's psychological system. Rather, the problematic reactions that occur must be understood in light of an interaction among subject variables, including history, psychodynamic considerations and nature of psychopathology, specific hypnotic techniques used, specific therapeutic strategy or experimental manipulation, and demand characteristics created by the setting. Both clinician and researcher must be prepared to handle problematic effects that arise during or following the use of hypnosis, and both can learn from examination of and research in this area.

IV

THE MECHANISMS OF CHANGE IN THERAPY

In her clinical writings, Erika Fromm always emphasized the inner coping resources of the patient, the mechanisms by which the patient gains access to, and the methods by which the therapist enables the patient to explore, these resources. She believed that the therapist provides a permissive context within which the patient becomes receptive to unconscious and preconscious material and then can draw on these in a creative way in an active attempt to resolve life problems. Fromm's interest in the mechanisms of therapeutic change, creative change as she viewed it, centers on the ego-psychoanalytic concepts of ego receptivity and ego activity, and on the shift from secondary to primary-process thinking.

These themes are echoed in the chapters in this section. Marlen Eisen's chapter, "From the Magical Wish to the Belief in the Self," applies these concepts to the treatment of psychophysiological illnesses. Eisen focuses on the mechanisms of change associated with the mind–body interface. Modern neurobiological research has shown that words and images can have a kind of "magic" to the extent that they activate neurobiological mechanisms associated with the mind–body interface. The patient's beliefs—whether belief in his or her own ability or the seeming "magic" of the therapist—have equal likelihood of activating the body's healing mechanisms. Initially if the patient seeks hypnotherapy out of a need to believe in the magic of the therapist, the skilled therapist helps the patient realize that healing comes from "magic" within. Fromm's ego-psychoanalytic approach to treatment in general, and in particular her work on the treatment of psychophysiological disorders (Brown & Fromm, 1987), has always emphasized the importance of helping the patient tap inner resources and come to believe in him or herself. Both Eisen and Fromm share this view. Both also believe that imagery serves as an important catalyst for mind–body change.

Peter B. Bloom (chapter 13) in "The Creative Process in Hypnotherapy" also explores the mechanisms of change in therapy. His work focuses on certain critical moments in therapy where genuine change occurs. Bloom considers these therapeutic moments between the patient and therapist as creative acts. He identifies six discrete steps occurring in rapid sequence in the patient or therapist that culminate in creative change.

Bloom's own thinking about creativity in psychotherapy resonates with Fromm's ideas. Both believe that altered states of consciousness like hypnosis provide fertile soil for creative change in therapy. Both see primary-process thinking as critical to creative change. In his work, moreover, Bloom argues for the importance of balancing therapeutic intuition with scientific discipline. His method for discovering and refining creative insights in therapy reminds us of Fromm's work on scientific intuition.

Whereas Bloom takes a microscopic view, Sexton and Nash (chapter 14) take a macroscopic perspective on therapeutic change. In "Hypnosis as a Tool for Facilitating Change in Short-Term PsychoanalyticPsychotherapy" the focus shifts from critical moments of change to the process of therapy unfolding over time. Sexton and Nash are interested in how hypnosis can be integrated with short-term therapy. They discuss three distinct components of short-term psychoanalytic therapy: assessment, identification of a core dynamic conflict, and resolution of the conflict. Sexton and Nash believe that hypnosis, when combined with short-term therapy models, can shorten the length of even psychoanalytically oriented treatment more than short-term therapy alone. Because hypnotized patients have greater access to unconscious material, primary-process thinking, imagery and affects, Sexton and Nash believe that hypnosis can enhance each phase of short-term therapy. Hypnosis helps in the assessment of a patient's appropriateness for short-term therapy, in the identification of the core dynamic conflict, and in its resolution. Sexton and Nash's view of the clinical efficacy of hypnosis builds on Fromm's own work, as outlined in *Hypnoanalysis and Hypnotherapy* (Brown & Fromm, 1986), and extends this line of thinking into a general model of short-term hypnotherapy.

Daniel Araoz's chapter, "The Problem-Solving Nature of Hypnosis: Its Use with Corporate Managers," focuses on the process of creative change outside the clinical setting, namely, in the area of management training. He describes a 3-year study in which group hypnosis was used with high-level corporate managerial personnel to identify communication problems within the corporate system and to find solutions to these problems. Managers learned to use hypnosis creatively to explore all possible solutions to designated problems and then to rehearse plans of action in fantasy. According to his experimental study those managers exposed to hypnotic methods developed more effective and lasting solutions to communication problems than those who did not use hypnosis. While Araoz views hypnosis from a cognitive–behavioral perspective his comments resonate with Fromm's ego-psychoanalytic perspective in his emphasis on the problem-solving nature of hypnosis. Fromm might view his guided hypnotic instructions on creative exploration of solutions to problems and on rehearsal of action plans as examples of ego receptivity and ego activity in hypnois, respectively.

Chapter 12

FROM THE MAGICAL WISH TO THE BELIEF IN THE SELF

MARLENE R. EISEN
Illinois School for Professional Psychology

How can I help being a humbug when all these people make me do things everybody knows can't be done?—Oz, in *Wizard of Oz* (Baum, 1960, p.199)

THE HEALING PROCESS FROM A NEUROPSYCHOBIOLOGICAL PERSPECTIVE

Healing takes place in the interplay between the functions of body and mind. Physicians find that placebos, medications that are deemed chemically inert, have a strong mediating effect on many patients. *Placebo*, from the Latin, "I will please," is a term used to describe an artificial medical intervention (e.g., a sugar pill) that presumably has only a subjective effect. Recent research has disclosed that nothing taken into the body accompanied by conscious thought is chemically inert. Every thought is accompanied by electrochemical change. If one takes a pill with the idea that it will bring relief, the pill will be metabolized in a very different environment than if it is believed to be harmful. When placebos are administered, the pain relief is a function of the increase in production of the body's own pain-relieving chemicals, the endorphins or enkephalins. The activating mechanism is the imagination of the recipient.

The effect is clearly not in the sugar pill, but in the patient's belief. "The wise doctor within each of us knows how to make pain disappear and tumors melt, all in the proper order and combination. It knows whether to call forth T-cells or histamines or endorphins. The placebo triggers the process" (Achterberg, 1985, p.85).

Simonton, Matthews-Simonton, and Sparks (1980) found that placebos were unnecessary if cancer patients were taught to image the healing processes of the autoimmune system. Pioneering investigations of Schneider, Smith, and Whitcher,(1983) and by Hall, (1983) also determined that the image is capable of controlling functions of the immune system. Barber (1978) suggested that images can elicit changes in blood glucose, gastrointestinal activity, and blister formation.

Neuropeptides present in the brain central nervous system serve as neurotransmitters in some cases and neuromodulators in others. The opiate peptides or endorphins bind opiate receptors and mimic the effect of morphine. It has been postulated that this family of peptides has a variety of functions; in particular, regulating mood, pain perception, and the organism's response to various forms of stress (Pincus & Pardes,1985).

Just as thoughts directed toward healing may stimulate physiological healing phenomena, strong emotions or acute stress may cause physiological processes leading to dis-ease. Acute stress results in the release of a variety of neurotransmitters (catecholamines and corticosteroids). These mediate important body changes such as smooth muscle responses, affecting in turn the size of blood vessels in hypertension and the size of air passages in asthma. Also affected are the histamine-mediated inflammatory response in inflammatory bowel disease, certain skin diseases, asthma, and headaches, as well as the pain threshold, making the individual more sensitive to pain in general and headaches in particular. Failure to experience emotions in healthy ways, especially anger, is implicated in the etiology or exacerbation of migraines, bowel disease, and some forms of cancer in some people (Brown & Fromm, 1987).

Rossi and Cheek (1988) introduced a psychobiological approach to understanding the molecular basis of mind, memory learning, and therapeutic hypnosis, which is based on the operation of the information substance (IS-receptor) communication system, utilizing the neuropeptides. Information substances, called *messenger molecules*, may be diffused through extracellular fluid between neurons and through other tissues. These substances are localized at important nodal areas of the central nervous system (CNS) and other parts of the body associated with emotions, pain, and sensory perceptual processes. There are potentially thousands of information substances interacting with hundreds of different kinds of receptors on the brain neurons.

The state-dependent neuronal networks are ever changing dynamic structures, as they would have to be to function as the psychobiological basis for the phenomenology of mind, emotions, and behavior. The constantly shifting somatotopic maps of the "mind-brain" that are modifiable by life experience provide particularly vivid experimental evidence for the psychobiological dynamics of neuronal networks (Kandel & Schwartz, 1985).

Kandel (1983) has proposed how these molecular genetic mechanisms could account for many of the classical phenomena of acute and chronic human anxiety and neurosis. "Moreover I have suggested that normal learning, the learning of anxiety and unlearning it through psychotherapeutic intervention, might involve long term functional and structural changes in the brain that results from alterations in gene expression" (cited in Rossi & Cheek, 1988 p. 1291).

Anticipatory anxiety, a powerful phenomenon related to the pain experienced with illness or emotional dysfunction, and highly resistant to therapeutic amelioration, may be conceptualized within this framework. On the basis of previous experience, folk beliefs, or comments made by doctors or friends and family, the individual expects to have certain reactions to upcoming sensations or experiences, and does so. A headache prone patient, dreading a migraine may, through stress, disregulate the vasomotor response and actually produce the headache. The patient with asthma may cause bronchial spasms by anticipating them. The cancer patient, expecting nausea with chemotherapy, becomes nauseated.

Research findings connecting the perceptions and experiences of the mind with physiological changes in the structure and function of the body give credence to our contention that what has hitherto been labeled *supernatural* or *uncanny* are simply natural phenomena awaiting technological sophistication sufficient to discover and explain them. Rossi's (1986) formulation of the psychobiological basis of mind–body therapy derives from the concept that

> state dependent memory, learning and behavior processes encoded in the limbic-hypothalamic and closely related systems are the major information transducers between the mind and body. All methods of mind–body healing and therapeutic hypnosis operate by accessing and reframing the state dependent memory and learning systems that encode symptoms and problems. (p. 55)

Research results on the effects of imagery on physiology imply that images:

1. do effect physiological states,
2. may precede or follow physiological changes (e.g., they may be causative or reactive),
3. may be spontaneous or consciously produced,
4. can be considered the hypothetical bridge between conscious processing of information and physiological change, and
5. can influence the voluntary (peripheral) nervous system as well as the involuntary (autonomic) nervous system (Achterberg,1985, p. 115).

Body image is generally lateralized in the right hemisphere of the brain. Research indicates that when damage occurs in the parietal lobe of the right hemisphere through stroke or injury, the patient may fail to recognize part of his or her own body. The right hemisphere is, in general, the locale for processing emotional nonverbal or imaginal communications. Images intimately connected with healthy physiology or disease are preverbal, without a language base. The right hemisphere also has a predominant role in processing emotional information and making judgments based on this information. A vast network of neural connections between the right hemisphere and the limbic system support the connection between the latter and the autonomic nervous system. Thus, accessing the imagery of the right side of the brain is the most direct medium of communication between consciousness and the internal environment of the body (Achterberg, 1985). It is through this communication channel that healing is promoted.

BELIEF IN THE HEALER: PERSPECTIVES FROM PSYCHOANALYSIS AND HYPNOTHERAPY

Freud (1933b) spoke of a primitive stage in man's development, the stage of animism, when the internal world was peopled with demonic beings resembling men. They inhabited and perhaps were identical to objects in the external world. Man defended himself against these demons through rituals to which he ascribed powers to drive them away, or to palliate them in order to influence nature. In the struggle against the powers of the world around him, man's first weapon was magic, the earliest forerunner of the technology of today. Reliance on magic came from an overvaluation of intellectual operations, a belief in the omnipotence of thoughts. Man attributed magic powers to words and actions, and in religion and healing practices of today, he still does!

When an individual experiences great physical or emotional pain, there is a regression to earlier states and strategies, leading to a search for a cure from some omnipotent source. Some turn to psychotherapy seeking a cure through words and images. Words have been considered the origin of life itself ("and in the beginning there was the word") and to this day words have sustained much of their power.

> By words one person can make another blissfully happy or drive him to despair; by words a teacher conveys his knowledge to his pupils; by words the orator carries his audience with him and guides their judgments and decisions. Words provoke affects and are in general the means of mutual influence among men. (Freud, 1912a, p. 17)

Milton Erickson captured the power of word magic in his work as a hypnotherapist. Using metaphors carefully tailored to the needs of a specific patient, Erickson is revealed as "a practitioner of a universal healing tradition based on his skill as a storyteller, a word magician who uses alterations of consciousness to amplify the evocative power of language" (Kirmayer, 1988, p. 158).

However, the thought of being invested with magical powers may be both appealing and frightening to the therapist. Perhaps it is because the magician, as portrayed in myth and fairytale, has enormous power to heal and power to destroy. Merlin, the quintessential magician of the Arthurian legends (White, 1958) used his powers to fulfill the destiny of the founder of Camelot. At times, however, his powers were destructively or mistakenly used, with disastrous results. In the end he could not change what the fates had decreed; the death of Arthur and the demise of the dream of Camelot. Is the magician the master or the tool of destiny?

In fairytales there is good magic, magic that overcomes giants and grants wishes; and bad magic, magic that cripples and destroys. Sometimes one is masked as the other. Magical gifts may come at a great price. Faust was granted eternal youth, at the cost of his soul.

Perhaps the idea that wishes may be granted but a terrible price exacted, comes from the fear, conscious or unconscious, that when one is favored by fate, those not so favored will seek retribution.

Underlying the fear of being seduced into the role of magician may be the therapist's grandiose fantasies about his or her healing powers. According to Freud (1912a), it is man's narcissistic investment in ego that leads to a sense of the omnipotence of his thoughts to affect the course of events through magic. There is always the temptation to play guru and purveyor of wisdom. Some may be loath to play out the imagined role of healer, because in that context, failures become serious narcissistic injuries, difficult to confront and integrate.

According to Freud (1919), we all pass through a period of libidinal narcissism, where our sense of omnipotence leads to a belief in the magical power of our words and actions that can be reactivated at other times in our lives. An uncanny effect is often and easily produced when the distinction between imagination and reality is effaced, as when something we hitherto regarded as imaginary appears before us in reality or when a symbol takes over the full function of the thing it symbolizes. Such an effect is affirmed when an authority figure gives it credence. The human craving for the strength and reassurance of the father, the ultimate authority who resolves ambiguity and irresolution, has been well documented by students of the human condition (Fenichel, 1945; Freud, 1919). People seek omnipotent beings whose help, comfort, and protection can be depended on. Loyalty toward the charismatic leader knows no bounds (Diamond, 1988). The hypnotist, in this role, encourages archaic involvement, becoming a kind of magician, savior, or sage. Such features of archaic involvement can facilitate psychological health, growth, and adaptation, as well as mediate physical healing.

ANCIENT HEALING RITES: MAGIC AND SHAMANISM

Webster's Encyclopedic Dictionary (v.s. Thatcher, 1971) defines *magic* as "the art which claims or is believed to produce effects by the assistance of supernatural beings or by a mastery of secret forces in nature . .. any seemingly occult power" (p. 508). *Occult* is defined as "being beyond the scope of understanding..using incantations" (p. 576). The word "magic" comes from the theology of the Magians, sages of the East related to the Zoroastrian religion (Oyle, 1976).

The concept of the magician as omnipotent healer is found at the beginning of man's recorded history and probably before. Shamanism, the belief in the magician/healer, is the oldest and most widespread method of healing using the imagination. Archeological evidence indicates that for at least the last 20,000 years the practices of shamans are remarkably similar in Asia, Australia, Africa, the Americas, and Europe (Achterberg,1985). The consistency in Shamanic practices exists because it works. "The ancient ways are powerful, and tap so deeply into the human mind that one's usual cultural belief systems and assumptions about reality are essentially irrelevant" (Harner, 1980, p. xii).

The idea that a single act or thought can change an individual's world may be a useful delusion if shared by the patient and the therapist because a firm belief in the efficacy of an endeavor invests it with power. In the Carlos Castenada books (1985) about his involvement with an Indian shaman, it was only when Castenada, an anthropologist, was able to share Don Juan's belief in "nonordinary reality," that the experiences Don Juan introduced him to could expand his own awareness. We know from stories of magical healing and voodoo inspired illness and death how true is the statement, "expectation shapes experience."

The case of an elderly Indian, suffering from what had been diagnosed as inoperable cancer, illustrates this point. He wanted to live "just a little longer," in order to arrange things for his teenage son. He was being treated in an experimental oncology program in hopes that some new radical interventions might slow the process of metastasis. He believed strongly in the magical healing powers of the hypnotherapist. The doctors were amazed when the tumors began to shrink and disappear, a phenomenon for which their treatment would not account. Suddenly, however, he took a turn for the worst. His older son had learned that a former wife was a witch who had put a death curse on his father. When the son shared this information with his father, the elderly man's condition worsened. Within weeks after he told the therapist that he could not believe her good magic could overcome the bad magic directed at him by the witch and her coven, he was dead. He had survived 8 months beyond what the oncologists had projected as possible.

Another dramatic example of the magical effect of belief on cure occurred when a former patient phoned from a hospital where she had been taken with hip pain so excruciating that she was immobilized. The medical staff could find no cause and heavy doses of pain killing medication put her into such a deep sleep that the immobilization was simply exacerbated. Her husband was furious at her "refusal" to get well and return home to take care of him and of their children. When she had been in therapy working on problems related to chronic anxious depression, to which she also responded by becoming immobilized, she had proven to be an excellent hypnotic subject. A second patient, suffering from a dissociative disorder, and also a good hypnotic subject, believed that she had healing powers in her hands. Calling the second patient, the therapist requested that she visit the immobilized woman and use her healing powers to cure the immobilized woman. Then, the latter was told that a person with strong healing powers would be sent to her, and that she would be cured, feel fine, and be able to return to her home and family. It all worked exactly as the therapist said it would and both the healer and the healed felt empowered by the experience.

Illness is regarded by shamanic healers as the loss of personal power that permits an alien force to intrude into the functioning body. Disease is classified as sorcery or magical power. A contravening power must be invoked. Therefore, shamanic treatment for all ailments emphasizes first augmenting the power of the sick person and only secondly counteracting the power of the illness producing agent (Harner, 1980).

ACCESSING THE HEALER WITHIN

People enter treatment because they sense, through physical or psychic pain, a sense of disequilibrium. "Our instinctive being constantly emanates from and seeks a state of mental, emotional, physical and spiritual equilibrium. All pain is a request or demand to us (our minds) to help restore this equilibrium. It is a positive process" (Ward, 1977, p. 18).

"The client, in projecting the archetype of the Healer, or Wise Old Man, is experiencing something within. He is becoming aware of that within him. Maybe, later on, he will see that it was always there" (Spiegelman & Vasavada, 1989, p. 22). The client, or patient, initially needs to project the role of the healer onto the therapist. Ultimately, the patient comes to accept the idea that healing comes from within. The elements of cure can then be sustained through recognition that the mind–body is invested with the very powers originally sought outside the self. Like Dorothy and her friends in the *Wizard of Oz* (Baum, 1960), the patient had the capacity to grant his or her own wishes from within all along.

The value of providing suggestions that activate the patient's capacity to visualize a meeting with the wise inner spirit, the healer within, can be illustrated by the case of a woman who came for support in dealing with chemotherapy for postoperative cancer control. Given the suggestion, in trance, that she go to a quiet place in the center of her mind where she would find her own spirit guide, she imaged clearly an old Indian woman. Not only was the spirit a healer, who helped the patient through her chemotherapy without the usual debilitating side effects, she was also a weaver, who demonstrated for the patient, also a weaver, ancient Indian patterns that greatly enhanced her skills. Three years later, this patient is still cancer free, and very successful in her craft. Such outcomes, not totally uncommon, are beyond the scope of our present understanding. They do, however, reinforce the power of belief as it shapes therapeutic outcomes.

The power of hypnosis may lie in this very process of guiding the patient into an altered state of consciousness that allows the full force of the magic power of words and images to work on him or her. Like the shaman, who evokes a receptive mood through rhythmic patterns of chanting, musical sounds and dance, the hypnotherapist alters the individual's external reality so that the focus is retrained onto inner processes. The individual thus becomes a spectator of his or her own life, a process that is essentially against our common nature.

Imagery is not only a natural concomitant to all healing, but is involved in every interaction health-care professionals have with their patients (Achterberg, 1985). When bodily sensations come to awareness, an image of an internal landscape is created. We form mental images through a cognitive assessment of symptoms related to past experiences with these sensations or a knowledge of what they might mean. A patient complains of awaking each morning in a state of panic. Her heart is beating fast, her mouth is dry, her breathing fast and shallow. She is afraid to get out of bed. In trance it is suggested that she find a memory of a time when she was pleasurably excited, anticipating a wonderful event. She is directed to focus on her physical state as she awaits the longed for moment. She reports that her heart is beating so fast she can hear it drumming in her ears. She can barely catch her breath. Suddenly she says excitedly, "this is exactly how I feel each morning!" She is then told that physical sensations are experienced according to the way we define them. The chemical response to anxiety is similar to the response for excitement. We can reshape the experience by redefining the sensations. Her morning panic attacks cease and she begins her day with a more positive mind set.

Cancer patients often experience the disease itself as less destructive than their feelings that (a) their bodies have betrayed them; (b) they are out of, or have lost control of their lives; (c) that they are being punished for not living more virtuous or less stressful lives; and (d) that they might as well give up because they are going to die anyway.

The decision to come to a hypnotherapist indicates a strong wish for magic. There is implied in this act at least a flicker of hope that can be fanned into a flame by the therapist's collusion with the patient in his or her belief in the omnipotence of thought and image. A strong message is given that he or she can regain control over bodily processes, that the body has built into it all that it needs to facilitate healing, and that working together with the medical team, the personal internal physician can orchestrate the healing process. The consensus of therapists working with cancer patients emphasizes the importance of deep relaxation, and ego strengthening through positive imagery, suggestions for altered perceptions and a reinforcement of the role of the patient as an active participant in the healing process (Margolis, 1983; Newton, 1983; Rosenberg, 1983; Simonton, Matthew, Simonton, & Sparks, 1980). Once the patient feels empowered, imagery to activate the body's autoimmune system can be effectively utilized.

Providing coping skills to overcome the debilitating effects of stress, anger, or pain can have a strongly positive mediating effect on these and other problems such as smoking, alcoholism, and overeating. The sense of personal control, or self-efficacy, may feel like magic to a person who has traditionally felt helpless in the face of suffering. Self-efficacy is essential to any therapeutic change (Bandura, 1977).

The French bag lady further serves to illustrate the importance of accessing the healer within. She came to me at 7 a.m., 3 hours before her appointment, unkempt, confused, carrying several bags. She had been sent by a local community health worker. Her story unfolded in a long, erratic monologue punctuated by long hesitations and signs of agitation. She had been an office manager in a nursing home for many years. Early in the year she had slipped and fallen, and struck her head getting on a bus. The doctors said she had a stroke, but she did not believe them. She had been cared for in the nursing home where she worked for 6 months. Now she was back in her apartment, alone, needing a job but unable to find one because, for a reason she could not understand, she could no longer type. She wanted to be hypnotized to regain her typing skills.

Concerned that her confused state would make hypnosis difficult, and could also be masking some more serious mental dysfunction, I suggested that she simply close her eyes and breathe herself into a quiet, relaxed state. She was told that she would be taught to warm her hands, and that if she could learn that, everything would soon be better for her. By the end of the session she announced proudly that her hands were quite warm. During the four sessions that followed, the hand warming ritual was repeated, with reassurances that from this all else would come. By the third session, the patient, now a well-dressed, well-organized woman, appeared promptly on her hour, reporting that she could now warm her hands and her feet, that she was sleeping well for the first time in years (because her hands and feet had always been terribly cold) and was practicing at her typewriter. By the fifth session, she had found an office job that did not require much typing, within walking distance from her apartment, and she was looking forward to using her new skill (self-hypnosis) to make other positive life changes. She now felt that because she was able to learn so quickly to warm her extremities through her own efforts, she could cope with anything.

This woman had gained a sense of her own self-efficacy. What began as an archaic involvement with the magician/healer (the therapist) shifted to a belief in her own "magic," the omnipotence of her thoughts and images. The degree to which a person perceives and reacts to stress depends to a large extent on the scope and adequacy of his or her personal coping skills. Hypnotically induced alterations in perceived physiological and emotional states provide a feeling of personal power over the vagaries of physical and emotional experience. This power can be mobilized to sustain and strengthen the individual's capacity to regain equilibrium in the face of experiences that threaten the quality of life.

CONCLUSION

While on a cross-cultural exchange in China I presented a paper on the use of hypnosis with children. During the discussion that followed, a doctor declared, "we do what you have described . . . we call it magic therapy." What a provocative label for hypnotherapy!

Mesmer was condemned over 200 years ago for his "unscientific, magical" approach to healing. How can we now embrace the thought that what we do as hypnotherapists might have anything to do with magic?

In the West, this connection between hypnosis and magic has condemned its practitioners as scientifically questionable for years. Yet, so often patients who seek hypnotherapy come asking for magic to cure their physical ailments, to take away their incapacitating fears, to assuage their emotional pain. In my own practice, I originally went to some lengths to assure these seekers that I was not a magician. Rather, I characterized myself as a benign guide and teacher, who could hopefully teach them to utilize the healing powers within themselves. For some patients that approach worked effectively, especially when issues of control were paramount, but others turned away bitterly disappointed. Once again they were being denied, abandoned in their search for trustworthy dependency. They desperately needed something to believe in outside of themselves. They needed magic.

Viewed in these terms, magic does not seem so alien to the work done by hypnotherapists. Although the idea that supernatural beings guide the hypnotherapist may be overblown, it can initially be of great help to the suffering patient to be able to accept the power invested in the therapist, who then transfers that power back to the patient, where it belongs, suggesting that a wise healer exists within the mind who knows how to activate and enhance the natural healing powers of the body.

Whether science or magic, healers from shamans to modern "medicine men" have known intuitively the connection between belief and body function, the power of words and thoughts to effect physiological change and of man's yearning for the wise authority figure who rescues him from the dangers of life and death. We are now beginning to understand this concept scientifically. In a world where validation is won through scientific proof, we seek to demystify our healing techniques and results in order to legitimate them.

The true magic of healing lies in the unquenchable power of the human spirit as it reaches for life. The indomitable courage of the agoraphobic whose clenched fist reminds him that he has the power to expand his "comfort zone," the cancer patient who, after multiple surgeries continues to visualize the T-cells of the immune system battling cancer cells, and continues to heal and live actively between bouts, the epileptic child whose "magic fingers" keep his seizures under control so he can play baseball and ride a bike, are all heroic examples of the force of the human spirit. The ultimate power of magic is a belief in the omnipotence of one's own thoughts and actions in the face of pain and emotional chaos, yes, even in the face of death. In short, the power of healing lies in a belief in the self.

Chapter 13

THE CREATIVE PROCESS IN HYPNOTHERAPY*

PETER B. BLOOM
School of Medicine, The University of Pennsylvania
Institute of Pennsylvania Hospital

In medical school and in the practice of medicine, as well as in graduate school, the emphasis is on acquisition of knowledge. However, sensitive clinicians may be dissatisfied with the efficacy of knowledge alone. Even without the sanction and support of colleagues, the therapist may feel a push for recognition and respect from his or her own hunches, instincts, and intuitive understandings. Enthusiasm and excitement for some of us stems from the sharing of experiences and insights into the psychological processes that so capture our interest and define our work.

A deeply inward examination of the processes that occur in ourselves during the actual moments of clinical change can stimulate our consideration of how growth occurs, and the nature of our creative process in hypnotherapy. My experience with this inner self-appraisal has confirmed to me what others have said about the therapeutic process—that the most successful interventions are serendipitous combinations of scientific and intuitive knowledge. The art of hypnotherapy is neither equivalent to intuitive expression alone nor the opposite of science. Each is a necessary but not a sufficient skill for the practicing psychotherapist. A cumulative harmonious process brings about clinical change in both patient and clinician.

*Adapted from Bloom, P. B. (1989). The art of medical hypnosis and therapy. *Hypnos* (pp. 64–75).

REVIEW OF THE RELEVANT LITERATURE

George Groddeck (1949), an internist and contemporary of Freud, has been called the father of psychosomatic medicine. In *The Book of the It* he suggested that each organ system has its own unconscious, whose forces influence the function of that organ and the person as a whole. He named these forces, using the German *das es,* which has been translated into English as "the it." He and Freud corresponded extensively. Freud acknowledged his debt to Groddeck (Grossman & Grossman, 1965), and used the concept of *das es* to identify some of the psychological forces of the unconsious. In Freud's writings, *das es* has been translated into the Latin, "id."

Using Groddeck's own terminology, change in psychotherapy occurs when the "It" of the patient transforms the "It" of the therapist so that the therapist becomes more useful for the patient's own purposes. He described the process of transformation as occurring through a therapist's "active passivity."

Don Juan, a Mexican Indian sorcerer described by the social scientist, Carlos Castaneda (1972), said that a man who wished to become a hunter after his own personal power, if successful, would become a man of knowledge. He named some of the processes and forces at play in the teacher–student, doctor–patient relationship "nagual," and suggested that one could stalk these powers as one might stalk a deer—remaining totally centered, aware, and prepared to seize moments of opportunity. One's path toward growth and knowledge requires taking these forces into direct account. Don Juan shared Groddeck's sense that these forces ultimately were unknowable. This also is consistent with Zen Buddhist literature, which uses koans (short phrases or instructions that must be demonstrated nonverbally to the teacher, such as "Show me the sound of one hand clapping," to alter rigid reliance on cognitive processes, and gives ultimate recognition to unknowable forces by silence (Reps, n.d.).

However, communication between any two people can be studied. In Philadelphia, Birdwhistell (1970) and Scheflan (1973) minutely examined 16-millimeter motion picture films of people talking. They studied every picture frame and noted in detail when eyebrows arched, hands postured, and bodies moved. These observations were fundamental in supporting the descriptions of experienced clinicians, such as Erickson (Haley, 1967b), who already were using this kind of information in therapy.

Erickson was the modern master of deriving clinical strategies from clinical data. In 1972 I asked him directly, "What one word should I carry with me for the rest of my life?" He immediately responded, "Observation!" He said that if I looked at the moment to moment transaction of words, tones, and behaviors, I would have all the data I needed. He also advised me not to strive to become an Ericksonian. "Don't become like me—you're already becoming like you." This is good advice for any age, but I was fortunate to hear it when I was young.

Whitaker and Malone (1953/1981) applied psychoanalytic principles to the treatment of psychotic patients and attempted to describe the forces inherent in therapeutic change. They concluded that these were mostly unconscious, and like Groddeck, they suggested that all therapeutic change occurs as a function of therapist change. They used a colleague as cotherapist to focus on the primary therapist during the actual therapy hours to insure optimal therapist functioning.

R.R. Pottash and J. Edward Taylor (personal communication, February 14, 1970), often stated that the difference between the art and science of psychotherapy was in pattern creating versus pattern finding. They stated that creative therapists and their patients together formed new patterns of thinking, feeling, and behavior out of old and familiar remnants.

In *Learning Psychotherapy,* Hilda Bruch (1974) defined psychotherapy as two people coming to an understanding of one another so as to be of help to the complaining person. In fact, the process might be more intense than that. In *The Power of Myth* (Campbell & Moyers, 1988) the following story illustrates the phenomena of being in direct primary process contact with another person.

> In Hawaii . . . there is a place called Pali, where the trade winds from the North come rushing through a great ridge of mountains. People like to go up there to get their hair blown about or sometimes to commit suicide—you know, something like jumping off the Golden Gate Bridge. One day, two policemen were driving up the Pali road when they saw, just behind the railing that keeps the cars from rolling over, a young man preparing to jump. The police car stopped, and the policeman on the right jumped out to grab the man but caught him just as he jumped, and he was himself being pulled over when the second cop arrived in time and pulled the two of them back. . . . Do you realize what had suddenly happened to that policeman who had given himself to death with that unknown youth? Everything else in his life had dropped off—his duty to his family, his duty to his job, his duty to his own life—all of his wishes and hopes for his lifetime had just disappeared. He was about to die. Later, a newspaper reporter asked him, "Why didn't you let go? You could have been killed." And his reported answer was, "I couldn't let go. If I had let that young man go, I couldn't have lived another day of my life." "How come?" Schopenhauer answers, "Our true reality is in our identity and unity with all life . . . a metaphysical truth that may become realized under circumstances of crisis." (p. 110)

In psychotherapy there are important moments of this kind of contact, this kind of acceptance, and complete involvement with our patients. We need not fear being pulled off the cliff, as there are lines we all draw and that is as it should be. However, the willingness to be open to that risk marks the substantive therapeutic alliance. "Better to maintain shallow, superficial affairs; that way the scars are not too deep. No blood is hacked from the soul" (Cleaver, 1968, p. 22). And of course, there will be no change.

CASE HISTORIES

In each of the three cases discussed here, a complete history and mental status was taken, and a trusting therapeutic alliance (with a fair share of bonding through humor) established.

Case 1

The first patient was an airline freight stewardess. She stated that each time she was about to sexually consummate her engagement she heard her mother's voice saying "no". The history and mental status was unremarkable except it should be noted that she had been raised a Roman Catholic, was strong minded, and full of life.

During one particular session in about the fourth month of therapy, she came into my office shaking and stated that two men at work were approaching her sexually. She was frightened and did not know how to say "no."

As she sat in her chair to my left, I turned to my right, away from her, and pretended I saw a ticker-tape machine. I said to her "here's a ticker tape" and, as I looked back to my left, I noted that she appeared to be staring past me to my right as if in a kind of a trance. I decided to continue with my imagination and, as I "let the tape come out further," I read, "the United States Public Health Service has notified all young women that these two men [by name] have the most virulent case of syphilis ever recorded. All young women are advised not to have any contact with them." While we previously had used hypnosis for relaxation, she was now clearly in a trance. I proceeded and with an imaginary pair of scissors, cut the "tape" off from the ticker-tape machine and held it up before her. She spontaneously opened her purse, I dropped the imaginary tape in, and she closed her purse again.

All this took place in the first 2 minutes of the therapeutic hour. What were we to do for the next 58 minutes? I decided to leave well enough alone and so we just shared coffee and talked about her free air tickets to go to Dallas from Philadelphia in order to shop for Christmas presents. Every time she started to come back to the topic, I diverted her away. We thus spent the balance of the hour on nontopics. However, as she stood by the door preparing to leave my office, she poignantly turned to me, patted her closed purse, and warmly said, "thank you." She then smiled, turned, and left.

I understood the patient's need to use the primitive defense mechanism of projection as follows. She simply could not say "no"herself, and mean it. She hallucinated her mother's voice to say it for her. The unconscious experiences opposites simultaneously. One needs to be able to say "no," if one is also to be able to say "yes."

One cannot express love without a genuine capacity for hate. We all know the strange feeling we experience in the presence of persons who only profess to love. The psychological balance is missing. I, therefore, felt this patient's obvious inability to say "no" except as her mother's hallucinated voice, indicated equally strongly that she couldn't say "yes".

The shared image of the ticker tape was a symbol for saying "no"—a symbol she accepted and received in her purse. As she abstracted this concrete metaphor, she could begin the process of internalizing the ability to say "no." Once she had the inner resources to freely say "no" to the two men at work herself, she now could tap these same inner resources freely to say the more desired "yes" to her fiancé.

Six months later my wife and I danced at her wedding. Twelve years later, the marriage was thriving and they were blessed with children. She called and asked if I had a recommendation for a pediatrician for one of her children. I said, "By the way, do you remember that time in the office with the ticker tape?" She replied, "You know, I don't remember much about what happened in therapy—just that I thank you very much."

Case 2

I was asked by a psychiatric colleague to see a 52-year-old schizophrenic woman who had been ill longer than I had been in practice. Her chief complaint was encopresis, or involuntary soiling by fecal contents. She did it in the marital bed, on the floors at home, in the state psychiatric hospital when an inpatient, in the Acme food market, and in the beauty parlor.

Not many people were pleased about her behavior. She had been evaluated by a surgeon for megacolon or other colonic disorders and none were found. I agreed somewhat reluctantly to see her, having some real worries about my newly reupholstered office chair. In creating a context for patient care, I wanted to maximize the opportunity for success while minimizing the likelihood that I might get into a frustrating long-term chronic care situation with little likelihood for significant results.

I agreed with everyone that I would see her for 1 hour—that was it. I would give her everything I had during that hour, and no matter what happened I would not see her again. She and her husband would pay at the time of the appointment, thereby leaving at the end of the hour with no loose ends.

During the initial interview she acknowledged how long she had been schizophrenic, and thus it was likely she had more views about her experiences of being schizophrenic than I did. She smiled when I accepted that fact and agreed to deal only with her then-current chief complaint of encopresis. It was as if she said, "Oh, good! We're not going to take that on and you're not going to try to do something that I know and you know you're not going to be able to do."

I proceeded to take a complete history of her bowel habit. She complied and, in the detail I requested, described her urge to defecate, getting up out of bed, the awareness of her stool hitting the floor, and stopping, looking back, and seeing it lying there.

In every patient with a psychosomatic illness, I examine the experience of the symptom moment by moment by moment. After repeated attempts, I did not yet have insight into her problem. The hour was rapidly progressing, nearly 40 minutes had elapsed, and I had no sense of what if anything was to come.

Suddenly, I realized she had never mentioned her underpants. Having raised three children, I shared every parent's experience of taking my children's underpants down, sometimes just in the nick of time, when they go to the potty. But I never heard that detail in her own history and so I said, "Where is your underwear?" She turned red, blushed, and said, "You are the only one who's ever asked me that. I do not wear any underwear!"

At that moment, an image came to my mind—a diaper. I remembered advertisements mailed to me by a surgical supply house for garments that can be worn following a variety of surgical procedures such as hernia repairs and the like. These garments come in many configurations. I told her my conclusion was for her to buy six of these underwear-like garments, always wear one and carry a fresh one in her purse. Then, if she had an accident, she could simply go to the ladies rest room and change. She would thus have her mobility by wearing these adult diapers. I almost said baby diaper but caught myself at the last moment. I collected my fee, shook their hands, showed them to the door, and wished them good luck.

This schizophrenic patient was knowledgeable about the process of her basic illness. She also knew that to accept an adult diaper literally and its obvious metaphor for a baby diaper, might fix her in a regressive infantile mode symbolically and experientially.

One can induce change by paradoxical intention. In general, people who are stuck can often be helped by being pushed psychologically forward or backward. Either way is acceptable. So, by experiencing my literal suggestion as psychologically regressive, she had only one option to regain control—she must become continent somehow. All patients who are treated paradoxically fight to regain personal control and do it by achieving a higher level of functioning. The intuitive image of the diaper in this case seemed to fit the dynamics of her primitive defense mechanism and offer the possibility of change.

I did not plan to call the woman. I had told them I never wanted to see them or hear from them again. This was to be 1 hour of contact only. Her husband called me 3 months later anyway for a financial statement for insurance purposes. I could not resist. I inquired, "How is she doing? Did she have any trouble finding that diaper?" He said, with surprise, "Doctor, don't you know, she hasn't had a single abnormal soiling since she left your office—she has been totally continent." "Where did you get the diaper?" I asked, and he said. "Doctor, she was so furious at you that, as she walked out your door, she said, 'I will never, never get or wear that diaper!'" Her creative solution and the only way she could avoid using a diaper was to give up soiling.

Case 3

This third and last case occurred very early in my training. I was treating a young woman also early in her training as a clinical psychologist. The issues centered on control. In addition, fortunately, there was a flexible therapeutic alliance and a playfulness throughout this therapy.

One day, she sat back, crossing her arms, and said, "Next week's my birthday." I responded, "Give me a present for your birthday." She came in the next week and stated, "I brought you two marbles for my birthday." She put the two marbles on my desk and with a glint in her eyes said, "There is your present for my birthday. Choose one."

There was a moment of intense thinking and feeling. Which one to choose? Either one I chose would be wrong. Her response would be "What's wrong with the other one?" and so on. Suddenly, with an inner experience I describe later, I reached out for both of them and put them in my mouth. She looked at me, I looked at her, and we both started a belly laugh that rose up in each of us.

Fortunately for me, she was more objectively alert at that moment than I and said, "Please take them out—you're going to choke." I followed that good advice and we continued to laugh and experience deeply what had happened there between us.

Finding two marbles in my mouth was a wonderfully humorous experience for both my patient and myself. Taking control within the context of a flexible therapeutic alliance is often difficult. Fortuitously, playfulness, humor, and metaphor intermingled with a conscious need to work through issues of control. The image, dynamics, and therapy converged on the precise moment of change.

I kept the two marbles and still have them somewhere. The issue of control between us was softened from that point on. She and I, both in training, spent rest of that session, as well as much of the next, trying to understand the process that had just happened from every theoretical viewpoint we could muster. This intellectual discussion, although enjoyable, did not, however, change the process of what had happened. From that session on, she remained more flexible in her relationship to me and others, and she is now an exceptional professional in her own field these 20 years later.

DISCUSSION

Creativity between the therapist and the patient has something to do with certain pivotal moments that occur between them. These moments have special qualities that can be examined. Every credentialed therapist goes through exhaustive training requiring secondary process evaluation. However, through the necessary and intimate exposure to other's pain, not to mention psychological theory, we develop an awareness of the vastness of our own unconscious life, which is rich in images, affects, intuitions, and conflicts. In short, we must become equally facile in using primary-process thinking. Secondary and primary processes can be considered as left and right brain perceptions, or as normal consciousness versus varied altered states of consciousness. No matter how they are characterized, in psychotherapy there are particular moments when everything falls together to create change for both the patient and therapist. Primary- and secondary-process experience fuse and content and context of therapy merge into a new unified whole.

Although I value control, even complete control, in the process of becoming a therapist, I have had to let go sometimes and allow creative mutual growth to occur. I have discovered that there must be a mutual attraction, or sense of personal chemistry, between therapist and patient. Each participant must accept the other as a person, willing and free to deal with issues of power, control, and intimacy.

THE CREATIVE PROCESS IN THE THERAPIST: MY OWN EXPERIENCE

We clinicians tend to do our thing behind closed doors. We are not used to looking at our introspective and subjective experiences and are even less likely to share them with our research colleagues. We therefore often miss the opportunity to apply methodological parameters and other insights to our work so that we as a group, clinicians and researchers alike, can form testable hypotheses on how therapy works. In the spirit of inviting such a dialogue, I present what I discovered during one evening of introspection on the process of suddenly imaging these interventions—the ticker tape, thinking of the diaper, and putting the marbles in my mouth.

There seem to be six characteristics during the creative process in my clinical practice, which occur in rapid sequence but nevertheless are identifiable as discrete. This is the moment-to-moment sequence of what I usually experience:

1. There has been *no preplanning and yet there has been full preparation,* and there is no awareness that something is about to happen. All the planning, studying, history taking, or consultation does not allow me one smidgen of insight into the process that is about to happen, or give any hint as to when or even what will happen. This seems to be an invariable and absolute fact that you cannot predict it and that you cannot plan for it. However, it is not likely to happen unless there has been maximal study, history taking, consultation, and careful, continuous observation. This paradox might be called the zen of psychotherapy. You cannot study for it, but if one does not study, the process will not occur.

2. The creative response seems *totally spontaneous.* It occurs and unfolds rapidly. There is a clear and complete image of a ticker tape coming out of a machine, a pictured adult diaper, or the putting of the marbles in one's mouth. It seems perfect and occurs with a complete sense of naturalness. These are primary process experiences, so the words used to describe them are only approximations of the experience. The process, however, feels flawless, fluid, clear, and effective, but it is real and there is no mistaking when it happens.

3. A *clinical problem has been posed and there is a need for a solution.* The therapeutic intervention seems to be a response to a need for tension resolution. A clinical problem or a challenge can be created by the patient, or we as therapists can create it in order to promote growth. Tension purposely or even inadvertently built can be seen to be emerging slowly in awareness, yet without any knowledge or conscious need to solve a problem until it appears somewhat unexpectedly during the course of therapy.

4. *There is an awareness of silence.* As I was considering what to do with the marbles, I experienced a moment of total silence. The silence probably is primary process, but there seems also to be a series of trial and error attempts at solving the problem. There is an observing ego with full secondary-process functioning. Which marble am I going to take, and how am I going to do it? These attempts punctuate the silence, float by, and my mind is again quiet. There seems to be a profoundly deepening and effortless concentrating; a kind of actively passive waiting to be moved by something from within. There is no awareness of me as the therapist and yet there is total awareness. This is truly an altered state in which time seems to stop and I, the therapist, feel fully free, alert, and passive, anticipating something and yet not anticipating anything. I can only describe it as a moment of fully experienced

experiencing. I know of no moment in therapy where life is so full of pure essence with no self-doubt or no self-consciousness, but yet with no sense of what is to come.

5. *A picture or image emerges in either myself or the patient.* It can happen in either of us. A response to the patient's problem occurs in the form of an image, a solution, a resolution, a behavior, or an action that begins and then flows fully and freely into consciousness with a feeling of release. The experience becomes even more exquisite and satisfying as shaping, focusing, and refining continually occurs. There has to be a willingness to integrate these experiences into the fabric of the patient's and therapist's own growth. Ones maximal degree of training is called on as the therapist uses all his or her training, experiences, and skills to transform and translate into therapy what has happened during the moments of creativity. I stopped to see if the woman was involved with me as I imagined the ticker tape, and I corrected my wording of baby to adult diaper. These critical uses of secondary process functioning refine the creative experience into a therapeutic one.

6. There is a knowledge that *something definite has happened.* As the tide of the process begins to ebb, it is not always intellectually understood or even verbalized, but it is known and felt as a permanent and complete change in that particular increment of growth.

CONCLUSION

Clinicians who use hypnosis in their practices are fortunate to feel comfortable working with altered states of consciousness. This comfort gives a great advantage and excitement in experiencing the creative process of hypnotherapy. This creative process depends on a balance created between scientific knowledge pursued with diligence, and intuitive understanding gained by expectant openness. These two modes of awareness, when forcefully yet easily fused, often create welcome changes in our patient's and our own thinking, feeling, and behaving.

Chapter 14

HYPNOSIS AS A TOOL FOR FACILITATING CHANGE IN SHORT-TERM PSYCHOANALYTIC PSYCHOTHERAPY: ON ALLOYING THE GOLD OF ANALYSIS WITH THE COPPER OF SUGGESTION

MARK C. SEXTON
MICHAEL R. NASH
The University of Tennessee

This chapter explores how and when hypnosis can be used to facilitate therapeutic change within the framework of short-term psychoanalytic psychotherapy. Hypnosis is a therapeutic tool that can contribute to effective treatment outcome when used in the context of short-term models of psychoanalytic psychotherapy. When used sparingly and judiciously, hypnosis can help patient and therapist resolve impasses in diagnosis and treatment. Freud (1981) first proposed that the benefits of psychoanalysis could be extended if: "The pure gold of analysis [might be] freely alloyed with the copper of direct suggestion" (p. 168).

Efforts to shorten the length of psychoanalytic treatment and extend its benefits to more individuals began early in the history of psychoanalysis. Such efforts, beginning with the work of Ferenczi and Rank (1925) and extended by the work of Alexander and French (1946), entailed a modification of classical psychoanalytic techniques. More recent attempts to develop comprehensive systems to shorten the length of treatment, while retaining the goal of modifying long-standing forms of psychopathology, have been undertaken by various researchers (Davanloo, 1978; Gill, 1982; Malan, 1963; Mann, 1973; Mann & Goldman, 1982; Sifneos, 1972; Strupp & Binder, 1984). Most often these therapists work with a select group of high-functioning patients, but sometimes with more resistant, characterologically disordered individuals.

The usual goal of these short-term models is to treat circumscribed neurotic level problems while still adhering to basic principles of psychoanalytic therapy. Strupp and Binder (1984) suggested that proponents of short-term therapies attempt to achieve these goals by three common methods:

1. selecting patients whose presenting symptoms and personality organization is such that relatively brief interventions produce positive therapeutic results,
2. selecting goals for therapy that are more focal, and
3. improving technical interventions to produce more rapid and enduring change.

This chapter is most relevant to Strupp and Binder's third point: We propose a further refinement of short-term psychotherapy technique. Specifically, we believe that hypnosis is a technical innovation which when used in the context of short-term psychoanalytic psychotherapy, can enhance the therapeutic effectiveness of this treatment modality.

Brown and Fromm (1986) in their comprehensive book on the clinical uses of hypnosis, suggested that when used judiciously, hypnosis can speed the course of symptom improvement in long-term psychoanalytic psychotherapy and psychoanalysis. Recent clinical and laboratory findings suggest that hypnosis enhances the process of uncovering dynamically important material by stimulating increased awareness of symbolic processes, memories, and affective states (Nash, 1987). Hypnosis also can produce cognitive and perceptual changes, offering new opportunities for insight and conflict resolution (Frankel, 1976; Orne, 1977). Hypnosis may also invoke transference feelings that are more intense, immediate, and accessible to interpretation (Fromm, 1968b; Nash, 1988).

The clinical efficacy of hypnosis as a tool for promoting therapeutic change in psychotherapy has been documented in cases in which the patient is at least moderately susceptible to hypnosis (Wadden & Anderton, 1982) and where the symptoms are relatively focal or circumscribed (Beutler, 1979). Brown and Fromm (1986) stated that therapists working in clinics with diverse patient populations can in many cases achieve important symptom improvement with relatively brief insight-oriented or supportive hypnotic interventions. However, the use of hypnotic techniques to facilitate change within the context of the most widely used short-term models has never been systematically explored. Specifically, how and when the clinician working within a short-term psychoanalytic model might use hypnosis as a useful therapeutic tool is described in this chapter. A successful combination of clinical hypnosis techniques along with the technical advances that have been developed within short-term models of psychotherapy, could result in more effective treatment outcomes. Hypnosis may be used only with certain patients. Like every other technical intervention, the use of hypnosis is strategic. When used at all with a patient in short-term treatment, hypnosis is employed for a specific reason, and then typically only on two or three occasions. Three general considerations in using hypnosis in short-term psychotherapy are described here.

One difficulty in integrating hypnosis and short-term therapy is that a unified model of short-term therapy does not exist. Short-term treatment models differ in criteria for patient selection, *and* conceptual focus of treatment, methods of handling resistance and the nature of interpretive interventions. To make the proposed uses of hypnosis more general and applicable, we distill short-term therapies into their essential components and propose how hypnosis might facilitate the achievement of therapeutic goals within each component of treatment. Although discussing short-term models in this generic vein may lead to a loss of specificity, hopefully, the astute clinician will be able to apply our recommendations to the specific model with which he or she works.

A review of the major short-term treatment models (Davanloo, 1978, 1980; Malan, 1963, 1979; Mann, 1973; Sifneos, 1972, 1979; Strupp & Binder, 1984) suggests that there are three relatively distinct components of short-term treatment. These include:

1. an initial assessment phase where patient history, interpersonal characteristics, and ego functioning determine the initial appropriateness of short-term treatment approaches;
2. the identification of the core dynamic conflict (sometimes part of initial assessment, e.g., Davenloo, 1978); and
3. the resolution of the core dynamic conflict.

Clinical examples illustrate how hypnotic techniques can facilitate the achievement of goals specific to each phase.

INITIAL CONSIDERATIONS IN USING HYPNOSIS IN SHORT-TERM PSYCHOTHERAPY

Some general considerations with regard to using hypnosis in any form of psychoanalytic therapy should be noted. These are the: (a) regressed nature of hypnotic experience, (b) relevance of hypnotic susceptibility, and (c) form of hypnotic intervention to be implemented. Hypnosis does seem to invoke a topographic regression (Nash, 1987, 1988). The nature of this regression can be characterized as a shift from secondary-process thinking to more primary-process, imagistic, and affect-laden thought and experience (Gill & Brenman, 1959). If this regression is not managed skillfully, neurotic patients can develop the kinds of iatrogenic infantile dependencies that Davanloo (1986) cited as anathema to therapies of brief duration. Addressing this issue, Brown and Fromm (1986) advocated the use of a permissive style of hypnosis where the emphasis is placed on the patient's discovery of inner resources to cope and effect change. Permissive hypnosis minimizes the patient's experiences of dependency. The patient's autonomy and capacity to make changes are encouraged to develop. Still, the therapist using hypnosis in a short-term intervention must titrate the regression with care. Skillfully modulating regression enhances the patient's access to affect-laden and conflictual material without engendering ego passivity and infantile dependency. It is this controlled and optimal level of regression that Kris (1972) referred to as "adaptive regression in the service of the ego." In turn, adaptive regression, sometimes achieved via hypnosis, facilitates the course of brief therapy.

A second consideration is the hypnotic susceptibility of the patient. Successful supportive hypnotic treatment for habit control (e.g., smoking cessation and weight loss) does not seem to require the patient to be highly or even moderately responsive to hypnosis, at least as measured by behavioral indices (Bowers, 1979). However, in the treatment of pain and in insight-oriented psychotherapy, it does seem that moderate to high hypnotizability is related to better treatment outcome (Brown & Fromm, 1986; Wadden & Anderton, 1982). Approximately 66% of patient and nonpatient populations fall in the moderate to high susceptible range of hypnotizability (Hilgard, 1965). As such, the patient's responsiveness to hypnosis usually will not be a grossly limiting factor in its application. However, Brown and Fromm (1986) suggested that a preliminary assessment of hypnotizability by either standard clinical scales or by informal induction might be undertaken as a way of disabusing the patient of any lingering misconceptions about hypnosis, and as a way of gauging their level of responsiveness.

A final consideration involves making an initial determination regarding the form hypnotic treatment will take. Brown and Fromm (1986) suggested that there are four treatment approaches with hypnosis: symptomatic hypnotherapy, supportive ego-strengthening hypnotherapy, dynamic hypnotherapy or hypnoanalysis, and hypnotherapy of developmental deficits. The decision to use one or a combination of approaches is dependent on the nature of the presenting problem and the form of treatment to be used. The short-term psychotherapy models discussed here strive to achieve change that goes beyond symptomatic relief, but do not attempt to resolve developmental deficits. Given the patient characteristics necessary for short-term treatment (neurotic level) and the focal nature of short-term therapy, the relevant hypnotherapeutic interventions for this chapter are supportive ego-strengthening hypnotherapy and dynamic hypnotherapy. Supportive ego-strengthening hypnotherapy emphasizes the facilitation of relaxation, while increasing self-efficacy, confidence, and automony. Dynamic hypnotherapy emphasizes uncovering conflicts and working them through via interpretation of defense and impulse.

HYPNOSIS IN THE INITIAL ASSESSMENT PHASE OF SHORT-TERM PSYCHOTHERAPY

The initial assessment phase of treatment is fairly consistent across short-term therapy models. It entails determining the suitability or unsuitability of candidates for treatment based on certain pre-existing guidelines that previous research has indicated are related to more successful outcomes in brief therapies. These guidelines concern the presence of major strengths or deficits in personality as suggested by past behavior, interpersonal characteristics, and ego functions. Although exclusion and inclusion of patients based on past behavior and interpersonal characteristics varies across short-term models, some consistency does exist. Malan (1976) offered nine criteria that would exclude patients from short-term treatment: psychotic involvement, serious suicide attempts, drug addiction, convinced homosexuality, long-term hospitalization, more than one course of electroconvulsive therapy, chronic alcoholism, incapacitating chronic obsessional symptoms or phobic symptoms, and gross destructive or self-destructive acting out.

Strupp and Binder (1984) suggested that certain patient characteristics are associated with greater outcome success in their model of short-term therapy and constitute criteria for *inclusion* in short-term treatment. These characteristics are emotional discomfort with symptoms, a capacity for basic trust, a willingness to consider conflicts in interpersonal terms, a willingness to examine feelings, a capacity for mature relationships, and motivation for the treatment offered.

In addition to these symptomatic or interpersonal patient characteristics, Davanloo (1978) considered an assessment of ego functions essential in determining the appropriateness of short-term treatment. Davanloo suggested that an assessment of ego functions include the quality of human relationships, the affective function of the ego, motivation, psychological mindedness, response to interpretation, and intelligence. Davanloo (1978) made a determination regarding the patient's developmental level by assessing the level of psychosexual adjustment and drive organization. He suggested that "the more the central core of the patient's conflict is at the oedipal level, the better the prognosis, despite the fact that in every neurosis there is usually some regression from genital to pregenital" (p.19).

The short-term therapist may have difficulty in obtaining or integrating the necessary assessment information from the clinical interview alone (Strupp & Binder, 1984). Particularly, questions may arise regarding specific ego functions of the patient. Hypnosis can be used in the initial assessment phase of short-term treatment to assist the therapist in determining the relative strengths and weaknesses of the patient's ego functioning. This would enable the therapist to make a more informed judgment regarding the patient's appropriateness for short-term treatment.

Hypnosis affords greater contact with unconscious, primary process material (Brown & Fromm, 1986). Because of this, the hypnotherapist is in a position to assess ego functions in a more direct and specific manner. In this evaluative phase of treatment, hypnosis is used as a projective tool to explore the patient's capacity to tolerate the fast-paced uncovering techniques of brief dynamic psychotherapies. Here the clinician's strategy is to fashion hypnotic imagery that supplies some structure, but invites the patient to construe the situation in whatever way it seems to unfold. This approach is one of the most effective tools for discovering the patient's ability to manage and later resolve unconscious conflicts and transference reactions (Horowitz, 1970; Kubie, 1943b; Reyher, 1963; Shorr, 1972). This is precisely because processing through imagery mobilizes less resistance and involves less censorship than secondary thought processes (Horowitz, 1970). Here we offer two examples of how hypnosis can be used to assess the viability of ego functioning.

Hypnosis in the Assessment of Affect Tolerance

Affect tolerance is an ego function that Davanloo (1978) considered particularly relevant to positive outcome in short-term therapies. The patient's capacity to mobilize, experience, and tolerate affective states such as anxiety, guilt, and depression is a necessary pre-condition for short-term treatment. Assessing this capacity may be a difficult task to accomplish in one or two interviews because most patients wish to avoid, and therefore do not always experience, intense or painful feelings.

Case Example. A 33-year-old man presented to an outpatient clinic with intrusive and obsessive thoughts about swallowing. His father had died 5 years before from cancer of the throat and larynx, but this was mentioned only incidentally. He had consulted various medical specialists about what he considered to be excessive mucus, coughing, and difficulty in swallowing. Despite numerous and thorough evaluations, no medical problem was evident. He was a relatively happily married man with two children, a fulfilling job, and a history of genuinely intimate relationships. In this sense he fit the profile for short-term dynamic intervention in that he presented with a circumscribed complaint, good motivation, and neurotic level functioning. However, this obsessive symptom with somatic preoccupation is considered problematic for such therapies because overly ideational patients are often quite limited in their ability to access and tolerate affect. Thus, despite some positive indications for a course of brief uncovering therapy, there was still the question of the availability of affect. If little emotion could be tolerated or acknowledged, a supportive, cognitively oriented approach aimed at symptom relief might have been most appropriate for this patient. Alternatively, if this patient could make use of emotion within the bounds of a therapeutic relationship, something beyond symptom relief might be attempted. To assess this patient's ability to tolerate affect, hypnosis was induced during the third intake session. Following some preliminary ideomotor suggestions that established him to be relatively responsive to hypnosis, the patient was given the following suggestion:

> In a little while I am going to stop talking, and when I do, you are going to have a dream; a real dream; just the kind you might have when you are asleep at night. But there will be two differences. First, this dream will be about your swallowing. This dream will be about what your swallowing means. Second, this dream will be dramatic; it will have some feelings involved. So, you are going to have a dream. A real dream. A dramatic dream about what this swallowing business really means . . .

The patient's dream was indeed quite complex and vivid. He dreamt that he was a little boy again, driving in his father's car, as he did many times as a youngster. The car was filled with cigarette smoke and his father would only open the windows briefly to spit out phlegm after coughing. As the patient described how sick he felt, and how irritating the smoke was, his eyes actually began to tear in the session. The car became so smoke filled that he could see nothing. He could only hear his father's cough; and feel his wet, irritated eyes and throat. He was angry, but he knew he was crying. After some post-dream questioning during hypnosis, it became quite clear that this patient's fairly circumscribed obsessional symptoms about swallowing reflected unresolved conflicts about being suffocated and even poisoned by authority figures, especially his father. Thus, it appeared that intense feelings (anger, grief, and an abiding attachment to his father) could be accessed by this young man, and could become available for use in a short-term intervention.

Hypnosis in the Assessment of Motivation

Short-term psychoanalytic therapies generally consider a desire by the patient to achieve more than symptomatic relief an important consideration for treatment (Davanloo, 1978; Sifneos, 1979). Davanloo stated that both conscious and unconscious motivation should be assessed. He suggested that a determination should be made between the patient's unconscious attitudes for entering treatment that are based on satisfying an infantile need and those based on a genuine desire for change. Sifneos (1979) placed special emphasis on determining the patient's motivation for change versus symptom relief. Hypnotic techniques may facilitate the task of determining unconscious motivation for change.

Case Example. A 26-year-old female patient presented with a phobia to thunderstorms. She was a recently married working woman who reported that her phobia had "come and gone" over the years, but it had become consistently worse since she married. She initially wanted a medication to rid her of her "nervous problem" during storms, and she was curious about whether hypnosis could cure her. Although the patient presented with hysteric symptomatology organized at a neurotic level, her motivation for change versus symptom relief was suspect.

Accordingly, during the second intake session hypnosis was induced. With some initial difficulty the patient was able to settle into a mildly relaxed state in which she responded to some, but not all ideomotor suggestions. To test the patient's personal commitment to change and insight, an age progression technique was used:

> In a little while I am going to count to five and as I count ahead, you will move ahead in time, and as I count, time will move ahead, at each count one month will go by, . . . so that by the time I reach *five,* it will be August. During all those months you will have been in treatment with me, and you will have overcome this fear of storms. You will be at peace because you will know what this fear of storms really means. When I reach the count of *five* it will be a stormy night in August. It will be a very stormy night in August when you are at home with your husband. It will be very stormy and you will have gone through five months of treatment with me quite successfully. You will have found out what all this fear of storms means. When I reach the count of five it will be a stormy night in August, but you will have gone through therapy here, and you will tell me all about what happens . . .

The patient described a moderately vivid experience of being with her husband at home on a stormy summer night. The lightening and thunder scared her, but she arose from her living room chair and went to the bathroom medicine cabinet. She took a pill, settled in her chair, and the storm seemed to go away. She looked at her husband and thought how petty and unfair she had been with him. The patient's age progression was judged to reveal little genuine motivation for the rigors of insight oriented therapy. A brief systematic desensitization intervention supported by pharmacotherapy was moderately successful in reducing levels of fear during storms. There were no reported changes in the problematic marriage.

HYPNOSIS IN THE IDENTIFICATION OF THE DYNAMIC FOCUS IN SHORT-TERM PSYCHOTHERAPY

During the course of the evaluation process the patient and therapist must come to a conclusion regarding which problem(s) treatment should address. Strupp and Binder (1984) suggested that the dynamic focus in short-term treatment approaches is commonly conceptualized as "a cardinal symptom, a specific intrapsychic conflict or developmental impasse, a maladaptive conviction about the self, an essential interpretive theme, or a persistent interpersonal dilemma or pattern of maladaptive activity" (p. 66). Short-term therapies consider the determination of a dynamic focus an important therapeutic component that maximizes the efficiency of brief or time-limited treatment (Armstrong, 1980; Davanloo,1980; Luborsky, 1984; Malan, 1976; Sifneos, 1972; Strupp & Binder, 1984).

Establishing a dynamic focus may be a difficult process due to patient resistances or the nature of patient pathology. Davanloo (1980) suggested that there is a spectrum of patients who can benefit from short-term treatment. He suggested that at one end of the spectrum are patients who are highly motivated, responsive, and who present with a focal complaint. Establishing a dynamic focus is a relatively easy process with such patients. On the other end of the spectrum lie patients with long-standing character neurosis in which establishing a dynamic focus is complicated by complex patient resistances.

Davanloo (1980) suggested that the patient's response to the trial therapy model of the initial interview is a sensitive and effective assessment method for determining the patient's core neurotic structure and for selecting patients for short-term treatment. The trial therapy model emphasizes a systematic pressure and challenge to patient resistances (Davanloo, 1980; Said & Worchel, 1986).

Some criticisms of this method for determining the dynamic focus of treatment have been raised. Strupp and Binder (1984) suggested that too much importance is placed on successful responses to trial interpretations in determining patient suitability for short-term therapy. They suggested that if the patient is not able to produce historical data enabling the therapist to rapidly construct a dynamic formulation, the patient may be wrongly deemed unsuitable for short-term treatment. In addition, Strupp and Binder (1984) proposed that the confrontive or anxiety provoking approach adopted by Sifneos (1972, 1979) and Davanloo (1978, 1980) to deal with patient resistances, although productive with many patients, may disrupt the collaborative therapeutic relationship and be experienced as overly coercive. Patients may not be willing or able to respond to direct challenges of resistances or transference feelings. A treatment stalemate may ensue. At such times, confrontive short-term approaches have no other treatment alternatives available to them to overcome this stalled process. The result would be a determination that the patient is unsuitable for short-term treatment. In the following portion of this section, we suggest ways in which the use of hypnosis might unblock such treatment stalemates.

Hypnosis can address some of the difficulties inherent in establishing a dynamic focus with neurotic and highly resistant patients. Patient resistances are less of a factor in the hypnotic state due to the positive transference feelings of the patient, which promotes cooperation with the therapist (Brown & Fromm, 1986) and the use of imagery and symbols that involve less secondary processes and censorship (Horowitz, 1970). Our aim is not to suggest how hypnosis might supplant the innovative confrontational techniques devised by short-term therapists. Rather, we wish to inform the reader that there are some hypnotic techniques that are compatible with the short-term paradigm, are effective in the uncovering of hidden feelings, and are less confrontational. Because hypnosis seems to "soften" or temporarily suspend certain ego operations without confrontation, it may prove more productive for patients whose defenses might become more entrenched or crumble when faced with a head-on attack.

The utility of hypnosis in helping to identify a core dynamic conflict resides in its ability to illuminate the process of resistance. First, hypnosis can enable the therapist and patient more quickly to address resistance to the awareness of the dynamic conflict itself. Second, hypnosis can clarify resistance to the awareness of transferential feelings. In short, hypnotic techniques can reveal the patient's dynamic conflict or "core conflictual relationship theme" (Luborsky, 1984) with more immediacy and emotional availability than might otherwise be the case

Hypnosis and the Resistance to the Awareness of Dynamic Conflict

For some resistant patients, identification of a core dynamic conflict can be quite problematic because the patient unwittingly employs defensive strategies that obscure emotion and meaning (e.g., intellectualization, isolation of affect, denial, reaction formation, and repression). We must first enable these patients to become aware that they are indeed participating in this obfuscation. Only then can the patient actively participate with the therapist in the lifting of these resistances as a first step in identifying the underlying dynamic conflict.

Hypnotic techniques enable the patient and therapist to associate meaningful and personal images to the resistance. When this happens, the process of resistance becomes more available to examination. While exploring issues related to the dynamic focus in hypnosis the patient may produce material that represents the resistance in symbolic form. Ego-supportive and strengthening suggestions can assist the patient to face painful unconscious material and make the use of such resistances less necessary.

Case Example. A 28-year-old man suffering from mild depression and an inability to establish trusting relationships with women arrived 15 or 20 minutes late for each of his first three sessions. Therapist interpretation of the patient's lateness as a manifestation of "mixed feelings about therapy" was unproductive until a metaphor for the resistance appeared during a hypnotic procedure. During hypnotic age regression to age 10 designed to explore dynamic material related to his family of origin, the patient looked down at his body and begun to laugh. When asked about this he states that his body "looks like it is 10 years old, but I am still thinking like an adult." When asked to close his eyes and report where he is at age 10, he stated that all he sees is "fog." He can see his father and his mother in the kitchen, but all is foggy. At this point the therapist recognizes the fog as a manifestation of the resistance and invites the patient to pay attention to this fogginess and this feeling that he is, and at the same time is not, age 10. "This fog, this feeling of being 10 and not being 10 in some way represents your mixed feelings about what this being 10 means. What would it mean to really know? Now watch this fog, feel it, and as you do it will lift somewhat, it will clear to some extent. There will undoubtedly be some obscurity because it may not be time for all the fog to lift. But soon the fog will become clearer and as it does you will see and know more about what it means to be 10 and to see mom and dad."

The reader should note that this work addressed the resistance, without attempting to eliminate it. Connecting the fog with the patient's mixed feelings about therapy and the patient's tardiness would be a sufficient accomplishment in itself. It attempted to address the patient's resistance to the awareness of the dynamic conflict. Lifting the fog, gently and carefully, is really movement toward *resolution* of the dynamic conflict, and is covered in a later section of this chapter. In the present case however, the patient was able to "lift the fog" somewhat. Mom and dad were having an argument of some sort (later work revealed it was an argument about his sexual experimentation with a neighbor's child). But more importantly at this phase in therapy, the patient was able to identify his resistance, thus making it available to change He was no longer late for sessions.

Exploring the patient's resistances in this manner respects the defensive function such resistances serve, yet, encourages the patient to gain a clearer understanding of the manner in which he or she avoids becoming aware of conflictual material. During hypnosis, the patient can be encouraged to find new ways to overcome these resistances, and later discuss these insights in the waking state.

Hypnosis in the Resistance to the Awareness of Transference

Utilizing transference reactions to elucidate the dynamic focus is emphasized by most short-term treatment models (Strupp & Einder, 1984). Patients who resist exploring transference feelings make the establishment of a dynamic focus difficult. Davanloo (1986) outlined a method for utilizing transference reactions to gain information regarding the patient's core neurotic structure. He suggested that repeated challenges to the patient's resistances provokes an intensification of complex transference feelings that contain a number of affective elements. He suggested that as a result of the therapist's pressure and challenge to patient resistances, the defenses become exhausted and the patient is able to experience the transference feelings directly. This results in a mobilization of an unconscious therapeutic alliance suggested by, increased motivation, positive feelings toward the therapist, and an unblocking of unconscious material often related to the patient's core neurotic structure (Davanloo, 1986).

As in working with patient resistances, difficulties may arise when the patient is unable or unwilling to examine transference feelings, despite the therapist's pressure and confrontive maneuvers. Hypnosis may be used in such instances to examine patient transference feelings in a different manner. Brown and Fromm (1986) suggested hypnosis brings into focus transference feelings related to unconscious conflicts and affects more rapidly and deeply than nonhypnotic approaches. In addition, hypnosis can be used to explore patient transference reactions and determine their relation to the patient's core neurotic structure and the eventual dynamic focus of treatment

Case Example. A 31-year-old single woman presented with depression, perfectionism, and unsatisfactory relationships with men. During the second intake session she told three stories about situations where men expected more from her than she could deliver: a teacher, her father, and co-worker. The persistent and strained quality of these stories seems to suggest that they might be references to the transference—that is, she experienced me as demanding and critical in our previous session. But invitations to consider this idea were met with pained denial.

In a later session hypnosis was attempted, in part, to challenge and highlight her resistance to the awareness that she was having important feelings about me. Accordingly, after an initial induction and series of ideomotor suggestions, the patient was instructed to have a dream about "hypnosis and me." "You will have a dream about me doing hypnosis with you and what it means. This might be directly evident from what you dream, or you may dream about this quite indirectly, but you will have a dream about me doing hypnosis with you, and what it means."

The patient reported that she is in the classroom where she has seen me teach. I am lecturing to her and the other students, but I never ask anyone else questions, only her. Soon she is unable to hear my questions or make sense of what I am saying. But I look angry with her because she does not know the answers. She feels humiliated.

This work with hypnosis proves pivotal. As we explored the meaning of this dream outside of hypnosis it became evident that her perfectionism was a desperate defense against intrusive fears of being shamed and humiliated by those she loved. She could now explore this dynamic material as it unfolded in the therapeutic relationship.

By assisting patients to explore the nature of their resistance and transference feelings, and by finding new ways to address these neurotic repetitions through ego-supportive and anxiety modulating suggestions, patients come to experience a "softening" of defenses. Because patients are encouraged to explore these defensive reactions outside hypnosis, a clearer picture of the neurotic core emerges.

HYPNOSIS IN THE RESOLUTION OF THE DYNAMIC CONFLICT

Of course the goal of all models of short-term dynamic psychotherapy is the interpretation and resolution of the core dynamic conflict. The preparatory interpretation of resistances is essential if enduring resolution is to follow. But it is the working-through process that most theorists identify as mutative.

Here too hypnosis can be of considerable value. However, caution must be exercised to avoid uncovering unconscious conflicts and piercing defenses too quickly. Just because the patient has revealed the nature of the unconscious conflict in hypnosis does not mean that he or she is able to recognize or acknowledge the material in waking state. The permissive therapist will not demand that the patient remember in waking state all the unconscious material that was uncovered during hypnosis. Rather, it is advisable to suggest: "When you return to the waking state, you will be able to bring up with you as much as you will be able to face" (Brown & Fromm, 1986, p. 143). Such a suggestion encourages the patient to remember previously unconscious material but respects the patient's defenses and unconscious protective mechanisms. Such safeguards should be used even with high functioning patients selected for short-term therapy. In the permissive form of hypnosis advocated here, the therapist should strive to enrich and expand the patient's ego capacities rather than prohibit or take away defenses and coping mechanisms.

Addressing patient resistances and transference reactions as they come up again and again constitutes the working through process. As such, the hypnotic techniques used in the establishment of the dynamic focus phase are equally applicable in the working-through phase. Two hypnotic techniques can be specifically helpful in the resolution of the dynamic conflicts phase of treatment and are described and illustrated here. The first is an abreactive technique originally articulated by Helen Watkins (1980). Here the therapist uses hypnosis not so much in service of insight per se, but rather in service of the further unfolding of intense emotion that must sometimes precede, and accompany, truly mutative insight. The second is a technique that can enable some patients to identify how, when, and where displacement or conversion of primitive emotions has occurred.

Hypnosis and Abreaction

The role of catharsis in facilitating emotional insight is sometimes underestimated. Abreaction, far from merely providing a relief from long repressed emotion, plays a role in the corrective emotional interaction between patient and therapist. Focusing our work on emotion heightens the immediacy of clinical material. After all, it is not only meaning and memories that must be enlarged and examined, but also emotions with all their nuances. A technique that can assist with the latter is the silent abreaction (Watkins, 1980) What follows is an example of its use in a long-term dynamic therapy case.

Case Example. A 28-year-old female patient with three children was referred for depression. Following nonhypnotic work on resistance it became plain that she expected men, including the male therapist, to dominate and abuse her. Unfortunately her usual response to this unconscious expectation was nurturance of, and submission to, the man in question. With the resistance thus illuminated the patient began to remember incidents of early sexual abuse (age 6) by the maternal grandfather. These brutal episodes were remembered with only limited emotional involvement. Feelings were still quite vague, although the memories were clear. Concomitantly, indirect signs of increasingly pressing rage emerged: irritability at family members, uncharacteristic sleep disturbances, conversion reactions, and motor agitation. But these signs of barely contained emotion remained quite unavailable for her use in the therapy hour. Accordingly, the therapist employed a hypnotic technique designed to bring emotion into the foreground of her awareness.

During hypnosis the therapist suggested that she go back to the bedroom where the brutal attacks took place. No one would be there but her. The door is closed and she would not make a sound . . . "not a peep." It was suggested that she "examine the bed very, very carefully, telling me every detail." She carried this out with vivid precision. I mentioned that soon she would find a very sturdy new oak baseball bat, and as we explored her feelings she began quietly, silently, but thoroughly to demolish the bed with the baseball bat. As she did, the tears streamed down her face as she whispered through her clenched teech how she hated him, his "ugly body," and his "sick mind." With every word she struck the bed. For over 15 minutes she raged quietly.

Here much of the important work occurred after termination of hypnosis, as the patient discovered words that could meaningfully articulate the enormity of her rage. Over the next month of working through this material outside of hypnosis, the patient's distress and agitation gradually lifted.

Hypnosis and Displacement of Affect

The following case illustrates the tracing of affect using hypnosis.

Case Example. A 37-year-old married female patient with three children presented with a long-standing untreated depression with recent acute suicidal features. This woman also suffered from serious pain for which she had undergone several courses of surgery over the past 5 years, with little success. The patient was a bright, but excessively submissive woman who had little capacity to be directly angry or assertive with her husband. She overidealized her husband and strived to be his "perfect little girl." During the initial intake session she reported that the previous evening she had placed a loaded pistol in her mouth: She had played with the idea of pulling the trigger. She was hospitalized for what turned out to be less than 10 days. While in the hospital the patient was seen daily for psychotherapy. The initial focus of therapy was the relief of her pain because this was her only conscious reason for wanting to commit suicide. The therapy proceeded quickly in two phases: the unraveling of her conversion of anger to somatic pain; and the emergence of the original interpersonal matrix in which this anger was embedded.

During the third session in the hospital the patient was hypnotized and found to be highly responsive. Accordingly she was asked to have a dream about what her pain meant. She vividly described a beautiful day on a beach in the Caribbean. She was alone, sunning herself on a white-sand beach. The noises of the surf and the gulls were soothing and peaceful. As she visually scanned the scene she chanced to glance at her own body. There she noticed that coming out of the right side of her abdomen was "a white cloth, half in and half out." When asked to describe this white cloth, she says, [it is] "white cotton; it emerges about 7 or 8 inches from my side; and it is gently waving in the breeze." She was bewildered by this, but certain that the cloth had something to do with her pain. Mindful of the patient's unconscious resentment of her submissive posture in important relationships, the therapist queried whether this white cloth might be "a flag of surrender." Stunned for a moment, she wondered aloud whether she could ever stop wearing "this thing." Out of hypnosis for several sessions the patient productively considered whether surrender and pain might be connected for her. Interestingly her pain began to recede as she articulated her husband's oppressive insistence on her having a recent abortion. During later hypnosis the "white cloth" gradually emerged entirely from her abdomen. She could now examine it much more closely. While she was entirely pain free for the first time in months, she was left with a raw anger at her husband that was quite frightening to her. When she returned home from the hospital she reported "blowing up" at her husband for seemingly trivial oversights.

The second phase of this therapy was entered when the patient was invited to examine this anger more closely, to follow its course to the very source. Accordingly, a hypnotic technique, the "affect bridge" (J. G. Watkins, 1971) was employed. Here hypnosis was used to magnify and intensify an important emotion (in this case anger). When the patient was experiencing the emotion with vivid intensity a rapid age regression was suggested: an age regression to an important time when this same intense feeling was in play. The somewhat atypical age regression settled on a relatively recent, but no less important incident at the age of 19. As the patient regressed to age 19, she coolly reported she was walking down the steps of her parent's home (where she lived at the time she was age 19). She was thinking about a very attractive young man she had met during the summer. A brief romance had developed, but he had to leave town for 3 months. When he left he promised to write. In the regression, as the patient walked from the stairs of her parents' home to the living room, she was wondering why he had never written. It had been over 2 months and she had not received a single word. As she somewhat glumly and silently entered the living room she noticed her mother standing by the fireplace with a sealed letter in her hand, about to pitch it into the flames. She realized that she had caught her mother in the act of destroying what turned out to be the seventh or eighth letter from the young man. What was exceedingly peculiar to the therapist about the patient's story was that she was not in the least bit consciously aware of being angry at her mother. She numbly submitted to her mother's explanation that the boy "was not really suited for you." She returned to her room feeling that what her mother did was probably wrong, "but she really is just trying to look out for me."

As the therapy shifted to a once-a-week, outpatient format we could now trace the demoralizing and humiliating surrenders she had made to the pathogenically intrusive mother: a mother who interpreted even the most innocent manifestation of separation/individuation as literal "sin." This patient's will had been crushed by her mother; as she began consciously to experience anger at a previously over-idealized mother, her depression lifted markedly. Just as importantly, a neurotic burden was lifted from her marital relationship. Couples therapy could now begin in earnest.

CONCLUSION

It has long been recognized that relatively brief hypnotic interventions can yield significant symptom relief for some patients via direct suggestion. But only since the 1950s and early 1960s with the work of John and Helen Watkins (Watkins, 1949), Gill and Brenman (1959), and Erika Fromm (1965) did clinicians begin to explore in earnest the value of hypnosis as a diagnostic and interpretive tool in uncovering therapies. These early clinical investigations found that a conservative and judicious use of hypnosis can quicken the pace of insight-oriented psychotherapies. All these theorists cited the ability of hypnosis to engender a relatively safe regression in the service of the ego. That is, hypnosis can facilitate a "softening" of defenses that enables patients to productively explore emotions, memories, and transferential reactions. These important properties of hypnosis dovetail quite nicely with the basic tenants of brief dynamic psychotherapies in their emphasis on addressing resistance and transference reactions

This chapter has summarized and illustrated how hypnosis can be integrated into short-term dynamic therapies during the assessment, focusing, and interpretive phases of treatment. It should be abundantly clear that we are not describing hypnosis as direct suggestion for symptom relief, but rather as an invitation to explore and examine images and feelings. When used in this way hypnotic techniques can yield new and helpful material that might otherwise be stubbornly unavailable to the clinical hour. Here hypnosis shares properties with dreams, fantasies, and other regressed states. The difference is that hypnotic regressions are more easily modulated and structured by the patient and therapist. When used appropriately in short-term therapies, hypnosis might be administrated on only two or three occasions. In our experience, hypnosis is rarely used more than 20% of the time in any therapy. In this sense we are proposing that hypnosis can be an exceedingly valuable adjunctive technique in short-term dynamic psychotherapies when used with the right patient, at the right time, and with a balanced respect for both impulse and defense.

Chapter 15

THE PROBLEM-SOLVING NATURE OF HYPNOSIS: ITS USE WITH CORPORATE MANAGERS

DANIEL ARAOZ
Long Island University/American Management Association

The use of hypnosis for problem solving, symptom reduction, and concrete goal attainment has appeared frequently in the professional literature, especially subsequent to the general acceptance of behavior therapy (Dengrove, 1976; Kroger & Fezler, 1976). Success may often be had in just one or two sessions outside of a clinical setting, and yet may have therapeutic value and bring about major life or systems changes. For example, a 42-year-old woman had suffered from insomnia for over 20 years in spite of prolonged use of medication. In the one hypnosis session she had with me I simply appealed to her unconscious, suggesting that if there was some reason for being awake, she could pay attention to it at some other time, instead of at night during sleep. I taped my hypnotic intervention and recommended that she repeat the hypnotic experience by herself at home every day. I did not hear from her again and, honestly, I forgot about her. At a lecture 5 months later, she approached me to inform me with gratitude and excitement that she "had been sleeping like a baby" since that single time we had met. More importantly, she told me that she had finally started therapy to work through issues of a painful childhood.

Because of this case and similar cases, and in line with extended uses of hypnotic techniques since the early 1970s (T.X. Barber, 1985), I became interested in applying hypnotic interventions outside of the clinical setting. In particular, I wished to find applications of hypnosis in the area of management training and development (Araoz, 1989a, 1989b).

RESEARCH METHOD

This is a brief report on a 3-year study conducted with corporate personnel at the executive/managerial level. The intent of the study was to find out (a) if hypnotic techniques enhance interpersonal communication during a 5-day workshop. If they do, (b) does the improvement generalize to other situations after that unique intensive experience? and (c) does the improvement last 6 months past the original learning and practice?

Fifteen teams of 9 to 14 executives each (156 subjects) were divided randomly into experimental (85 subjects) and control (71 subjects) groups. Ages ranged between 35 and 57. The discrepancy in numbers between control and experimental groups was a result of separating certain personnel who already worked very closely together and/or were in exactly the same type of work (e.g., accounting), to better balance and mix the groups. The 15 teams participated in intensive 5-day workshops conducted in a resort. Eight teams used hypnotic methods and seven used nonhypnotic techniques. This study presents a brief overview of the way human systems in the corporate world can benefit from an hypnotic approach, although not so named, in this because setting the term *hypnosis* is confusing and misleading when used with executives. A caricature of hypnosis is predominant for most lay persons, including high-level corporate personnel. Therefore, I used instead the terms *relaxed state of mind, self-suggestions, right-brain management*, and *dynamic mental imagery* (Araoz, 1989a, 1989b).

Working with human systems is eminently solution and goal oriented (Araoz, 1984; Araoz & Negley-Parker, 1988). Because human systems are communication networks, the purpose of the interventions in this study was to make communication more effective by giving the members of the system the opportunity to learn and practice improved communication skills and techniques. Work was conducted generally with two or more members of the system whose communication was in need of improvement. The rare occasions in which one member was seen alone were in order to reinforce the new communication skills so that the whole system could work more effectively for the benefit of each of its members. Although the controls employed ordinary conversation of the so-called "left-hemispheric" type, the eight experimental groups were taught to practice "right-hemispheric" or hypnotic techniques.

The research method used consisted of four steps:

1. define objectively the team communication "problem";
2. determine a solution or remedy for the communication problem as the goal to be achieved by the team;
3. decide on concrete actions to be taken by the team in order to attain their goal; and

4. evaluate both behaviorally and affectively the efficacy of actions taken to attain the goal.

Communication Analysis

The first step was to define the team communication problem. This involved a communication analysis comprising five diagnostic areas: communication style, frame-of-reference, motivation, intentionality and perception. Each will be described briefly in terms of how the experimental teams received the material. The control group was presented with the same information didactically with plenty of opportunity for discussion.

Communication Style. The first element in this analysis uses Satir's (1972) models of communication (four defective styles: blamer, placater, computer, and distracter; and one effective style, congruent). The communication style was uncovered hypnotically by asking the members of the experimental teams to recall in as much detail as possible a single typical situation of verbal communication in the group and to "get into" that situation as much as possible mentally, so as to awaken the feelings belonging to that interaction. It should be noted that participants were not asked to think of a difficult or problematic situation, but merely of a "typical situation." They were instructed to take time in order to "relive" that situation in great detail, noticing any circumstances or influences affecting it, such as the place where it happened; possible interruptions or distractions; other people's interventions or contributions, both negative and positive; and the like. After this hypnotic exercise, they returned to the ordinary mode of thinking (from "right-hemispheric" activity to "left-brain" thinking), comparing notes and discussing their previous experience. This "left-hemispheric" discussion continued until they all agreed on a particular situation involving communication that was especially difficult or taxing for them as a system or group. Then they went back, hypnotically, to again review and relive it. This was done silently and individually, without interaction among the team members, for about 15 minutes. As before, once this practice was finished, they spent some time talking about it as a group and giving each other new ideas from what came to mind doing this mental exercise.

After this repeated practice, it became possible to identify the defective elements in the communication style of each member, as well as the *congruent* aspects of it, and to begin to make sense of the conflicts arising from the differences in communication styles that clashed within the group.

Frame-of-Reference. The second diagnostic element of the initial communication analysis refers to a person's inner or outer orientation: "Do I enjoy the feelings from having done what I consider to be right, or do I depend on other's approval?" Once more, the system members relived hypnotically past situations, or projected themselves into future ones, in order to discover this tendency of their "frame-of-reference," on which many differences in communication depend. The procedure followed loosely the same format described for the definition of communication style. This began with the hypnotic experience, followed by rational discussion, which led back to another hypnotic mental rehearsal in order "to try on" new possibilities mentally. Further discussion ended in a decision arrived at by the whole system to work toward identified goals.

Intentionality. This item refers to goal orientation: "Do I generally want to obtain (reach, get) something in my communication, or do I want to avoid (stay away from or out of) something?" The "something," incidentally, may be very concrete or rather diffuse and be positive (e.g., recognition) or negative (e.g., rejection). Hypnotically, the members of the system placed themselves mentally in different situations and checked their spontaneous inner reactions and feelings. The repetition of this exercise made them aware of their "intentionality." Once aware of their inner "movement," either *away from* or *toward* goals, as their natural habitual tendency, they were able to review their communication style to check if it was congruent with their conscious goals, values and lifestyle. This they did, as before, through discussion with other members of their team.

Motivation. Motivation analyses people's action orientation: "Must I do (say, avoid) something, or do I have choices and options?" Once more, a particular scenario was constructed mentally by the members of the group, based on their experience as a system, although the natural, unrehearsed feelings elicited by that scenario were noted. This was done in a relaxed way, activating imagination, while being aware of the physical reactions in different parts of the body as the mental scenario was being reviewed. Communication style can be modified and improved simply by becoming aware of being in a position to choose, as opposed to feeling bound to respond in particular ways.

Perception. The final diagnostic area in the communication analysis focuses on one's tendency to view situations and people in benign or threatening ways; to perceive things as familiar or strange. This is an essential element in communication, because it affects how people listen to each other, how they receive the messages that others send them, and in general, how open to differences and how tolerant and respectful of them they are. For example, effective cross-cultural communication greatly depends on this sort of perception. In order to get quickly in touch with their feelings and inner reactions, the members of the experimental group were led in hypnosis through situations that could lend themselves to both *familiar* and *strange* reactions. At this stage it was sufficient that they became aware of their inner reactions. Once the analysis provided a fairly clear idea of the communication *problem* in all its complexity, it was possible to move on to the next step of determining a solution or solutions for it.

Goal Setting

The members of the system were asked to get into their "inner minds" hypnotically, and to allow their imaginations to bring up any and all possible solutions, regardless of logical or reality considerations. Although they were engaged in this practice they were not interacting with each other, and the leader encouraged them to review mentally all the possible ways in which the problem could be resolved. This exercise lasted about 15 minutes. After it was completed, the experimental group members were asked to exchange their hypnotic experiences until they were able to decide unanimously what solutions they wanted and felt comfortable with. When attainable goals began to emerge out of the group discussion, they were prioritized and made very concrete so that they could become measurable, and progress toward their achievement could be monitored. At this point, participants hypnotically "tried on" these goals by means of time progression and hypnotic mental rehearsal until all the members of the system felt comfortable and pleased with the concrete goals they envisioned. It must be emphasized that a practice of mental rehearsal was one of the essential elements in the process of change herein described. By means of it, the group creates its own vision of what will be their reality (at least in the area of communication) in the future.

Action Plan

The next step was to decide on the *actions to be taken in order to reach the desired goals*. The experimental group members were guided into mental rehearsal once more, paying special attention to affective states (i.e., what emotional reactions were elicited by the mental images related to the attainment of the goals desired?) This practice was repeated several times until each person was able to produce and experience an inner state appropriate and conducive to attaining the agreed on goals. At this point, when what they wanted was vivid in their inner experience and had become something for which to earnestly strive, the members of the system were asked to let their imaginations take over and break loose, as it were, regarding the steps to be taken in order to make those goals real. When done in this way, rather than logically or "left hemispherically," the members of the system became very creative.

This was the time when each was given the freedom to speak out loud *while in hypnosis*, and to say what came to mind. This produced a fruitful cross-fertilization of ideas to the enrichment of every member of the team: Many suggestions were proposed by the people involved in this exercise and each person was able to sort things out in a relaxed, naturalistic, state of mind. One person took an idea from another and embellished it, thus giving the others the opportunity to continue to enrich the first thought proposed. While they were engaged in this type of communal hypnosis, they were told to let images, fantasies, memories, or ideas connected with attaining their goals together as a system-in-action into their minds, using the talents and resources of every member of the system. After this practice, which usually took from five to eight tries, they discussed logically the actions needed for the attainment of their goal.

They were emphatically told to spend about half an hour daily in the type of self-hypnosis work that they had learned during the 5-day workshop. This they were supposed to do individually, but because these people saw each other daily at work, they were asked to have a weekly meeting to discuss their practice and to monitor the progress toward the goals they had agreed on.

Evaluation

The final step in the process described here took place after the 5-day workshop. Participants were instructed to keep a written record of their daily practice and to keep notes on the weekly group meeting to evaluate behaviorally and affectively the efficacy of their concrete actions in attaining their goals of improved communication. Once a month after the 5-day workshop, for 6 months after its completion, the workshop leader attended both experimental and control meetings and answered any questions that they might have had. At this monthly meeting, they were also asked to write a brief paragraph evaluating the progress made in interpersonal communications, as each perceived it. However, the main purpose of the leader's presence was to reinforce the hypnotic practice in the experimental group.

RESULTS

The comparison between the experimental and control subjects (who had not been exposed to hypnotic methods during the workshop) was rather dramatic. All the experimental subjects assessed the whole experience (workshop and weekly and monthly meetings) as very positive, productive, educational, and enriching. They unanimously claimed "to be now more to the point," "to use words that are more appropriate," "to express ideas much more clearly and without ambivalence," to use more effective speech, not just at work, but with family and friends as well. By contrast, throughout the monthly meetings with the leader, the controls were unclear about their goals as a group, spent much time arguing, and made little or no progress in communication both as evaluated by the leader and by their own self-reports. They showed confusion about the practical steps to be taken in order to attain their goals. Intellectualization and power plays were common, even after the leader pointed them out. Less than 10% of the controls kept a daily log writing their thoughts about the influence of the workshop on their day-to-day communication, whereas there was 98% compliance in the experimental subjects. "Weekly" meetings were held on an average of one every other week among the controls, whereas the experimental group did not miss one single week. Over a 6-month period original control participants were all present only once at the weekly meeting. Attendance at the weekly meetings consistently was close to 90% in the experimental groups. Overall, hypnotic methods engaged participants more than nonhypnotic techniques. Experimental subjects were more productive than controls with respect to defining problems, setting goals, and taking practical actions to reach these goals.

CONCLUSION

It may be concluded that the (a) hypnotic techniques learned during the original workshop enhanced interpersonal communication significantly more than nonhypnotic techniques; (b) hypnotic techniques were generalized after the workshop to other communication situations; (c) improvement in interpersonal communication learned during the workshop lasted at least 6 months after its completion. However, the benefits of hypnosis, regardless of the designation, can become very real if applied in a structured program that people, oriented toward planning, action, and results, can accept as "making sense" to them. Once they understand where these mental exercises and practice will lead them, they are receptive to "right-hemispheric" methods and, precisely because they are new to them, they give hypnotic techniques a fair chance. As a consequence, a vast majority benefit. Management consulting, which recognizes, teaches, and utilizes hypnosis, can be highly effective to enrich the lives and communication of individuals in a corporate social system.

V

CLINICAL APPLICATIONS AND NEW DIRECTIONS

Erika Fromm has always been a pioneer in her clinical work. In the last decade, for example, she made significant contributions to hypnotherapy for post-traumatic stress disorders, severe psychopathology, and behavioral medicine. Her initial work in each of these areas has served as a catalyst for many clinicians who have since begun more systematic exploration of the use of hypnosis in each of these areas.

Fromm's interest in post-traumatic stress disorders (PTSD) began in the 1980s exemplified in her most detailed published case study, the case of Jessica (Brown & Fromm, 1986). In that study she outlined 11 stages for the treatment of a woman suffering from a borderline/narcissistic condition and chronic PTSD subsequent to childhood sibling incest. Because the patient had thoroughly repressed the trauma, Fromm illustrates her systematic approach to the symbolic and direct uncovering of the memories and feelings associated with the sexual victimization.

Fromm also engaged in a collaborative dialogue with some of her colleagues regarding the treatment of PTSD. Several of the chapters in this section are the result of that ongoing exchange. In "The Variable Long-Term Effects of Incest," Daniel Brown addresses some important issues in the understanding and treatment of PTSD that were not emphasized in Fromm's study of Jessica. Jessica is an example of chronic PTSD in the denial phase (Horowitz, 1976), where slow and systematic uncovering and transference interpretation is indicated. However, many PTSD patients are referred for treatment during the intrusive phase of post-traumatic recovery, when they are flooded with memories and/or feeling about early traumatic experiences. In his case study of Jane, Brown uses Fromm's view of hypnosis as a process of creative coping and problem solving to illustrate how the clinician can help the patient effectively cope with such intrusive experiences and integrate traumatic experiences without being overwhelmed.

Brown also explores in some detail why some adult incest survivors manifest DSM-III Axis II (structural pathology), as did Jessica, and others Axis I PTSD symptoms, as did Jane. He argues that the long-term sequelae of incest are multidetermined, presents a model of the main determinants of long-term sequelae to childhood sexual victimization, and helps us understand why the clinical pictures of Jessica and Jane seem so different.

Onno van der Hart and his associates continue the dialogue about hypnoanalytic treatment of PTSD in their chapter, "Writing Assignments and Hypnosis in the Treatment of Traumatic Memories with Directive Therapy." Van der Hart is especially interested in extending our understanding of methods for use with PTSD patients. He makes a distinction between nonhypnotic techniques, specifically writing assignments, and the kind of hypnotic techniques described by Brown and Fromm (1986) in *Hypnotherapy and Hypnoanalysis* for use with PTSD patients. He discusses various ways clinicians can structure therapeutic writing assignments to help the patient translate traumatic memories into a personal narrative. He also reviews a variety of hypnoanalytic methods that can be used with such patients. Moreover, the chapter includes a valuable discussion about criteria for deciding when to use either writing assignments or hypnotherapy techniques with traumatized patients. Writing assignments are useful for patients who have some degree of awareness of their trauma history and can see a connection between their past experience and present symptoms. Hypnotherapy techniques are especially useful for patients who have repressed traumatic experiences and suffer from strong dissociative symptoms. Van der Hart and Fromm share a caution about the use of abreaction wth traumatized patients. Both favor a stage model of treatment that emphasizes stabilization and systematic integration.

In "Ego-State Transferences in the Hypnoanalytic Treament of Dissociative Reactions," Jack and Helen Watkins focus on another dimension of clinical work with PTSD patients, namely the transference. Like van der Hart, the Watkins are interested in the strong dissociative reactions characteristic of many traumatized patients. They draw on Federn's ego-psychoanalytic theory of ego states as a way to understand the variety of transference reactions a given traumatized patient may manifest in treatment, even within a single treatment session. In some respects, the Watkins' view of ego states differs significantly from Fromm's Gestalt emphasis on the total personality of the patient. The Watkins see personality not as a unity, but as a complex aggregate of separate and differentiated ego states, each of which has its own characteristics, associated memories and affects, and transference manifestations. Although differing in point of view from Fromm, the Watkins extend our understanding of the phenomena and treatment of severely dissociated patients, especially patients with multiple personality disorder. In several cases they illustrate the vicissitudes of ego-state transferences in multiple and nonmultiple personality disordered patients.

Arnold Wilson's chapter, "On Silence and the Holocaust," continues the discussion about the clinical sequelae to traumatization. Wilson and Fromm (1982) collaborated in a study of the intergenerational transmission of PTSD. Specifically, they studied the psychological consequences to children raised by parents who had survived the Nazi death camps. They noted that not only the parents, but the children of Holocaust survivors also suffer psychological damage. The extreme traumatization suffered by camp survivors can affect their parenting ability, and therefore their children's psychological development. Drawing upon Kohut's concept of the self-object transference, Wilson and Fromm discussed the surviving parents' use of a child as a "restitutive self-object," in which the parent unconsciously evokes, or attempts to avoid evoking, images, memories, feelings and identifications regarding the Holocaust in the child, in an attempt to undo and repair their own psychological damage subsequent to the death camp experience. The parent's use of the child in this manner can affect the child's normal development. In this chapter Wilson extends these ideas. He focuses on the impairment of affect tolerance in some children of Holocaust survivors. Wilson believes that the adult child's construction in psychotherapy of an historical narrative which includes the Holocaust legacy is an essential ingredient of effective treatment of children of survivors, because it enables the patient to integrate heretofore split off intolerable affects. Although this chapter is not about hypnotherapy, we have included it here, nevertheless, because it extends some of Fromm's thinking about the integration process in the treatment of PTSD patients, and because its essential ideas could very well be applied to the hypnotherapeutic treatment of trauma.

The last chapter in this section illustrates ground-breaking work in the treatment of the severely disturbed patient. Elgan Baker pioneered the use of hypnosis with severely disturbed patients (Baker, 1981). Erika Fromm was influenced by his outline of the stages of hypnotherapy designed to facilitate healthy internalization, integration of split-off self- and object representations, and the development of object constancy in the severely disturbed patient. She modified and extended his outline of treatment (Fromm, 1984a) and illustrated its use in the case of Jessica (Brown & Fromm, 1986). In the chapter here, "Hypnoanalysis for Structural Pathology," Baker gives an overview of his current thinking on the topic. He discusses the hypnoanalytic treatment of the severely disturbed patient with particular reference to fostering the development of a positive, cohesive, functional, and stable self-representation. Because many patients with structural psychopathology lack a cohesive and/or stable self-representation, the successful correction of these developmental failures has significant value . He shows us how hypnosis is well suited to address structural psychopathology, provided that the hypnoanalyst is able to modify the hypnotic methods for use with this patient population.

Chapter 16

THE VARIABLE LONG-TERM EFFECTS OF INCEST: HYPNOANALYTIC AND ADJUNCTIVE HYPNOTHERAPEUTIC TREATMENT

DANIEL BROWN
The Cambridge Hospital/Harvard Medical School

THEORETICAL BACKGROUND

Defining Incest

Although clinicians come to appreciate incest as a widespread social problem, little agreement has been reached on defining it. Most experts advocate a "broad and encompassing definition of child sexual abuse" (Haugaard & Reppucci, 1988, p.29) that takes into account competing perspectives.

The legal definition of incest emphasizes the ineligibility of the sexual partners because they are family members—either because they are blood relatives, in the case of parent–child incest, or because of prohibitive social ties, in the case of stepparent–child incest (Benward & Densen-Gerber, 1975). Nearly every state in the United States has a law prohibiting marriage or sexual relations between blood relatives when at least one is a child. Although state laws differ considerably in the age under which sex is prohibited (ranging from 11 to 17 years of age), these laws generally agree that sex between family members and a child is considered a crime.

Incest has been defined with reference to: (a) parties involved (b) the type of sexual or violating activity and (c) motive. According to recent surveys of the parties involved, the most common type of incest occurs across generations (i.e., between a child and a parent, stepparent, in-law, grandparent, or aunt or uncle; Courtois, 1988; Russell, 1986). Studies have been conducted on each of these forms of incestuous involvement: father–daughter incest (Herman, 1981; Herman & Hirschman, 1981; Justice & Justice, 1979; Meiselman, 1978, Parker & Parker, 1986; Spencer, 1978); mother–daughter incest (Finkelhor, 1984; Goodwin & DiVasto, 1979; Goodwin, McCarthy, & DiVasto, 1981; Groth, 1982), father–son incest (Dixon, Arnold, & Calestro, 1978; Lew, 1988; Mrazek, 1981), mother– son incest (Margolis, 1984; Meiselman, 1978; Shengold, 1980; Ward, 1985), grandparent–child incest (Bass & Thornton, 1983; Courtois & Hinckley, 1981; Forward & Buck, 1978; Goodwin, Cormier, & Owen, 1983), Uncle–niece incest (Kinsey, Pomeroy, Martin, & Gebhard, 1953), and multiple incest (Courtois, 1988; Doron, 1982). Peer incest (i.e., occurring between a child and an older sibling), has not been studied as extensively and may be more common than is generally appreciated (Cole, 1982; Finkelhor, 1979; Forward & Buck, 1978; Laredo, 1982; Mrazak, 1981; Russell, 1986; Smith & Israel, 1987).

Type of activity

Definitions of incest that focus on the parties involved have been criticized because they focus on who is involved in the sexual act rather than on what they are doing (Courtois, 1988; Ward, 1985). The type of sexual activity considered incestuous is seldom agreed on by experts in the field. Most experts have adopted Burgess and Holmstrom's (1974) conception of some kind of continuum of sexual contact between the child and the adult (e.g., Brant & Tisza, 1977; Rosenfeld, 1979; Sgroi, 1982; Summit & Kryso, 1978). One end of the continuum pertains to nonsexual contacts required for normal caretaking, such as affectionate holding or contact occurring while changing or bathing the child. Further along the continuum are noncontact sexual acts such as nudity and disrobing in front of the child. Still further along the continuum are sexual acts involving contact, such as fondling. At the other end of the continuum are genital finger penetration and intercourse. Some experts include noncontact acts such as exhibitionism while others limit the definition to genital contact. Most at least agree that nongenital sexual contact such as fondling should be considered incestuous.

Definitions that fail to take motive into account and focus on the sexual activity per se also have been criticized in that they do not give an accurate view of the motive involved in incest. Feminist clinicians, beginning with pioneering work by Burgess and Holmstrom (1974) have emphasized that incest is not primarily sexual in nature, but rather is an act of aggression and dominance. Some experts believe that incest is more correctly viewed an "aberration or disorder of power" (Sgroi, 1982 , p. 2).

Finkelhor (1978) defined incest by the three standards of consent, meaning, and community. The relationship is abusive if (a) the child does not have the understanding about the sexual activity involved to consent freely (b) the child's experience of the activity is negative despite whether or not the child discloses the event, and (c) the age difference between the child victim and adult perpetrator is great enough that the perpetrator is in a position of authority and has primary responsibility for the relationship.

The distribution of power in the relationship between a child and a parent is inherently unequal. The child cannot freely consent to such a relationship (Finkelhor, 1979) that is generally one-sided (Meiselman, 1978) and in which the child submits to the sexual activity largely in response to the overwhelming power and authority of the adult (Ferenczi, 1949). The inequality in power also is inherent in the relationship by virtue of the age difference between the victim and perpetrator. Most perpetrators including siblings are at least 5 or more years older than the victim and are perceived as knowing whether the act is right or wrong (Finkelhor, 1979). Feminist clinicians remind us that this dynamic of dominance and violation, typically by an older male, is common to patriarchal families (Herman, 1981, McIntyre, 1981; Rieker & Carmen, 1986). The same power distribution exists even in cases of mother–daughter incest, wherein the mother abandons the maternal role for an exploitative relationship (Goodwin & DiVasto, 1979).

The aspect of exploitation is emphasized by many authors, because when incest occurs, the adult imposes his or her needs on the child. This act constitutes a kind of exploitation. Incest is defined as "a sexual act imposed on a child who lacks emotional, maturational, and cognitive development" (Sgroi, Blick, & Porter; 1982, p. 9) or "when a child of any age is exploited by an older person for his own satisfaction while disregarding the child's own developmental immaturity and inability to understand the sexual behavior" (Steele, 1986, p. 284). Some feminists therefore consider incest to be a kind of rape (Brownmiller, 1975; Ward, 1985). Exploitation is likely to occur by men who feel weak and powerless in other areas of their lives and compensate by dominating their families and exploiting their children (Meiselman, 1978). Such men often feel "entitled" to exploit family members (Herman, 1981).

THE PREVALENCE OF INCEST

Since Freud abandoned his seduction theory (Masson, 1984), Western mental health entered into an "Age of Denial" (Armstrong, 1978) regarding incest that lasted until the late 1970s (Summit, 1982). The shift toward greater sensitivity about incest began with the ground-breaking study by Kinsey and his associates (1953) on female sexual behavior. Since then, clinical, scientific, and forensic interest in child sexual abuse has flourished and our current understanding of the incidence of childhood sexual victimization is based on extensive scientific surveys; case reports from mental health; social service and legal agencies; and first-hand accounts of adult survivors who, largely influenced by the women's movement, have found an increasingly permissive climate to tell their stories (Bass & Davis, 1988; Herman, 1981; Rush, 1980).

The prevalence rates for incest vary greatly across numerous survey studies of adults' childhood sexual experiences (Courtois, 1979; Finkelhor,1979; Fritz, Stoll, & Wagner, 1981; Fromuth, 1986; Gagnon, 1965; Haugaard, 1987; Kinsey, Pomeroy, Martin, & Gebhard, 1953; Landis, 1956; Russell, 1986; Sedney & Brooks, 1984; Wyatt, 1985). This variance in part is due to type of sexual activity defined as incestuous and in part to sampling biases.

Fraser (1981) argued that we should distinguish more carefully between acts without physical contact (e.g., exhibitionism), nonviolent sexual contact (e.g., fondling), and aggressive contact (e.g., intercourse). Most of the surveys in question define incest in terms of some form of physical contact between the child and an older individual in the family (5 years in Finkelhor, 1979), but generally neither restrict the inquiry to sexual intercourse nor expand it to include acts not involving contact. Obviously, incidence rates are higher with broader definitions including both contact and noncontact experiences.

There is some consistency in prevalence rates. About one fifth to one third of all women in the United States have had some sort of childhood sexual encounter with an older individual (primarily adult males) by the age of 18 (Herman, 1981; MacFarlane & Waterman, 1986;. Mrazek, 1981; Schetky & Green 1988). The only genuinely random sample reports 38% of all women in the United States being victimized by some form of sexual contact with an older adult by age 18 (Russell, 1986). A recent national survey in Holland gives remarkably similar results, reporting 32% of all women there having been sexually victimized by age 16 (Draijer, 1988). Prevalence rates for peer incest (brother, sister, and cousin) vary from 3% to 18%, although these rates are probably underestimated (Weinberg, 1955).

Although these figures may seem high, many authorities in the field believe that the current estimates are still conservative (Herman, 1981) because not all victims report their sexual victimization experiences, especially in surveys. However, prevalence rates derived from the surveys are nearly always considerably higher than the number of cases actually reported to mental health, social service, and legal institutions, because most cases are not professionally identified. The number of institutionally documented cases is believed to be 5 to 10 times lower than estimates from national surveys, which more closely reflect a "hidden incidence" of incest (Tsai & Wagner, 1978).

From agency and institutional reports, the incidence of incest is known to be especially high in certain risk populations: runaways (McCormack, Janus,

& Burgess, 1986), delinquents (Burgess, Hartman, & McCormack, 1987), prostitutes (James & Meyerding, 1977; MacVicar & Dillon, 1980; Silbert & Pines, 1981; Vitaliano, James, & Boyer, 1981); substance abusers (Benward & Densen-Gerber, 1975), borderlines (Stone, 1981), and psychiatric inpatients (Beck & van der Kolk, 1987; Bryer, Nelson, Miller, & Krol, 1987; Husain & Chapel, 1983).

TYPICAL PROFILE OF THE INCESTUOUS FAMILY

In most studies the victims are primarily female (e.g., Russell, 1986) and the perpetrators are primarily older males (Herman & Hirschman, 1981), with an age difference greater than 5 years (Browne & Finkelhor, 1986). In most cases, the perpetrator is known to the victim, who typically is a preadolescent child (Finkelhor, 1979; Husain & Chapel, 1983). The first sexual victimization occurs on the average around age 10 for girls and slightly earlier for boys. Although nearly 60% of incestuous acts are single occurrences (Finkelhor, 1979), in almost half the cases of incest, the victim is involved in two to many more sexual incidents with the same adult over an average duration of 4 years (Courtois, 1988; Draijir, 1988; Russell, 1986). It is also not unusual for incest to involve more than one perpetrator in the nuclear or extended family over time (Courtois, 1988; Doron, 1982; Russell, 1986; Walsh, 1986). The reason for this has been explained clearly by Courtois (1988):

> Once the incest barrier is breached, there is little to disinhibit additional incestuous activity; incest becomes the "normal" way to interact and seems to become unconsciously embedded within the family, even though the abuse is commonly kept secret. (p. 26)

The first sexual experience commonly involves nongenital or genital fondling in 33% to 66% of the cases (Haugaard & Reppucci, 1988) and often follows a progressive pattern from the establishment of a special relationship to the eventual sexual boundary violation with increasing sexualization of the relationship, to fondling and then to finger and/or genital penetration (Meiselman, 1978; Sgroi, 1982). Incest usually does not involve physical violence. If force is used it is more likely to be used by stepfathers (Russell, 1984) or grandparents (Draijer, 1988) where blood ties are weaker. Moreover, it nearly always involves some sort of inducement on the part of the perpertrator to keep the child silent. The child usually responds to this authority without question. This typical "conspiracy to silence" (Butler, 1978) is the main reason why so many incest cases remain unreported and untreated.

Considerable research has been devoted to understanding the structure and dynamics of the families and sociocultural context in which cross-generational incest is likely to occur (Lustig, Dresser, Spellman, & Murray, 1966). Many family therapists have emphasized the long-term dysfunction in the marital relationship between the husband and wife (Courtois, 1988; Gelinas, 1983; Paulson, 1978). Typically, such dysfunction is manifested in the sexual relationship between husband and wife (Westermeyer, 1978). Unable to communicate in direct ways, the partners become increasingly estranged and distant, especially sexually (Draijer, 1988). It is common for one more of the children to become triangulated into meeting the needs of the incestuous parent while the other parent becomes distant from both (Rist, 1979) and often depressed (Browning & Boatman, 1977). The "special" relationship develops to compensate for the lack of intimacy in the couple's relationship until, eventually, when the boundaries in the progressively close relationship are violated, the increasingly distant mothers often collude with the incestuous involvement by denying that is it occurring (Meiselman, 1978). Typically a "role reversal" occurs (Meiselman, 1978) in which the child becomes increasingly "parentified," that is, assigned parental roles and functions (Gelinas, 1983).

Cross-generational incest is most likely to occur in families where one adult, typically the father or stepfather, is the patriarch (Lustig et al., 1966). Patterns of dominance may vary. Kempe and Kempe (1984) described "chaotic" and "outwardly stable" family patterns. The "chaotic family" is usually of lower socioeconomic status and is characterized by unstable and stormy relationships or substance abuse. The adult offender in this case compensates for his weak position by dominating his children. "Ideas of persecution and grandiosity" are often prevalent in such fathers (Goodwin, 1989). The "outwardly stable family" is often of high socioeconomic status and high visibility in the community (e.g., successful businessman or professional). The father is dominant as head of the household and other family members are subordinated. He may seem well adjusted in many areas of his life and manifest a kind of "restricted psychopathy" with respect to sexual behavior with the child (Wells, 1981). In either case it is likely that the male adult is less involved or emotionally invested in the caretaking of the children (Parker & Parker, 1986) and maintains his dominance by patterns of shaming and subordination (Fossum & Mason, 1986).

RISK FACTORS FOR INCEST

The factors that increase risk of incest include:

- less involvement in the caretaking by the father (Parker & Parker, 1986);

- less emotional attachment to the child by a stepfather due to lack of blood ties (Finkelhor, 1980);
- emotional distance or depression of the mother (Browning & Boatman, 1977);
- absence of mother from the family due to illness (Finkelhor, 1980: Herman, 1981);
- isolation from the wider community or enmeshment of the family with ignorance about social norms regarding acceptable contact between family members (Cooper & Cormier, 1982; Gelinas, 1983; Weinberg, 1955);
- isolation of children from peers (Finkelhor, 1980);
- cultural sanctioning of incest in certain isolated religious or rural groups (Justice & Justice, 1979);
- previous history of incest (Goodwin, McCarthy, & DiVasto, 1981);
- a pattern of substance abuse or alcoholism within the family (Gelinas, 1983);
- situational stressors (Meiselman, 1978);
- poverty (Finkelhor, 1980); and
- excessive life-change stress (Meiselman, 1978).

An excellent study by Finkelhor (1980) demonstrates that each risk factor present in a family increases the probability of incest in a cumulative and linear fashion. Families with no risk factors had virtually no incest. Two thirds of the children in families with five risk factors present were sexually victimized. The presence of each additional risk factor increased the child's risk by 10% to 20%. Families with six to eight risk factors were likely to be incestuous close to 100% of the time.

SHORT-AND LONG-TERM EFFECTS OF INCEST

There has been little agreement in the literature on the psychological effects of incest, varying from reports of few symptoms or aftereffects to severe psychopathology (Conte & Schuerman, 1987; Koch, 1980). Early clinical literature tended to minimize the effects on the victim, whereas later literature may have exaggerated harm (Bender & Blau, 1937; Constantine, 1980). Aside from clear biases in interpretation of aftereffects, it is probably true that the effects of incest are highly variable not only in intensity (Herman, Russell, & Trocki, 1986), but in type. Mrazek and Kempe (1981) listed over 60 reported effects.

These have been broadly categorized. Typically the categories include: (a) emotional effects, for example, anxiety, phobias, depression, anger, guilt, and shame; (b) somatic effects, for example, nausea and vomiting, pain, sleep and eating disturbances; (c) behavioral disturbances, for example school problems, running away, delinquency, substance abuse and alcoholism, self-mutilation, early marriage and pregnancy, and the repetition of traumatic abusive relationships; and (d) sexual problems, for example, confusion of sexual orientation; problems of desire, (including inhibited sexual desire or promiscuity), and failures of satisfaction, arousal, and climax, such as vaginismus, frigidity, or impotence, anorgasmia, or pre- or postmature ejaculation (Browne & Finkelhor, 1986; Courtois, 1988; Draijer, 1988; Gomes-Schwartz, Horowitz, & Sauzier, 1985; Lew, 1988; MacFarlane & Watermanetal 1986; Maltz & Holman, 1987). Although these symptoms commonly are observed in incest victims, no general pattern of aftereffects is identifiable. Most experts agree that incest does increase the risk of psychological damage. It is not a sufficient condition for such damage to occur (Herman, 1981). Most incest victims report that incestuous involvement was subjectively experienced as a negative emotional experience, but not all perceive themselves as harmed by it (Draijer, 1988; Herman, 1981). Incest, a "potentially traumatic experience" (Goodwin, 1985, p.165), creates a "predisposition" to psychological disturbances (Meiselman, 1978).

It is useful to distinguish between the short-and long-term impact of incest (Browne & Finkelhor, 1986). Initial effects are defined as occurring within 2 years after the termination of the abuse and long-term effects as persisting after 2 or more years. Initial effects of the experience typically meet the DSM III criteria for a diagnosis of PTSD (Armsworth, 1984; Courtois, 1988; Donaldson & Gardner, 1985; Draijer, 1988; Finkelhor & Browne, 1985; Frederick, 1985; Gelinas, 1983; Goodwin, 1989; Horowitz, 1976, 1986; Krener, 1985; Lindberg & Distad, 1985a; van der Kolk, 1984) that includes such features as:

1. an event outside the range of usual human experience;
2. persistent re-experiencing of intrusive recollections, dreams, and feelings regarding the trauma;
3. persistent avoidance of thoughts, feelings, and stimuli associated with the trauma; and
4. persistent symptoms of arousal such as an exaggerated startle sensitivity yor physiologic reactivity to situations associated with the trauma.

Although PTSD symptoms can vary widely across individuals there are some classic signs that are likely to indicate a history of incest. These include disturbances in thought content such as recurring nightmares, obsessions, phobias, and dissociative phenomena, and perceptual disturbances such as illusions and hallucinations (Ellenson, 1986).

Long-term effects of incest are also variables and may not become apparent for many years (Draijer, 1988; Gelinas, 1983). A significant subgroup of adult incest survivors meet the DSM III criteria for delayed or chronic PTSD years after the childhood sexual incidents (Gelinas, 1983; Lindberg & Distad, 1985a; Wooley & Vigilanti, 1984). Many experts believe that incest may result in a developmental arrest along one or several lines of normal development (Brown & Fromm, 1986; Gaddini, 1983; Rosenfeld, 1979). Sgroi (1982) best summarized this position. She said incest is an:

> interference with the accomplishment of normal developmental tasks. The progression of mastery of one's self, environment, and relationship with others is significantly disrupted by the child's permanently altered awareness and new role vis-à-vis the perpetrator. (p.35)

Areas of normal development most likely to be affected include sexual development, relationship to others, self, and self-esteem development, affect, cognition, and character development.

Sexual Functioning. This is most likely to be adversely affected in the survivor population (Draijer, 1988; Finkelhor, 1979; Gelinas, 1983; Maltz & Holman, 1987; Molnar & Cameron, 1975). The frequency of sexual problems is significantly higher in abuse victims than in the general population (Lukianowicz, 1971; Meiselman, 1978; Weeks, 1976). Incest is a form of premature sexual stimulation that interferes with phase-specific sexual fantasies and impulses in normal sexual development (Lewis & Sarrel, 1969), and also with the normal dating patterns of adolescence (Maltz & Holman, 1987). Depending on the circumstances surrounding the incest and the level of development of the child, incest may increase vulnerability to the variety of sexual problems in adult life already described. Even when sexual functioning appears normal incest survivors may suffer from impairment in sexual self-esteem (Finkelhor, 1979) or from unpleasant flashbacks during sexual activity (Bass & Davis, 1988; Maltz & Holman, 1987).

Relationships With Others. The relationship incest victims have with others is also likely to be impaired. Incest is a betrayal of trust in a significant relationship in early development. The long-term effects of such betrayal on the capacity for attachment relationships is only just beginning to be understood. Because incest is primarly an relationally based form of abuse (Gelinas, 1983), some sort of impairment in object relations is likely to become manifest over time (Rosenfeld, 1979). Common difficulties include mistrust (Kempe & Kempe, 1984), difficulty forming relationships, maintaining detachment, or keeping a distance from intimate involvement (Herman, 1981; Lindberg & Distad, 1985b). Incest survivors who seek intimacy often quickly sexualize the relationship because they confuse intercourse with closeness (Kempe & Kempe, 1984; Yates, 1982). All too often they easily see themselves as having no needs or rights in the relationship (Gelinas, 1983).

It is common for adults abused as children to experience repeated victimization in relationships (Russell, 1986; van der Kolk, 1989; Wooley & Vigilanti, 1984). They may internalize the inequality of power in the child-victim/adult-perpetrator model. Men, particularly abusing men, may be overvalued and idealized (Herman, 1981). Moreover, because acquiescence to incest as a child may impair the normal development of self-protective mechanisms (Herman, 1981), incest survivors can easily fall into a repeated pattern of unconsciously selecting abusive relationships or failing to use good judgment regarding dangerous situations. This impairment of self-protection may be one reason that incest survivors are significantly more at risk for abusive relationships or other types of traumatization like rape.

Body Image, Self, and Self-Esteem. Incest can interfere with body image and self and self-esteem development (Bass & Davis, 1988). Some types of childhood incestuous involvement, especially when complicated by sadistic aggression (Kluft, 1985) or an excessive need to deny the reality of incest (Rieker & Carmen, 1986), can interfere with the normal development of a cohesive sense of self and leave the victim vulnerable to fragmentation (Soll, 1984/85). Self-fragmentation occurs along a continuum from individuals who report the experience of separate parts of themselves to the formation of stable, bounded separate selves (Price, 1987), as in the case of multiple personalities (Allison, 1947; Braun, 1986; Coons, 1980; Goodwin, 1989; Kluft, 1984; Putnam 1985b). Although self-fragmentation represents the more extreme case of self-pathology following incest, self-esteem impairment is very common (Finkelhor, 1979; Gelinas, 1983; Herman, 1981). Many incest survivors see themselves as somehow different from others (Bass & Davis, 1988; Krener, 1985). Women survivors experience themselves as "damaged goods" (Sgroi, 1982), men as "less than a man" (Lew, 1988). Self-development is inhibited. Parentification common to incest (Gelinas, 1983) can lead to a kind of pseudomaturity (Lustig et al., 1966; Meiselman, 1978). This interferes with normal play and active exploration of interests necessary for children as vehicles of self-exploration and self-development. The range of potential interests and ambitions becomes restricted.

Affect. Incest can also interfere with the normal development of affect (Krystal, 1984; Lindberg & Distad, 1985a). The intense stimulation of sexual and aggressive impulses may lead to long-term dysregulation of these, characterized by extreme behaviors. Incest survivors may fluctuate between promiscuity or manifestations of inhibited sexual desire, but rarely demonstrate appropriate sexual expression. They may be passive and nonassertive or highly irritable and rageful, but selfom are appropriately angry. The normal capacity for affective tolerance is likely to be impaired (Brown & Fromm, 1986).

Cognitive Deficits. A variety of cognitive deficits may be sequelae of incest. These are often specific to the age at which incest occurred (Fish-Murray, Koby, & van der Kolk, 1987). Intrusive thoughts that interfere with attention and concentration are quite common. These intrusions and ruminations constitute a kind of "unfinished business" in the incest survivor's attempt to integrate and make sense out of the trauma (Silver, Boon, & Stones, 1983; van der Kolk & Kadish, 1987).

Excessive stimulation intensifies sexual and aggressive fantasies specific to the child's age (Lewis & Sarrel, 1969). Both bisexual and homosexual fantasies are often intensified by incest (Soll, 1984/85). Grandiose fantasies are a common accompaniment to the shattered self-esteem associated with incest (Ullman & Brothers, 1988). Such grandiose fantasies are often accompanied by fantasies about the need to be punished (Shengold, 1980).

Survivors lose any sense of belief in a just and fair world. The common attributional style is to expect bad events to happen (Gold, 1986). "Illusions of invulnerability" to harm and the capacity to reasonably predict how life unfolds have been shattered by the incest trauma. Survivors have difficulty feeling safe and feeling that they can reasonably predict life's events (Janoff-Bulman & Frieze, 1983). Once it occurs, such trauma is no longer unthinkable and the world is never the same again (Meiselman, 1978). Early trauma initiates a lifelong search for meaning that is infrequently fully resolved (Silver, Boon, & Stones, 1983).

Character Pathology. Because the effects on normal development can be (but are not always) pervasive, incest can result in the development of long-term character pathology. Numerous studies have appeared recently in which patients meeting the DSM III diagnostic criteria for borderline personality have been interviewed for possible trauma histories. The majority (from 60% to 80%) of borderline patients have a clear history of incest, which raises the question as to whether sexual trauma in childhood can contribute to the development of borderline personality organization (Herman, Perry, & van der Kolk, 1989; Gross, Deorr, Caldirola, Guzinski, & Ripley, 1890/1981; Gartner & Gartner, 1988; Stone, 1981). Parson (1984) coined the term "fluid character pathology" to emphasize how trauma can impact on a variety of lines of development, so that survivors of trauma may appear to be indistinguishable from patients given the diagnosis of personality disorder. Why severe pathology occurs in some incest patients and not others is not always clear, but a combination of pre-existing pathology in the mother–daughter relationship associated with a failure to successfully negotiate separation/individuation, along with a history of incest, is highly predictive of borderline personality development (Gartner & Gartner, 1988).

DETERMINANTS OF THE LONG-TERM EFFECTS OF INCEST

Clearly, a variety of factors come into play to determine whether incest results in mild, moderate, or severe long-term psychological harm, (Hartman & Burgess, 1986; Trepper & Barrett, 1986). Major factors implicated in the development of the long-term effects of incest include: (a) pre-existing condition; (b) the nature of the traumatic involvement; (c) the pre- and post-traumatic adjustment; (d) the crisis of disclosure; and (e) the post-disclosure adjustment (see Fig 16.1).

Some authors have argued that pre-existing conditions contribute as much if not more to the long-term psychological harm than the incest itself (Lewis & Sarrel, 1969). The parent–child relationship may be dysfunctional prior to the incestuous involvement. A disturbed mother–daughter relationship (Brooks, 1983; Draijer, 1988; Forward & Buck, 1978; Justice & Justice, 1979; Machotka, Pittman, & Flomenhoft, 1967; McIntyre, 1981) may predispose the child to a variety of preoedipally based forms of developmental psychopathology (Gartner & Gartner, 1988) and may undermine the normal separation/individuation phase of development, which serves as the basis for healthy self-and object relations development (Gutheil & Avery, 1977; Wooley & Vigilanti, 1984). The father–daughter relationship is disturbed by the father's excessive detachment in the early years of childrearing (Herman, 1981) and later over involvement with the child incest victim (Finkelhor, 1979).

Many experts have viewed incest as a symptom of an underlying family dysfunction during the child's developmental years prior to incest (Gelinas, 1983; Pelletier & Handy, 1986; Paulson, 1978) with inadequate communication between the partners, triangulation of the children into the parental conflicts, role reversals between children and parents, and poor boundaries. Conflicts over sexuality are characteristic of such families (Avery-Clark, O'Neil, & Laws, 1981).

The parents sometimes also bring considerable psychopathology into the family, not the least of which is their own personal history of physical and sexual abuse (Cooper & Cormier, 1982; Goodwin, McCarthy, & DiVasto, 1981; Kaufman & Zigler, 1987). Incest is often transgenerational. Having been victims of childhood trauma themselves, some parents are more predisposed to unconsciously set up the same dynamic in their family and thereby repeat the victimization with their own children (Avery-Clark, O'Neil, & Laws, 1981). Many abuse substances and alcohol, which serve to dysinhibit

Pre-Existing Conditions	The Traumatic Situation(s)	Post-Traumatic Adjustment	Disclosure Crisis	Post-Disclosure Adjustment
• Parent–child relationship • disturbed mother–child relationship • disturbed father–child relationship • Pre-existing family system pathology • Psychopathology within the parents (e.g., • trauma history • substance abuse • restricted psychopathy)	• Type of sexual act • Degree of Force • Intensity of stimulation • Age of onset/developmental level • Victim characteristics • perceived difference • resilience • Perpetrator characteristics • Sibling relationships	INITIAL ACCOMMODATIONS: • Defenses & coping strategies • Encapsulation of the trauma • Post-traumatic play • Denial of trauma reality FURTHER ACCOMMODATIONS: • Cumulative trauma • Role as participant • Conditional hypermaturity & hypersexuality • Loss of self-protection	• Family response • Agency response	Recovery vs Secondary Elaboratives: • Substance abuse • Eating disorders • Self-mutilation • Delinquency • Prostitution

FIG. 16.1. The determinants of the long-term effects of incest.

sexual and aggressive impulses and increase the risk that parents will act on these impulses with their children.

The traumatic sexual involvement itself also contributes to the overall risk of the development of psychopathology. When incest occurs, the initial boundary violation produces an acute psychological crisis in the child-victim. The severity of this crisis is determined by the type of sexual act (e.g., fondling, finger penetration, genital intercourse) the degree of force used (Conte & Schuerman, 1987; Geiser, 1981; Groth, 1982; Herman, Russell, & Trocki, 1986); the intensity of the emotional and impulse stimulation; the role of the victim during the initial sexual involvement (e.g., passive and submissive, or behaviorally resistant through fighting, or internally resistant through withdrawal into fantasy; MacFarlane & Korbin, 1983; Meiselman, 1978); the age of onset and developmental level of the child (MacFarlane & Waterman, 1986; Schetky & Green, 1988); the meaning attributed to the event by the child (Hartman & Burgess, 1986; Lindholm, 1984; MacFarlane & Waterman, 1986); and the duration of the traumatic involvement (because incest is often progressive and the trauma therefore cumulative; Groth, 1982; Russell, 1986).

Certain characteristics of the victim are also associated with the long-term outcome. For example, victimization is more likely to occur in children who are perceived as somehow different from other children. Mentally retarded, premature, and handicapped children are especially at risk (Friedrich & Boriskin, 1976). Because such children are likely to have pre-existing self-esteem problems, their selection as incest victims compounds their psychological difficulties in comparison to healthier children. On the other hand, some children are remarkably resilient and survive even the most severe trauma without long-term psychological scars. Unfortunately, the characteristics that contribute to resilience against the effects of trauma are not well understood (Benedek, 1985).

Certain characteristics of the perpetrator are also associated with long-term adjustment. The abuse is twice as likely to be very serious if done by a stepfather rather than a biological father (Russell, 1984). Presumably, blood ties more often than not have a palliative effect on the impulse to violate a child.

The child-victim's relationship to other siblings also effects the psychological outcome. Many siblings consciously or unconsciously know that incest is occurring. The jealousy and resentment they feel toward the incest victim who has a special relationship with the offending parent further serves to isolate the incest victim in the family (Conte & Schuerman, 1987; De Young, 1981). Moreover, because of the typical isolation of the incestuous family from the community, and the special relationship that develops between the child-victim and the offending parent, the child is likely to have limited peer involvement outside the home relative to normal children. Loss of an available peer group during a critical phase of childhood, especially during latency and preadolescence, can contribute to the overall pathology (Ganzarain & Buchele, 1986).

Once the incestuous involvement has begun the child enters into a period of post-traumatic adjustment. The nature of the child's coping strategies and the quality of the response given by the family also contribute to the long-term adjustment. Summit (1983) has described the "child sexual abuse accommodation syndrome" in which the child develops stereotypic coping mechanisms in an attempt to reconcile the emotional impact of the incest with the strong pressure to deny the reality of abuse within the family. The stages of post-incest adjustment that are typically observed are secrecy, helplessness, entrapment and accomodation, delayed or conflicted disclosure, and retraction.

The first burden placed on the child is the "conspiracy to silence" (Butler, 1978; Lister, 1982). The child realizes or is threatened to believe that disclosing the secret of incestuous involvement will have negative consequences for the victim and the entire family system. Fearing such negative consequences, the child will often comply with requests not only to keep the secret but to submit to subsequent incest (Conte & Schuerman, 1987). A deep sense of resignation and helplessness follows.

The child accommodates adult reality by adopting a variety of psychological defenses and coping strategies—what have been called *survival skills* (Hartman & Burgess, 1986) or *protection skills* (Maltz & Holman, 1987). These may include repression, fantasy, dissociation, denial and projection, splitting, fantasy, numbing, hypervigilance, withdrawal, somatization, and the adopting of special roles within the family like the martyr or the parentified child (Bass & Davis, 1988; Draijer, 1988; Gelinas, 1983; Lew, 1988; Summit, 1983). Most of the child's initial adaptive strategies are palliative in nature (Lindholm, 1984) and attempt to encapsulate the trauma internally by means of defenses such as repression and dissociation, and externally by isolating the incident(s) from everyday family involvement (Burgess, Hartman, & McCormack, 1987). The child may attempt to work through the negative impact of the incest in fantasy and play. Although serving as a warning signal of trauma, such post-traumatic play is seldom effective in helping the child to work it through (Green, 1985).

Many experts have noted that the necessity to deny the reality of the trauma may contribute more than other factors to the overall long-term psychological harm (Rieker & Carmen, 1986). Moreover, as the child becomes withdrawn he or she is likely to become increasingly isolated from contact with siblings and peers. Terr (1983, 1925), in her work with terrorized children, noted their tendency to avoid contact with peers for some time after the incident.

Beyond these initial coping attempts further accomodations must be made if the incest continues. Because the average duration of incest is 4 years the incest trauma is often cumulative (Gelinas, 1983). The child who is made to submit to incest more than once takes an increasingly active role as a participant in the sexual relationship (Gruber, 1981; MacFarlane & Korbin, 1983) and participates in more elaborate sexual activity (Browne & Finkelhor, 1986). The child also learns or is conditioned to be over-sexualized and hypermature in the relationship (Yates, 1982). Moreover, the child's capacity for self-protection has been severely eroded by abuse by a familial authority figure. This lack of capacity for self-protection combined with poor social controls within the family predisposes the child to multiple victimizations (Doron, 1982).

Hartman and Burgess (1986) described four characteristic patterned responses to incest over time: (a) learned avoidance, as if nothing had happened; (b) chronic symptoms of depression, anxiety, and behavioral difficulties appear; (c) identification with the abuser in which the child masters the trauma by exploiting other children; and (d) early psychosis.

Disclosure becomes its own kind of acute crisis, usually because the negative response by the family and by the social and legal agencies constitutes a kind of re-traumatization of the child. Disclosure often occurs because of accidental discovery, or because the child has reached an age where the press for independence from the incestuous involvement reaches crisis proportions, so that the adolescent acts out or sometimes voluntarily discloses the incest. Regardless of the means by which the incest is revealed, disclosure to agencies outside the family nearly always becomes a major crisis for the entire family (Geiser, 1981; Kennedy & Cormier, 1969; Molnar & Cameron, 1975; Simrel, Berg, & Thomas, 1979). Disclosure threatens to disrupt the structure and ongoing functioning of the entire family unit, a system that is likely to be disorganized even prior to the disclosure crisis (Geiser, 1981; Pelletier & Handy, 1986). As a consequence, the disclosure crisis evokes the family's pathological defense mechanisms (Meiselman, 1978; Pelletier & Handy, 1986). The usual family response is to deny the reality of the abuse by threat of withdrawal of support to the child. The child rarely receives an understanding response (Solin, 1986; Summit, 1983). In fact, the greater the severity of the abuse and the duration of the sexually abusing relationship, the less likely the child will receive support from the family upon disclosure (Russell, 1986). Moreover, disclosure is likely to evoke jealousy in the siblings (De Young, 1981), which further contributes to the child's perceived lack of support and increased isolation at a critical time. The fate of the family seems to rest entirely on the child. The child is threatened with the possible and sometimes very real collapse of his or her world (Frederick, 1985). An intensification of separation anxiety and world destruction fantasies are common. The child is likely to feel considerable pressure to deny the reality of the abuse and maintain the delusional image that the abusing parent(s) are all good and all knowing and that the abuse never really occurred (Pelletier & Handy, 1986). Faced with all this, the child is likely to sacrifice him or herself by denying the reality of the abuse internally through repression, and externally through public disconfirmation of the abuse. Retractions of abuse allegations are quite common unless the child receives special support (Summit, 1983).

A severe lapse in reality testing and self-perception lays the foundation for the subsequent development of psychopathology, by which the child victim is transformed into an adult patient (Rieker & Carmen, 1986). Although a pathological response can fix the trauma, healthy parental response can offset the long-term negative effects of the incest trauma (MacFarlane & Korbin, 1983). One should not underestimate the powerful role of the victim's support system particularly the critical parental response in ameliorating the effects of trauma (Conte & Schuerman, 1987).

Re-traumatization may be repeated by health-care and legal professionals if they become involved in the case (MacFarlane & Korbin, 1983). Investigative child protection and legal professionals, while trying to establish the facts of the incest allegations through interviews, often do not provide the kind of support needed by the child in a form that the child can comprehend. Fortunately, guidelines are being established for sensitive and supportive clinical inquiry of the child and family (Josephson & Fong-Beyette, 1987; Sgroi, 1982), and innovative methods have been implemented in some courts to minimize the traumatizing effects of a court investigation on the child victim (Haugaard & Reppucci, 1988). However, the response of both family and professional agencies to the disclosure of incest often contributes to a "second injury" (Symonds, 1980) compounding the trauma of incestuous involvement itself. On a positive note, however, involvement with professional agencies, however flawed, serves to undercut the isolation characteristic of many incestuous families and may constitute a kind of "resocialization" of the family into the community and its social norms (Phelan, 1987).

Once the pattern of pathological coping strategies develops within the victim and the family milieu, the child is vulnerable to the further development of "secondary elaborations" (Gelinas, 1983) such as a re-traumatizing or deviant lifestyle. Victimization can take on a life of its own, quite apart from the original family involvement. For example, the victim, left vulnerable to intense and often intolerable affects, or coping with a generalized numbing of affect, may turn to substances or alcohol as a means of attenuating or generating affective states. Although initially serving as an adaptive strategy, the use of substances and alcohol can become self-reinforcing (Burgess, Hartman, & McCormick, 1987). The same is true of secondary eating disorders or self-mutilative and suicidal behaviors. Their original adaptive function may have provided the victim with a sense of control (Briere & Runtz, 1986; Lindberg & Distad, 1985b; De Young, 1982), but become conditioned and take on a life of their own. If the child learned to actively participate in the sexual involvement and discovered that submitting to sexual victimization was a means to other ends such as affection or monetary rewards, delinquency and prostitution may develop. The child learns to exploit others to gratify such needs (Hartman & Burgess, 1986). Thus, the single or cumulative experience of childhood sexual victimization becomes transformed into an active lifestyle of deviance.

In summary, although it may be difficult to predict the severity and extent of long-term harm in any given case, several themes have emerged consistently from the research. First, it is clear that the likelihood of long-term damage increases if the incest trauma is compounded or multiplied by one or more other risk factors, such as: pre-existing pathology in the parent–child relationship (Gartner & Gartner, 1988); the family structure (Gartner & Kelly, 1983; Pelletier & Handy, 1986), the child (Friedrich & Boriskin, 1976) or in the parent (Avery-Clark, O'Neil, & Laws, 1981); cumulative or progressive sexual traumatization (Sgroi, 1982); or re-traumatization at the time of disclosure (Pelletier & Handy, 1986; Rieker & Carmen, 1986). Second, the probability of psychological damage is increased when the child's coping resources are severely challenged by the need to make excessive accommodations to the pressure of the family to deny the reality of the incest at the expense of the child's own psychological development (Reiker & Carmen, 1986). Third, severe long-term pathology seems directly related to the amount of sadistic aggression and force accompanying the incest (Kluft, 1985). Fourth, even when a number of such risk factors are present, a supportive familial environment can contribute considerably to alleviating the otherwise likely long-term psychological harm from the incest (Hartman & Burgess, 1986). Studies on the impact of the other kinds of trauma on children have shown that the quality of the familial response to trauma is more predictive than the trauma itself to the long-term psychological adjustment (Arroyo & Eth, 1985; Summit & Kryso, 1978). Fifth, the final psychological outcome is likely to be determined by a number of contributing factors. For example, the dual diagnosis of PTSD and character pathology is probably a function of both the incest trauma and the pre-existing pathological family environment (Gelinas, 1983).

Perhaps the single most consistent predictor of the particular nature of long-term effects of incest is age at the onset of the incest. Several empirical studies have recently appeared that demonstrate differential psychological adjustment according to age of onset (Adams-Tucker, 1982; Gomes-Tucker, 1982; Gomes-Schwartz, Horowitz, & Sauzier, 1985; Tsai, Feldman-Summers, & Edgar, 1979). Preschool incest victims typically are less symptomatic than school-age victims (Adams-Tuckes, 1982; Gomes-Schwartz, Horowitz, & Sauzier, 1985), and therfore previously thought to be less psychologically harmed. Experts now believe that problems of preschoolers may go unnoticed because they are less likely to manifest symptomatically, and of course, are less likely to be seen by outsiders. It is becoming increasingly clear that incest trauma occurring during the preschool years is more likely to be associated with pervasive developmental delays and increased social withdrawal than with behavioral symptoms (Browne & Finkelhor, 1986; Cohen, 1981; Gomes-Schwartz, Horowitz, & Sauzier, 1985; Simrel, Berg, & Thomas, 1979). Thus, the real psychological harm of incest for preschoolers may not appear until much later in life, in the form of damage to self and self-esteem development, the capacity to form object relations, and affect regulation (Brown & Fromm, 1986) and overall mental organization (Cohen, 1981).

School-age incest victims are more likely to manifest a variety of obvious internally based (autoplastic) symptoms, such as anxieties, phobias, situational fears, dissociation, and conversion symptoms, and externally based (alloplastic) symptoms, such as learning difficulties and conduct problems. Adolescents manifest the greatest amount of acting out (Sloane & Karpinski, 1942) and subjectively report the greatest suffering from incest, presumably because of their greater intellectual development. Adolescents relative to younger children have a greater capacity to understand the meaning of incest and are more aware of social norms. Therefore, adolescents usually feel a greater sense of responsibility for the incest, are more disturbed by its having occurred (Finkelhor, 1979; Tsai 1979), and are likely to express their distress through running away, promiscuity, substance abuse, and suicidality (Goodwin, 1989). They are also far more sensitive than younger children about how the incest may be viewed by peers (Goodwin, 1989; Kempe & Kempe, 1984).

TREATMENT

Abreaction

Treatment approaches to adult incest survivors have generally adhered until recently to an abreactive model of treatment. According to this model, it is generally assumed that the goal of treatment is to remember completely and to encourage the full expression of feelings associated with the incest trauma (Breuer & Freud, 1955). Many contemporary models for the treatment of incest are still based on assumptions about the value of abreaction, although emphasis has shifted from remembering and expression per se to the integration of the traumatic memories.

Although there may be no dispute that integration of the memories and affects associated with the incest trauma is therapeutically useful, some caution is indicated for those who adhere to a strict abreactive approach to therapy. Abreaction alone may be harmful to the incest survivor. Many incest survivors present to therapy in the denial phase of post-traumatic recovery. They are likely to present with so-called disguised PTSD (Gelinas, 1983), wherein the only manifest symptoms are anxiety-related symptoms or depression. It is well known that direct inquiry about suspected trauma during an intake can itself make the patient symptomatic (Gelinas, 1983). Iatrogenic symptoms are likely to be even more severe if the therapist has a clear bias and believes that successful treatment rests on expression of the feelings associated with the trauma. The therapist's encouragement of too rapid uncovering of the memories and affects associated with presumed trauma may overwhelm the patient's defense. The patient may shift rapidly from denial to an intrusive phase of post-traumatic adjustment. Distressed and fearful from this rapid shift, the patient is at risk for dropping out of treatment. Because the therapist has inadvertently contributed to the patient's undue distress by emphasizing uncovering too early in the treatment, even if the patient returns, therapy is characterized by a re-traumatizing rather than an emotionally corrective relationship.

Multimodal and Stage-Based Treatment

As understanding of incest has increased, more sophisticated multimodal and stage-based approaches to treatment have been developed and used. For child incest victims the integration of individual play therapy for the child, family therapy for the mother–daughter, offender–victim, and entire family, and a self-help parental support group seems to be the best combination of treatments (Sgroi, Blick & Porter 1982). For the adult survivor of incest, a multimodal treatment plan consisting of long-term individual psychotherapy; adjunctive structured group therapy or self-help groups; and sometimes adjunctive family therapy (Courtois, 1988), and/ or adjunctive cognitive behavioral therapy is used (Elsenga & Emmelkamp, 1989; Flannery, 1987; Jehu, Gazan, & Klassen, 1985).

Individual Psychotherapy

Sgroi and her associates (1982) have clearly identified 10 typical treatment goals for adult incest survivors to work through affects and self-perceptions including:

1. the "damaged goods" syndrome;
2. guilt;
3. fear;

4. depression;
5. low self esteem and poor social skills;
6. repressed anger and hostility;
7. impaired ability to trust;
8. blurred role boundaries and role confusion;
9. pseudomaturity coupled with failure to accomplish developmental tasks; and
10. self-mastery and control.

Other treatment approaches stress the value of uncovering and integrating affects and memories associated with the incest itself. This entails a validation of the reality of the trauma by the therapist. The therapist must strive to empower the patient rather than reinforce his or her status as a victim (Lamb, 1986). The therapist also helps the patient make sense out of the trauma, to construct meaning (Silver, Boon, & Stones, 1983) and to put its occurrence into proper perspective ("recontextualizing" the trauma; Rieker & Carmen, 1986). Integration also entails some safe means to gain access to and integrate the memories and feelings associated with the incest trauma (Butler, 1978; Courtois, 1988).

Scurfield (1985) has described five stages of individual therapy with adult for adults with an incest history:

1. the establishment of a trusting relationship;
2. education regarding the recovery process;
3. stress management;
4. regression back to re-experience the trauma; and
5. integration of the trauma.

Compared to stage-models used in the treatment of other sorts of trauma (Brende, 1984; Brown & Fromm, 1986; Harris, 1986; Parson, 1984), these stages for treatment of incest may not be adequately detailed. An alternative description of the unfolding process includes:

1. stabilization;
2. systematic uncovering and integration of the memories and feelings associated with the trauma or cumulative traumas;
3. integration of the split off parts of self and object representations (e.g., the perpetrator self representation);
4. self and self-esteem development through playful exploration of interests and activities and through realistic self-evaluation;
5. alleviating the psychophysiological reactivity resulting from the trauma; and

6. working through the feared consequences of consciously acknowledging sexual and aggressive impulses and associated wishes and fantasies (e.g., fear of being sexual or aggressive even when appropriate; (Brown & Fromm, 1986).

Hypnotherapy of Incest

Because hypnosis is a means to gain access to memories and affects not consiously available, it is the treatment of choice for various types of trauma (Brown & Fromm, 1986). However, the hypnotic literature on the treatment of PTSD pertains to the abreactive treatment (Balson & Dempster, 1980; Buchenholz & Frank, 1949; Fisher, 1943; Grinker & Spiegel, 1945; Kubie, 1943a; Leahy & Martin, 1967; Silver & Kelly, 1985; Simmel, 1944; Watkins, 1949; Wolberg, 1948), and sometimes to the systematic uncovering and integrative treatment of war trauma (Brende & Benedict, 1980; Silver & Kelly, 1985; Spiegel, 1981).

Very little has been written on the use of hypnotherapy with incest. Informed clinical literature on the treatment of incest makes little mention of hypnosis, in contrast to lengthy discussions of other clinical modalities (Courtois, 1988; Haugaard & Reppucci, 1988). Likewise, the hypnosis literature makes scant references to the hypnotherapeutic treatment of incest (Breuer & Freud, 1955; Gross, 1979; Peters, 1976; Schneck, 1966). To my knowledge, the only recent clinical reports on the hypnotherapeutic treatment of incest utilizing some sort of stage-model are the case of Jessica reported by Erika Fromm (Brown & Fromm, 1986) and the case of Jean reported by a colleague of Brown and Fromm (Miller, 1986b). In the spirit of these pioneering studies the case of Jane follows.

Although the overall progression of Jessica's and Jane's treatments followed a similar sequence of discernable states (Brown & Fromm, 1986), Jane's case in many respects is different from that of Jessica. Jessica was an incest survivor with a dual diagnosis of borderline pathology and chronic PTSD. With Jessica's case, Erika Fromm eloquently illustrated working through the transference in long-term hypnoanalytic treatment of a patient with structural pathology.

In Jane's case there was less underlying psychopathology and therefore the transference was less salient. Jane struggled with a variety of debilitating symptoms and the emphasis of the treatment was accordingly on symptom management. These typically include anxiety and panic, sleep disturbances and nightmares, dissociative symptoms, and somatic complaints. Moreover, if the patient is shifting from a denial to an intrusive phase of post-traumatic recovery (Horowitz, 1976; Brown & Fromm, 1986) she may fear being overwhelmed by intrusive memories and feelings. I discuss the first few stages of Jane's treatment in some detail as a way of illustrating the technical problems of working in hypnotherapy with adult incest survivors who experience such debilitating symptoms and intrusive experiences.

Jane: A Case Illustration of Adjunctive Hypnotherapy for Incest

Jane grew up in a Catholic family in a small New England town. She was the third youngest of four children: a brother 3 years older; a sister 1 year older; and a brother 3 years younger than she. Her father was a businessman. Both her mother and father were very active and visible within their community. Her family fit the profile for the "outwardly stable family" in which incest occurs (Kempe & Kempe,1984).

At the time of the referral for adjunctive hypnotherapy by her primary therapist of 3 years, Jane was a 43-year-old college-educated mother of three children in a stable marriage of 20 years. She was referred by her therapist of 3 years for adjunctive hypnotherapy for a chronic pain syndrome. Five years previously she began experiencing frequent and intense headaches. She was treated successfully for these in a behavioral medicine program. Two years later she injured her back while sledding with her children. Since then she experienced a reoccurrence of her headaches as well as the development of continuous low back pain. She sought the consultation from numerous physicians but no clear-cut medical cause was found for her pain and she found no relief. Episodic use of muscle relaxant and anti-inflammatory medications did not help, and she complained of "bad experiences" with physicians by whom she felt "traumatized ." She tried to maintain a relatively normal lifestyle, and continued, for example, regular consultation and teaching. However, she had to modify her work day so that she did not have to sit for extended periods of time, and her greatest difficulty with this was the "unpredictable" nature of pain episodes.

A muscle scan conducted at the time of the consultation revealed significant chronic bilateral muscle spasm in the mid- and lower thoracic areas (T6-T10) and significant left-biased chronic muscle spasm in the frontalis and cervical perispinal areas. The pattern of chronically elevated muscle tension was consistent with her report of unalleviated low back pain and headache. Through daily self-monitoring of her pain experience over the next weeks, she discovered that certain stressful situations were consistently associated with an increase in pain reports, notably her childrens' fighting, talking with her parents, and being "scared" when confronting unfamiliar situations. The diagnosis of psychogenic pain was clear. Few other symptoms were apparent. Her memory for childhood experiences was quite sparse and she seemed out of touch with her feelings. As the treatment developed, it became more evident that her initial presentation was consistent with a diagnosis of disguised PTSD (Gelinas, 1983). She had a generalized numbing of responsiveness, and amnesia for major portions of her childhood. Although she reported that her marriage was stable, in many respects sexual involvement with her husband was very infrequent. Initially she attributed this loss of interest in sex to her chronic pain but it became increasingly obvious that she had inhibited sexual desire, a common adult sequelae to childhood sexual victimization. Her sister previously had recovered memories of incestuous involvement with the older brother in therapy. Although Jane was aware of her sister's experiences and had discussed it in her own therapy, she had no awareness of her own incest background at the onset of the hypnotherapy.

Phase I: Stabilization. The initial goal of treatment of the suspected adult incest victim is not to uncover the feelings and memories associated with childhood sexual victimization, but rather to enable the patient to achieve some degree of stabilization. Hypnosis is sometimes contraindicated in the initial stages of treatment, but if used, hypnotic exploration first proceeds around the themes of safety and protection on the one hand, and soothing and comfort, on the other. The goal is to enable the patient to explore these themes through scene visualizations so as to generate the actual experience of safety and soothing in the context of the hypnotherapeutic relationship. Second, the hypnotic relationship also is structured to give the patient an increased sense of perceived control and self-efficacy at each step of the unfolding hypnotherapeutic process. Thus, if intrusive images, memories, or feelings, or dysphoric somatic sensations arise in the early sessions, which is often the case with trauma victims, the goal is to help the patient dismiss these intrusive experiences and thereby gain a sense of mastery over them. The patient learns skillfully to switch the unfolding experience in the direction of increased stabilization. Moreover, hypnoprojective methods are used to explore coping strategies for effectively dealing with intrusive experiences. Third, the initial goal of treatment is to help the patient manage concrete symptoms that she suffers from in her everyday life.

In the case of Jane, the primary emphasis of the initial stage of treatment was her chronic pain syndrome, not the suspected incest history. The objective was to help Jane learn pain-coping strategies to reduce her pain experience and thereby reduce effects of her distress in everyday life.

The goal of the first hypnotic session was to give Jane a positive experience of hypnosis. No attempt was made to work with her pain directly. Hypnosis was induced through eye fixation and waves of relaxation. The staircase method was used to deepen the trance. The patient then imagined floating in clouds and settling into a safe place. She went to a special park she remembered from her college days. She reported feeling "very calm and away from everything." She then spontaneously reported, "my back doesn't seem to hurt as much." The trance was terminated. Although it was clear that Jane was quite hypnotizable based on her positive response to every suggestion, she reported "lots of control issues." It is quite characteristic for PTSD patients to suppress their trance ability during initial hypnotic inductions out of fear that intrusive memories and feelings associated with previous traumatic experiences might emerge.

It is also quite common for patients with disguised PTSD to have untoward reactions to initial hypnotic experiences due to the emergence of intrusive experiences. The next session (Hour 2) was illustrative of such experiences. Jane came to the hour saying that she practiced self-hypnosis at home. She was concerned that "painful childhood scenes" would emerge so she stopped self-hypnosis. We proceeded cautiously with the hypnotic induction. Considerable time and care was spent having Jane imagine herself in safe and protected places. Despite these efforts she reported, "I'm getting dizzy. I can't stop the spinning." She opened her eyes out of fear. She was given suggestions to control the dizziness by breathing slowly and regularly. Then she was told, "some way will occur to you that will help to stop the spinning." She "visualized pleasant things" and told herself, "slow down", until the spinning subsided. She ended the hour pleased that she had gained control over the intrusive experience.

The next hypnotic hours (Hours 3–11) focused primarily on practicing pain-coping strategies in hypnosis and self-hypnosis and also on self-regulation of intrusive experience as they occurred. As is characteristic of trauma victims, Jane needed each session to be very predictable. She said, "I get very nervous thinking about the hypnosis because I don't know what you'll ask me." Therefore, I began each hour reviewing exactly what would be done in trance that day. Jane was also afraid that painful memories and feelings would emerge if she went "deeper" into trance. She learned to modulate the depth of trance using the elevator technique (Brown & Fromm, 1986), or if "nervous about going deeper" she imagined "climbing up a ladder" to a more comfortable state. She entered trance the same way each time, by imagining floating off to a safe place. After finding a level of trance that seemed safe (usually a light trance), she spent the remainder of the hypnotic session attempting to modify her pain experience. First, she scanned her body to identify discomforting and painful areas. Then, she practiced one or several pain-coping strategies such as imagining transferring numbness to the painful areas; imagining loosening each muscle group as if she were loosening separate strands of very tight rubber bands (Hour 3); changing the pain to some sensation other than pain (Hour 4) (Brown & Fromm, 1987). She continued to experience dizzy spells, but the frequency of these spells diminished as she became confident about using the coping strategies she had discovered to stop the dizziness. Each time she was able to significantly reduce the pain during trance and eventually to wake up from hypnosis free of pain. In Hour 6, she responded successfully to a pain challenge in which hypnotic suggestions were given to increase the pain, following which she was instructed to use the pain coping strategies she had mastered to alleviate the pain to her satisfaction.

Although she said, "I don't feel too much of anything...no pain," upon awakening she was nevertheless worried about being given a suggestion to "bring back the pain." The transference dimension of the hypnotherapy was becoming increasingly evident as she spoke about having being previously "traumatized by people in the medical community," namely male doctors.

At the onset of the next hour (Hour 7) she spoke of an incident of sexual harassment by a physician she had seen sometime earlier. She also spoke for the first time about her "chaotic childhood," specifically mentioning her sister's story about molestation by the older brother. As she became able to speak increasingly directly about her mistrust of men, she also acknowledged that her "pain was getting better" and that she was "exercising more." These changes helped her trust me as much as she was able. She continued to alleviate her own pain during hypnosis. In response to a future time-orientation suggestion she was able to imagine herself at some point in the future free of pain.

Over the next few hours, she experienced a number of "setbacks," ostensibly because she had been sitting for longer and longer periods of time. In my view, the setbacks were associated with the press of intrusive memories and feelings following the disclosure of her sister's incest (a displacement) and a sexual harassment episode (a screen memory). Hypnoprojective methods were used to explore "ways of coping with the setbacks." She imagined someone comforting her saying, "it's O.K.. Don't let it bother you" (Hour 8) and "feeling real strong" (Hour 9) when "in the midst of the kid's fighting," and "being able to step back" (Hour 10). She resumed practicing pain-coping strategies in daily self-hypnosis sessions, including the pain challenge. She reported increased pain-free intervals during each day. By the end of Hour 11 she was relatively pain free and reported "feeling good about myself."

Phase II: Systematic Uncovering (Hours 12-28). During the next stage of the recovery process, memories and feelings associated with the incest spontaneously return. The patient, however, is now better prepared than earlier to cope with the traumatic material because she has learned to cope effectively with symptoms and earlier intrusive experiences. Moreover, the patient has an increased sense of perceived control and is less fearful than earlier about loss of control. From a solid base of coping skills and perceived control, the hypnotherapy proceeds with the task of uncovering and integrating the memories and feelings associated with the incest (Brown & Fromm, 1986). It is best to recover traumatic memories slowly and to allow the patient first to uncover material in a symbolic manner through systematic exploration of guided fantasy. Each successive sequence reveals more and conceals less until the patient is able to recover clear memories of the episode(s) of sexual victimization and to integrate the memories and feelings associated with these traumatic experiences. Hypnotic techniques used to set the pace so the patient is not overwhelmed include protective imagery, hypnoprojectives of coping, and stop-action and split screen video, and an affect dial to regulate the intensity of affect (Brown & Fromm, 1986).

Once the patient is able to tolerate uncovering traumatic memories and feelings, the affect bridge (Watkins, 1971) and age regression are used to bring the traumatic experiences fully into consiousness. Uncovering typically proceeds in a stepwise fashion. Symbolization of traumatic experiences emerges first, actual traumatic experiences next, memories of multiple sexual victimization within the family, and finally memories and feelings regarding the post-incest adjustment. The latter includes recall of coping strategies used during and after sexual victimization, feelings, and self-perceptions subsequent to victimization and memories of conflicts precipitated by the use of force, the experience of sexual arousal, or active participation during the sexual victimization.

In Jane's case the transition to the uncovering/integration stage of recovery was marked by the re-emergence of intrusive memories and feelings. Hypnoprojective methods (e.g., the video method) were used to explore "the reasons for experiencing setbacks" (Hour 12). One scene was about "someone going to church and going to confession." Following this she experienced a spontaneous age regression. She said, "I see myself as a little girl. My (older) brother is telling me I'm no good." Upon termination of the trance she said, "I didn't realize you can go back and see your childhood in hypnosis. These feelings are sort of upsetting." She continued to explore scenes from her childhood with self-hypnotic practice that week. She said, "I guess I put this out of my mind for a good reason. I know my sister was victimized by my brother growing up but I've had no conscious memory of myself being victimized." Because of her need for control she used self-hypnosis in my presence to induce trance "in my own way" and to settle into a safe place. A suggestion was given to watch a television program about "what contributed to her not feeling she deserved to be well." She saw a scene about a cowboy getting off his horse to make a camp fire. In the next scene she saw a baby playing with pots and pans. In the subsequent scene she saw herself as the baby playing. Her brother approached. At that point she got "scared." In the next scene she said, "It's sort of dissociated. I'm lying in bed. I don't have my clothes on. My brother is touching me. It doesn't seem real." She reported being "numb" to her feelings at the time. She was about 7 years old.

In subsequent sessions (Hours 13–17) she used the video method and the affect dial to recover successfully the memories and feelings about the sexual victimization by her older brother. She recalled a scene wherein she was attempting to hide from her brother. She was discovered and dragged by her hair. She did "not feel any fear" because she was "numb." (Hour 14). Next, she recalled a scene of her brother "putting his thing inside me. I can see him but I can't feel in those parts" (Hour 15). In a symbolization of her rape by her older brother she was able to become aware of some of her terror. She imagined a woman making a expedition to a tomb in the Egyptian desert. On the way a man threatened her with a knife. Later the group discovers a tomb. Once inside the tomb the man is "angry and out of control" when he discovers there are no jewels. The woman is fearful. The man throws the woman to the ground, rapes her, and leaves her for dead, all alone in the tomb (Hour 16). In the following session the affect bridge method was used to induce an age regression. At around 7 years old she reports, "He's pulling me down. I hear myself saying, 'no!' 'no!' He is screaming at me. He is rubbing up next to me, holding me tight. He's rubbing his thing next to me." A suggestion is given, "notice what you are feeling, the feelings will become clear and you will be able to experience this feeling as much as you are able at this time." She responds, "I'm just trying to bring back the fear just a little bit at a time. Now I've got a lot of it back. I'm not numbing out. Now I'm real confused. I'm afraid and I have some feeling of warmth and pleasure, too. That's what's confusing."

Hours 18–28 concerned the recovery of memories and feelings related to the post-incest adjustment. She came to the next hour saying she was "feeling better" (Hour 18). She realized that the stress in her body was associated with the feeling of being pinned down. She relived the rape scene, this time adding material on the development of the conspiracy to silence:

> He gets up and puts his pants on. He says, "Didn't you like that? Wasn't it fun? Don't tell anyone or I'll get you again." He goes away. I'm sitting there. I don't know what to do. I get up and pull myself together. I have a headache. [Therapist: the scene will somehow change] I'm sitting over breakfast later that day. I can't say anything. I know we'll get in trouble. I don't feel very good so I don't eat very much.

The remainder of the hour was devoted to alleviating the patient's headache.

Jane reported at the onset of the next hour, "I'm doing a whole lot better. I'm not using a lot of energy to hold things back." Her memories now were of her teenage years. In one scene her family was sitting around the dinner table. She recalled feeling "sad" and "very alone" and wishing that her family were happy. She also recovered a memory of her primary coping strategy. She called this "getting away from it all" by going over to a friend's house or later by driving around alone in the family car to think about things (Hour 19).

From Hours 20 to 22 she had another "setback." Her "back [was] not doing well." She also had trouble with "flashbacks" and "sexual arousal" during self-hypnosis. In Hour 23 an affect bridge was used to explore this sexual arousal. She recalled being in her parents' bedroom with her mother. She notices feeling sexual and then gets afraid when her father walks into the room with only a towel on. Both parents leave the room. She is alone.

In the next hour (Hour 24) the stop action video is used to explore memories associated with her father. She sees herself lying on the bed. She rewinds the videotape and re-plays the scene with greater detail. Her father walks into the room and lies on the bed. She rewinds and re-plays the scene again. She sees him "rub me down the front of my chest." She is about 4 years old. In the next scene "he's pushing my shirt up and touching my breasts. I feel sexual down there but he doesn't touch me there. I'm confused." Over the next few hours she recalls feelings and self-perceptions subsequent to sexual victimization by her father. She has a fantasy of a "big metal dumpster full of trash inside holding all the garbage that doesn't want to come out." In the next hour (Hour 26) she is able to trace the origins of "feeling dirty." In an age regression she says, "He's saying something scary. Something to do with not telling. He makes me afraid as if it's my fault. I'd be punished." Later she adds, "I can't believe he told me it was my fault!" (crying).

In the next 3 hours (Hours 27–29) she recovered many memories of recurrent sexual victimization by her father that included attempts at vaginal penetration and a memory of her mother standing outside the bedroom door calling to her husband asking, "what's going on?" The mother did not enter the room nor attempt to intervene. She also recalled examples of her primary mode of coping with this abuse, by "freezing up." She completed this phase of the work saying, "I don't know how many pieces of this I need to remember. I don't know if what I recall is absolutely accurate, but I don't want the facts to get in the way of the truth. At this point I feel capable of dealing with the emotional part of this" (Hour 28). At the onset of the next hour she said, "I feel very proud of myself as a kid for being able to withstand all of this." The "feeling of strength" she developed during the earlier pain treatment had returned (Hour 29). This phase of the treatment came to a close (Hour 33) with the recovery of a memory in hypnosis of her father bruising her thighs and lacerating her vagina during an attempted intercourse. She told her mother she got hurt running into a table. Her mother took her to the doctor. Jane sensed that her mother and the doctor suspected the sexual abuse. Although her mother never directly spoke about it the sexual abuse by her father stopped abruptly after that incident at age 7.

Although the treatment continued beyond that point Jane rarely complained again of debilitating symptoms such as chronic pain or of intrusive experiences. She began to feel stronger and more confident in herself.

A Comparison of Jessica and Jane

A comparison of these two cases of Jessica and Jane is useful in appreciating the interaction of a number of determinants of the long term effects of incest, only one of which is the sexual act itself. Both Jessica and Jane came from seemingly "outwardly stable" families. At the onset of her hypnoanalysis Jessica suffered from structural psychopathology (borderline personality organization) as well as a variety of symptoms associated with chronic PTSD. At the onset of her adjunctive hypnotherapy Jane did not manifest signs of structural psychopathology and did not complain of intrusive PTSD symptoms. Her main symptom was chronic pain. Both Jessica and Jane suffered from a long-standing inhibited sexual desire in their marital relationships. After years of significant repression and 4 years of hypnoanalysis, Jessica recovered memories of a single incident of sibling incest. After 4½ years of psychotherapy concurrent with 1½ years of adjunctive hypnotherapy, Jane recovered memories of multiple incest with her father (ages 4–7) and with her older brother (ages 7–10). In Jane's case her sexual involvement with her father was progressive, beginning with being fondled in the bathtub (age 4) to repeated forceful attempts at vaginal penetration (ages 6–7). Were the long-term psychological effects of incest determined by the sexual act (s) alone, we would predict that Jane, not Jessica, would have been more damaged. Because the opposite apparently is true, a number of variables in addition to the sexual act itself must predict the long-term outcome of incest.

As discussed previously, age of onset of incest is one of the most important predictors of long-term negative effects. Jessica reported that her mother physically abused her and gave her regular enemas as early as age 3, although this probably occurred earlier. Incest with her brother occurred somewhere between ages 3 and 4. The pattern of progressive incest with Jane's father began at age 4 and occurred primarily in her early latency years. Sexual abuse occurring during the formative years is usually associated with pervasive developmental delays and long-term structural psychopathology, whereas sexual abuse occurring during the latency years is usually associated with the manifestation of a variety of observable symptoms. The differences in outcome between Jessica's and Jane's incest are in part attributable to the difference in the age at which the incest occurred.

Pre-existing conditions also make an important contribution to the overall effects of incest. Jessica suffered from a variety of respiratory illnesses as a child. She also grew up in a very strict household and reported being beaten everyday by her mother. It is well known that handicapped children are at greater risk for abuse than normal children. Jessica is likely to have been treated differently because of her physical condition. Because physical more than sexual abuse is associated with fragmentation of the representational world and structural psychopathology, we would expect more severe long-term effects in Jessica, even though Jane's sexual abuse was cumulative.

When the sexual act is considered independent of other factors, cumulative and multiple sexual abuse of this nature is usually quite damaging, In Jane's case her ability to draw upon healthy coping resources and her fortune to find a partially supportive familial environment alleviated the otherwise expected long-term negative effects. Jessica coped with her abuse primarily through dissociation and the adamant denial of the reality of the abuse. These defenses have been implicated in long-term negative adjustment following incest (Kluft, 1985; Rieker & Carmen, 1986). Jane coped with her abuse through somatization and seeking support, for example, "going off with friends." Those who actively seek support have a better long adjustment subsequent to traumatization than those who do not (Koss & Harvey, 1987). Both Jessica and Jane suffered from the "conspiracy to silence" (Butler, 1978) but each differed in their ability to find support. Jessica could not find anyone in her "concentration camp(-like)" familial environment to serve as support other than her brother, the perpetrator. Jane's mother appears to have taken some appropriate steps to stop her husband's abuse of her daughter (although not her son's abuse of her) upon discovering it when Jane was 7 years old. Jane also reported a "warm and supportive" relationship with her paternal grandmother throughout her childhood and a supportive relationship with her older sister, who was also abused, even though they never spoke about the abuse as children.

CONCLUSION

The *chronology* of the incest—the age of onset and its progression; the pre-existing *conditions,* the availability and effectiveness of the victim's *coping* resources, learning or *conditioning* of a maladaptive coping style and the *context* of both the familial environment and the extra-familial environment pre- and post-disclosure contribute as much to the overll long-term outcome of incest as does the sexual *contact* itself. These are the six "Cs" of incest and its aftermath. The possible combinations of these determinants, as in the cases of Jessica and Jane, help us to appreciate the great variablity in the long-term effects of incest, in the approach and response to hypnotherapy, and in the overall length of treatment as well.

Chapter 17

WRITING ASSIGNMENTS AND HYPNOSIS IN THE TREATMENT OF TRAUMATIC MEMORIES

ONNO VAN DER HART
Instituut voor Psychotrauma, Utrecht, The Netherlands

SUZETTE BOON
Regionaal Instituut voor Ambulante Geestelijke Gezondheidzorg, Amsterdam, The Netherlands

GHISAINE B. VAN EVERDINGEN
Redondo Beach, CA

There exist a number of therapeutic approaches, each with its own arsenal of techniques, for the exploration and working through of events from the past when memories of these happenings continue to disturb the patient in the present. In directive therapy, writing assignments and hypnotic techniques are important tools in such exploration and processing, leading to the integration of the patients' traumatic memories into their consciousness.

Writing assignments are a form of homework. For example, one much used form in mourning therapy is the writing of the so-called continuous leave-taking letter (T. Rubinstein, personal communication, 1977). Another form is the written narrative of past experiences. Although writing is done at home by the patient, hypnosis is usually done during the session with the therapist.

In hypnosis one of the first goals is to teach the patient to relax and to develop a sense of safety before any confrontation with the past is attempted. In directive therapy hypnosis is an important tool to bring to consciousness seemingly forgotten events and to integrate the memories of traumatic experiences.

Because many problems can be treated by either writing assignments or hypnosis, usually the choice is based on the therapist's personal preference. However, in our opinion there are situations where more specific criteria may be applied. These concern patients who have developed serious psychiatric complaints and complicated disorders due to the severity of their traumatization. In these cases a writing assignment, hypnosis, or a combination of the two may be especially indicated, or one or the other may be contraindicated. An answer given here is based on our clinical experiences with patients who in their childhood or adolescence were the victims of physical or sexual violence.

THE CONCEPT OF TRAUMA

Generally the word, "psychotrauma" is used as a synonym for extreme stress. According to Eth and Pynoos (1985), however, we can only define *trauma* in the case of an overwhelming event that results in a sense of helplessness in facing unbearable danger and fear and, we may add, pain. These authors recognize trauma when a child witnesses the murder of a parent, but do not when members of a family suddenly receive an unexpected notice of the death of one of them. In other words, being the recipient of some unexpected terrible news, not merely being the direct witness to or victim of an atrocious or horrible act, causes the trauma. Although Eth and Pynoos made an important distinction between trauma and stress (not all stress is the result of trauma), we believe that they over-accentuate the objective aspects of a traumatic event. As Janet (1904) noted already many years ago, objective criteria only partly determine if an event is experienced as traumatic. Some people are definitely traumatized when they receive sudden notice of the death of a beloved person (Janet, 1893, 1898). A number of events that are not experienced as traumatic by most people may certainly be experienced as such by a particular individual. Therefore, the subjective aspects are just as important as the objective ones (Van Dantzig, 1986); for Janet (1909) it is primarily the *intensity* of the subjective emotional reaction that in turn may lead to secondary reactions such as dissociation.

TRAUMA AND DISSOCIATION

Not all traumatic experiences are equally overwhelming. Thus, Krystal (1978) distinguished between what he called "catastrophic psychic trauma" and "partial trauma." In the first case, the threat emanating from the event is completely overwhelming; this occurs more often with children than with adults, the latter having learned to react to most traumata with defense mechanisms and symptoms.

The more overwhelming the traumata, the stronger the reaction of *dissociation* in individuals who are prone to react in this way (Putnam, 1985a; Spiegel, 1986). Dissociation is the escape of a specific idea, or even a complex of ideas, together with associated feelings and bodily movements, from the control and sometimes even the knowledge of the personal consciousness (Janet, 1889; van der Hart, 1986)

Sacks (1984) gave an instructive example when in a fall he broke his leg. Sacks was amnestic for the fall itself, possibly due to dissociation. Although soon he realized that in fact he himself had had the accident and subsequently corrected his perception, his initial determination was that the accident happened to someone else, whom he as "the doctor" had to examine. This too is an instance of dissociation, in Fromm's (1965) terms, between observing ego and experiencing ego. Moreover, Sacks dissociated the panic-laden thought that his leg was paralyzed and that he could not stand on it. This thought did *not* get corrected at the time, but continued to exist as an unconscious *idée fixe*: Sacks had no notion of it nor could he control it (Janet, 1894, 1904; van der Hart, 1986). The result was that the leg remained paralyzed, even after medical treatment had restored it into good working order; this dissociative symptom is labeled *conversion* (rather incorrectly, cf. Nemiah, 1974).

Traumatic memories may be dissociated to the extent of complete or partial amnesia (Putnam, 1985a). A concentration camp survivor may recall all sorts of camp experiences, but exactly not whatever has been extremely traumatic for him or her personally (Jaffe, 1968; Braber, 1987).

Traumatic memories often present in the form of nightmares, flashbacks, and completely dissociative episodes in which the trauma is as-it-were relived (Henlin et al., 1985; Jaffe, 1968; Janet, 1889). Often flashbacks are triggered by situations that have some resemblance to the original traumatic event. The reliving of a traumatic event in flashbacks, nightmares, and dissociative episodes implies that for this person this event still exists in the imperfect tense. A traumatic memory must be translated into a *personal narrative* with which the event gets a place in someone's life history and thus translates into the past perfect tense (Janet, 1904, 1935). Those who succeed in doing this have realized not only cognitively, but also emotionally and physically, that it happened to them personally; they have accepted it and are aware of the effects it has had on the course of their life. They are no longer persecuted by its memories and have adjusted to the changes the trauma caused in their life circumstances.

The personal narrative mentioned here has to be distinguished from the talking-about-the event from a distance as if it concerns someone else (Janet, 1919). This is usually how victims of sexual violence tell their story, dissociated from emotional and often also physical reactions (such as pain) to the event in question. The dissociation often occurred already during the experience itself. Thus, a victim of incest or rape may experience "floating to the ceiling and observing from there" (Gelinas, 1983).

If patients are completely amnestic of traumatic events they experienced, various dissociative phenomena can indicate to the therapist that such is the case; for example, if the patient regularly "loses time," complains about "blackouts," or finds notes he or she obviously wrote but does not recall or recognize as such. In addition to these memory gaps, there may be a disturbed sense of self. For instance, patients may hear *in* their own head voices that give a running commentary on what they are doing; they sometimes feel they are doing things against their own will or liking—as if they are being pushed into it by another person inside themselves.

It is important to know that patients who have such dissociative phenomena happen to them usually keep it to themselves for various reasons, among them the fear of being considered crazy. It is often easier for someone to report feelings of depersonalization and derealization (which occur frequently when other dissociative phenomena do not or hardly ever occur). In any case, the therapist will have to inquire about the patient's personal experiences. Several questionnaires and structured interview protocols have been developed over the last few years (e.g., Bernstein & Putnam, 1986; Sanders, 1986) to systematically assess the phenomenology of individual patient's symptoms.

THE CHOICE BETWEEN WRITING ASSIGNMENTS AND HYPNOSIS

When patients ask therapists for help to work through events that happened in the past, this does not always or exclusively concern traumatic experiences. However, the suspicion on the part of the therapist that traumatic memories are at play is, in our experience, one important factor in determining the choice between writing assignments and hypnotherapy. Is there reason to assume the unrecognized presence of traumata, for example, because of dissociative phenomena in the patient? Another factor concerns the degree of awareness patients have of traumatic experiences. Are they able to talk about them clearly; are they bothered by flashbacks, or nightmares; or do they only have a vague sense that the present difficulties have to do with unprocessed experiences from the past?

All three factors may be present independently of each other, but often they also seem to be related. There are indications that more extreme traumata get dissociated to a greater degree and are associated with deeper amnesia than less extreme or partial traumata (Putnam, 1985a; Spiegel, 1986). Besides the two factors already mentioned as important in determining the choice of writing assignments, hypnotherapy or a combination of the two, there is a third factor that is especially important in the timing of the processing of traumatic experiences, namely *the ego strength* of the patient. A person with low ego strength quickly feels anxious and nervous and has a limited degree of self-control. The smallest thing can trigger a tantrum. Exhaustion sets in quickly and the smallest task is experienced as an impossible assignment. Involvement with the environment is limited. Adjustment to actual reality is poor and the feeling of living in the present is faint (Bleich, Garb, & Kotler, 1986; Janet, 1903, 1909). Ego strength is often negatively influenced by insomnia, due to the occurrence of nightmares (in which the traumata are being relived), flashbacks, and the anxiety thus provoked. Some patients do their utmost to deny these traumatic memories, whereas others worry about them almost constantly.

How these three factors influence the choice between writing assignments and hypnosis is reflected in the following hypotheses.

Hypothesis 1. In therapies aimed at working through traumatic experiences, writing assignments are indicated if: (a) there is a cause in the past, which is clear to the patient; (b) its memories are not extremely traumatic, and (c) the therapist considers the situation to provide a relatively safe framework, because the patient did not respond to the original event with distinct dissociation.

In our experience the writing assignment makes sense if patients know about what and why (and to whom) they have to write, and if they can accomplish this task in a reasonably independent manner. This is, for instance, the case when patients have traumatic memories of the sudden death of a partner or a child. When the memories are too traumatic, however, they may get too anxious or suicidal and at the least may avoid the writing. If a high degree of dissociation seems present, it is desirable to be reticent with writing assignments. Often the writing will not remove the dissociation and thus the processing will stagnate. In case the dissociation (e.g., amnesia of the trauma) does get removed during the writing, the patient may get overwhelmed by the traumatic memories with their associated emotions and sensations, and be traumatized anew.

Hypothesis 2. In cases where the present complaints cannot be sufficiently explained on the basis of present circumstances and the patient is not aware of a clear cause in the past, exploration by the use of hypnosis is indicated. After such hypnotic exploration one can still consider continuing therapy via writing assignments and/or hynosis.

As is discussed later, hypnosis usually works faster and is more efficient than writing assignments.

Hypothesis 3. Hypnotherapy is indicated when: (a) the memories of past events are very traumatic for the patient, or (b) the patient shows dissociative symptoms. Hypnotherapy assumes direct guidance and support by the therapist during the exploration of traumatic memories. It also offers possibilities to the patient for handling these memories in such a way that they become manageable rather than overwhelming. An important advantage of hypnosis in the exploration of traumatic memories that were until then dissociated is the ability to give posthypnotic suggestions for amnesia after the exploration. If the patient is not yet ready to admit these memories into his or her personal consciousness, much additional distress (such as suicidal reactions) can thus be prevented.

Hypothesis 4. Support and reinforcement of skills are indicated for patients with low ego strength at the beginning of treatment. These patients often present with well-described syndromes, such as panic disorder, hyperventilation syndrome, and limited depression. These syndromes have to be treated adequately before exploration and processing of traumatic memories are initiated.

THE PREPARATION PHASE

It is self-evident that a preparation phase has to precede the exploration and processing of the past. Even in relatively easier tasks, such as when complaints relate to the fact that a patient has not worked through the death of his or her partner or a family member, and finds the connection between the two plausible, the opportunity to talk about the deceased and the loss eventually presents itself. Only when the time seems right, the therapist discusses with the patient (or the family) the reason or causes why the loss has not been worked through yet, and the manner in which this can still be accomplished. In the context of a therapeutic leave-taking, the patient is then informed, for example, about the writing of the continuous leave-taking letter and, of course, about its attendant difficulties (cf. van der Hart, 1983, 1984, 1987). Extensive attention is also given to the support patients may expect to receive from family and friends in the period in which the writing assignment in carried out. This preparation phase is rounded off when the patient declares him or herself ready to take leave and a definitive agreement about the subsequent treatment is made.

In more difficult cases, especially where there is low ego strength, the patient will have to get assistance first to be able to function at a higher level before tackling the exploration and processing of the past. The literature on PTSD states that a certain level of stabilization has to be reached first (Brende, 1984; Brown & Fromm, 1986; Parson, 1984). For patients with poor ego skills, the exploration of traumata via hypnosis or writing assignments is contraindicated. Overwhelming anxiety could cause further decompensation and/or termination of treatment prematurely. In this phase the patient must be assisted in gaining more control over symptoms such as anxiety, flashbacks, angry outbursts, and so forth (Keane, Fairbank, Caddell, Zimering, & Bender 1985). Relaxation exercises and ego-strengthening suggestions can play an important role here. If writing is indicated at all, in this stage it is for monitoring of symptoms only. If hypnosis is used at all, it is for relaxation and for providing ego-strengthening suggestions, aimed at increase in self-control and self-confidence (Silver & Kelly, 1985), or at pain reduction. Facilitation of premature emergence of traumatic memories by the use of hypnosis must be avoided in these cases.

The preparation phase may last for months and in cases of chronic complicated PTSD, sometimes even for years (Brown & Fromm, 1986). Anything enhancing ego strength, self-confidence, and self-control, not only enables patients to better tackle the assignments of the next phase, but it also helps them to trust the therapist more. Trust is a necessary condition for the exploration and processing of traumatic memories. If patients continue to be bothered by traumatic experiences such as flashbacks and nightmares, it will be necessary to help them resolve these in a later phase of the treatment. Taking the necessary time in the preparation phase will often shorten the duration of the overall treatment.

Many patients with chronic PTSD wish to consider the therapy as ended, if the goal of the preparation phase, coping with life a little better, is coming within reach. If at a later time in their life, for one reason or another things do not go as well, they may re-enter therapy at that time. Of course, this is a choice often supported by the directive therapist. Sometimes therapists themselves indicate that therapy can best be limited to this partial goal.

WRITING ASSIGNMENTS

Hypothesis 1 states that writing assignments are particularly indicated, if (a) the patient sees a clear cause in the past for present complaints, (b) memories of this event are not extremely traumatic; and (c) the therapist is convinced that the patient has reacted to the event with, at the most, a slight degree of dissociation.

Of course, writing has to appeal to patients. This does not mean, however, that the therapist necessarily must take a patient's initial reticence at face value, and abandon the idea. One patient wrote on top of his first written homework, "I do not like writing assignments," underlining this statement heavily. With gentle persuasion the therapist motivated him to discover the value of such writing. Soon his "yellow pad" became an important link to buried feelings, and eventually to trauma. Patients do have to be able to handle such a writing task in a relatively independent manner. Van Doorn and Aelen (1986) added that patients have to be willing to change, and to exert themselves to affect such change; to possess a reasonable ego strength;

to have the willingness for self-confrontation; to have a reasonable sense of responsibility vis-à-vis their own actions; to have the capability to discriminate between different emotional responses, and to associate them with different stimuli.

A Clear Cause

Often the cause of the complaint is related to the death of the partner or another family member, to separation or divorce, or to an accident. When the writing can address a concrete well-defined event, but provokes an array of emotions, specific instructions are in order from the start. One example is the *Three-Letter-Advice* (Hoogduin, 1980; Lange, 1977, 1987). When the cause concerns the death of a family member or a divorce, the actual moment of loss is preceded by an entire prehistory. In such cases the writing may be done rather in the form of a *continuous leave-taking letter*, and the initial instructions should be open rather than specific. Patients get the advice to write down everything they have to say to the person in question before they can actually take leave (van der Hart, 1983, 1984). Once the writing is in progress, the therapist may give the patient more specific advice, for example, to work out a certain theme like guilt or anger towards the deceased, or to also write to some other person in his or her past.

Even though the event that leads to the present complaints and the seeking of help may be clear, the specific underlying reasons for the connection are not always that clear. The writing in which patients are involved on their own and the sessions with the therapist can help them get a better perspective on those reasons and to work through the underlying experiences. In short, within the context of processing the past, writing can also serve the exploration of it.

Van Doorn and Aelen (1986) consider a writing assignment in order also when there are only vague complaints that may be assumed to be traceable to still unknown events in the past. They recommend writing about that past by reviewing year upon year in reverse sequence to give the patient the opportunity to get a better understanding of these events. To us this seems a somewhat roundabout approach without the assurance of a successful outcome. In our view exploration via hypnosis is probably a simpler alternative.

No Extreme Traumatization and Few Dissociative Phenomena

In our opinion, writing assignments are in order in the treatment of people with problems that are not based on extremely traumatic memories. Writing offers the patient the opportunity to focus systematically on pertinent events, to express the associated feelings, and ultimately to realize that these events have arrived where they belong—in the past perfect tense.

When the patient is bothered by intense flashbacks, hallucinations, or nightmares that refer to the trauma, writing at home is often too heavy an assignment; the possibility is ever-present that the patient will be overrun by even more traumatic memories and their associated feelings, will get panic reactions, or will respond with even more dissociation.

Especially when patients have been physically and/or sexually abused over an extended period, they may have dissociated intense feelings of pain, anger, and rage. A writing assignment has then the drawbacks discussed here.

In the first place writing can be insufficient and inappropriate to process intense, threatening, physical experiences. The remark of a patient, who felt very alienated from her body, provides a good illustration of this point. The patient loved to write and already had written a lot about her incest past, but she had not gotten much out of it. Upon inquiry by the therapist it became obvious that writing had been a purely distant, cognitive occupation for her. She had not been able to make her emotional reactions and physical sensations part of the experience, and had remained alienated from her body.

Second, as mentioned before, if the writing eliminates existing dissociations, the patient may lose self-control and get into a serious crisis. Many patients experience much anticipatory anxiety about this. A patient with an incest past got the advice to write at home about the rage she felt toward her stepfather. Once there she realized she could not do it: She was afraid she would kill her stepfather if she would allow herself to fully experience her rage against him. She wrote a letter to the therapist in which she remarked among other things: "not yet. Only when he's dead can I write."

In our opinion, in cases in which the elimination of existing dissociations may lead to serious crises, hypnosis is the treatment of choice, because in hypnosis amnestic barriers can be reinstated. If, for whatever reason, writing would still be a consideration, then every precaution has to be taken to prevent further traumatization. Fairly early in her treatment a woman, who had experienced serious incest in her past and who had dissociative symptoms (initially not recognized by her therapist), got the suggestion to write a continuous letter to her father. Her immediate reaction to this suggestion was an intense anxiety attack, during which she crawled into a corner of the therapist's office. After he had managed to finally calm her down somewhat, he changed his suggestion and told her to write to him after the session. This writing was to provide an overview of their discussions on her father. Each new step during the sessions continued to cause intense emotional reactions. However, the subsequent writing at home now enabled the patient to deal with the same material in a more cognitive way as well.

A Safe Framework for Writing Assignments

When patients start to write at home about difficult, anxiety-provoking matters, they may need help with it on the spot. Therefore, they have to be able to call between sessions, or in some other way consult the therapist or a colleague. Support from the spouse, family members, and friends is also important. To assure an optimal delivery of such support the therapist is well advised to include the significant others in the treatment process, at least during explanation of the writing assignment and the possible difficulties to be expected. Agreements have to be made about when and how such support is to be given. For example, patient and partner are to discuss the writing only when the patient takes the initiative; other family members are to take over specified tasks, such as household chores during the writing period (Ebbers, 1988). In addition, during difficult periods psychotropic drugs may be considered for symptomatic relief.

Besides providing these safety provisions, there are two instructions about the writing assignment that can give the patient support and a relative sense of safety. The first concerns the *ritulization* of the writing of a continuous letter or narrative. The ritual offers a context or stratum within which patients enter the confrontation with potentially threatening experiences and express their feelings about it. Writing at the same place, at the same time, and for a preset period of time, can protect against overwhelming emotions and prevent loss of control (cf. van der Hart, 1983, 1984), if the rules are adapted to the ego strength of the patient.

Some patients are motivated and able to write five times a week for 1 hour; others may have to settle for twice a week for 45 minutes. Gersons (1988) considered this freelance approach unsuited for among other, persons with a borderline personality structure. However, we have had some positive experience with writing assignments for borderline patients. For example, one man harboring unresolved mourning about his mother, had good results with writing for 10 minutes three times a week. Initially, when the time period lasted longer, he indeed got overwhelmed by intense, almost uncontrollable feelings. However, writing for only 10 minutes would allow him to just keep his affect within bounds. Although after this phase of his therapy there were various other problems that were dealt with later, he was able to process the death of his mother after all and was free from a number of related complaints. Thus, he got rid of the chronic headache that originated after his mother's death when he was 13, and that he himself connected with the fact that she died of a brain tumor. The borderline personality structure had not changed as a result of the writing, but an important problem was solved and associated complaints disappeared.

Nevertheless, we acknowledge that the structuring of a writing assignment for borderline patients can be tricky. We have known patients who, in spite of all the therapist's efforts to contain the writing, filled tomes of paper without much progress. In such cases we now set limits and encourage boundaries by instructing patients with that inclination to use a timer and to condition the end of their writing to its ringing.

The second instruction for the continuing letter concerns the fact that patients have the freedom to a greater extent to determine themselves when to write about what, which provides a built-in safety factor in most cases. As a rule initially the less loaded, less anxiety-provoking themes or events are described; the more traumatic experiences are explored later. In the context of mourning therapy the experiences around the death and burial often are expressed last.

Appropriate instructions for writing the continuous letter gives patients the opportunity to arrive at their own speed at the memories that are most difficult for them to process and that pertain to events that require the greatest adjustment. Such instructions thus serve to reduce anxiety.

The interplay between ritualization and freedom needs to be monitored by the therapist. One of the aims of writing at a set time and for a set period is for the patient to let an array of emotions surface. Van der Hart (1983, 1984) mentioned the well-known example of a young woman to whom specific instructions for ritualization were not given. There was no progress at all due to the fact that apparently she wrote her mother only when aware of positive feelings toward her. After the appropriate instructions were given, the patient started to also write about her anger and then indeed began to show improvement.

WRITING ASSIGNMENTS PLUS HYPNOSIS

In spite of all the support from therapist and others, the ritualization of the task, and a slow tempo, patients may still hit on traumatic experiences that they experience as too overwhelming and threatening to confront on their own. At such a point the use of hypnosis during the session with the therapist may be indicated, after which the therapist may encourage the patient to talk about his or her experiences and feelings before closing the session. In addition, the patient may be asked to afterward elaborate further in writing about what transpired during the hypnosis session.

Another circumstance where writing can get into an impasse and hypnosis may offer help, is the case when patients have strong physical reactions—such as pain—that "make it impossible for them to continue writing. Writing about that pain, rather than about what the patient had set out to address, may sometimes help" (van der Hart, 1983, 1984), although this is not always the case.

Closing the Assignment by a Leave-Taking Ritual

The termination of a certain activity is often regarded as an easy task, which does not require much time and attention. However, many people appear to have much trouble with it (Janet, 1903, 1919). Therefore, it is important that the therapist give careful attention to the closure of a writing assignment such as the continuous leave-taking letter. In our experience the so-called *leave-taking ritual* is an appropriate form for this closure.

Much has already been written about form and content of parting ceremonies and the associated cleansing and reunion rites (Ebbers, 1988; van der Hart, 1983, 1984, 1987). That literature indicates in what ways patients take leave of, or change their way of relating to, the written material and possible other objects (core symbols or *linking objects*), which are connected with the person addressed in the writings. Here we only want to point out that the timing, form, and content of the leave-taking ritual has to be negotiated and determined together with the patient. It has to be the patient's ritual, not the therapist's.

HYPNOSIS

Writing assignments have proven to be a good tool in directive therapy for working through many kinds of traumatic and other unassimilated memories. When, however, the memories concerned are of an extremely traumatic nature, or when the patient shows various dissociative symptoms, there are drawbacks to writing assignments aimed at exploration and processing of the past. In such cases the initial use of hypnosis seems to be a better indication—provided a number of conditions are met. At a later stage in the treatment hypnotherapy may then often be successfully combined with writing assignments.

Hypnosis for Further Exploration

Where feelings of free-floating anxiety, abandonment, irritation, and so forth exist, which cannot be totally explained on the basis of present circumstances, the so-called *affect bridge* is fast and effective (Edelstien, 1982; Watkins, 1971). This exploratory hypnotic technique is also sometimes indicated in cases of physical tension, somatoform pain disorder, and other complaints that manifest themselves physically. An alternative technique is *ideomotor response* (Cheek & LeCron, 1968; Cladder & Lens, 1985). *Ego-state therapy* (Edelstien, 1982) and so-called *reframing* (Grinder & Bandler, 1981) are also good techniques for hypnotic exploration of the function and origin of such complaints. Many patients succeed in becoming aware of an event of which they have not thought in years, but that still exerts an important influence on their life. In our opinion this concerns a dissociated memory, of which, for example, only the affective component (such as a feeling of abandonment) did become part of the personal consciousness. Even if this hypnothesis is not always borne out such approaches still turn out to be for patient and therapist reliable and effective tools in the reduction of complaints.

However, hypnotic exploration may bring to light more or less traumatic events. In the case of less traumatic events, which sometimes get described as bothersome, or annoying, rather than traumatic, a writing assignment may then form a fitting sequel, sometimes as a series of (or continuous) letters to the persons involved, sometimes as a narrative in the form of a diary. If in the hypnotic exploration we come upon extremely traumatic memories, further use of hypnotherapy seems indicated.

If the therapist a priori expects the existence of extreme traumata, the use of the affect bridge is to be discouraged. As mentioned before, the danger in such cases is that amnestic barriers are broken down too quickly, and overwhelming images and emotions are evoked prematurely.

Suggestions of Posthypnotic Amnesia

If there is reason to assume that amnesia for possible traumatic events has to be maintained for the time being, the therapist needs to assure that posthypnotic amnesia can be effectively suggested. This is not difficult in patients with serious dissociative disturbances as they are proven experts in the realization of hypnotic phenomena.

In general, it is good to give permissively formulated suggestions for amnesia at the end of exploratory hypnosis sessions. For example: "take along from hypnosis whatever is good to take, for which the time is right, and just leave in hypnosis whatever is better to leave there for the time being." However, when extremely traumatic memories come up it would be better for the therapist to behave in a more authoritarian manner. It should not be left to chance that patients take along memories surfaced in hypnosis with which they are not yet ready to cope.

Specific safety measures may sometimes be developed during a hypnosis session in deliberation with the patient. The advantage is that the focus is placed on letting the patients use their own capabilities rather than letting them depend solely on the therapist.

Astrid, a 32-year-old woman with a past of extreme child abuse, had devised under hypnosis her own imaginary ritual with which she closed off each session. During the last 10 minutes of the session she would in her imagination go to a safe in which she put one by one the memories with which she did not want to be burdened outside hypnosis. She would then lock the safe and give herself the suggestion that she could remember the combination of the safe only in the presence of the therapist. Other patients have developed similar closing rituals. It seems important to help patients create some kind of format for posthypnotic amnesia before continuing with exploration.

Protective Imagery

We described earlier how patients in the preparatory phase of treatment may be helped to increase their ego strength. We cannot assume offhand that a patient's ego strength is sufficiently high to let traumatic memories emerge safely in hypnosis, or that patients are capable of protecting themselves adequately against such memories in case of premature emergence.

If hypnosis is going to be used for the exploration of partially or completely dissociated traumatic memories, after completion of the preparatory phase the therapist would do well to train patients in creating positive, protective imagery. A good example is to instruct patients in hypnosis to imagine a place or spot where they feel safe and protected. The procedure may be recorded on a cassette tape during the session, so that, if the recording is successful, the patient is asked to listen to the tape and practice daily with it for the next 1 or 2 weeks. With this technique we recommend the use of general or vague expressions, such as "a safe place or spot," instead of specific and concrete expressions, such as "room," which might have gotten an unpleasant connotation for certain patients, especially victims of sexual violence. Rooms have shown to be far from safe in the past, especially for many incest victims. Hannah, a 30-year-old woman who was sexually abused as a child, built a beautifully camouflaged treehouse, because nowhere in a house did she ever feel safe anymore. Other examples are a bunker for the soldier with traumatic war memories in which he is safe against mines and snipers (cf. Brown & Fromm, 1986), or a cave in a mountain. Images of people whom the patient really trusts and with whom he or she feels safe are also useful. According to Brown and Fromm, hypnosis induction with the aid of this kind of imagery also gives the implicit message that hypnosis is a safe rather than a scary experience.

With this initial kind of experience in hypnosis, patients are best prepared to approach their traumatic memories. If the confrontation turns out to still be too much to handle at a certain point in the process, they can return to this safe place instead of going out of hypnosis. Moreover, the instruction of the "safe place" may also be a good way to round off a hypnosis session, for example by having the patient store in an imaginary spot the memories that are still too difficult to handle (like the safe in Astrid's example).

Brown and Fromm (1986) mention still another variant of the safe place : They have patients in hypnosis watch a safe scene on an imaginary television screen. When they are ready, they may switch to the channel where the traumatic event in question can be watched. When that becomes too much, they can switch back to the safe program. Patients may also imagine that the trauma is recorded on a videotape, which they can stop, rewind, and so forth, via remote control (Silver & Kelly, 1985). A variant developed by Spiegel (1981) contains a two-part television screen: The patient may watch safe images on the one half, and on the other half the traumatic event. Some patients will find viewing two TV sets more convenient in this setting.

It may happen that during the confrontation with traumatic experiences patients find themselves unable to return to a safe spot, or to switch the imaginary TV set to another program. Therefore, in addition to the aforementioned techniques we have developed the following technique, which we call *the General Store* (*de Winkel van Sinkel* in Dutch), where patients may buy themselves special gear. In hypnosis they are asked to imagine a store where they can get anything they want. In that store gear may be collected that will satisfy the following criteria: It is very light, always very easy to take along, and if needed it can be put on without effort within a few seconds. Moreover, the gear can ward off and keep away from the body anything that is not permitted to enter at that time. Because in this way patients can determine themselves how much pain, feeling, or emotion is permitted at each occasion, they appear better able, for example, to watch projected images than otherwise would be the case.

Of course, it is advisable to always test the gear in connection with less traumatic memories to determine if it offers sufficient protection. If necessary, the general store may be visited several times until the outfit is exactly to the patients' liking and fits their individual needs.

Techniques for Processing and Integration

When patients are well prepared, they may start in hypnosis with the activities that are aimed at integrating the traumatic memories into their personal consciousness. As with the writing assignments, it is important to grant patients time to confront these memories at their own speed. At times, it may be necessary to slow a patient down. Processing and integration are activities that take place by bits and pieces. Among other things, this may mean discussing outside of hypnosis, when the time is right, something that came up during hypnosis. Although this happens frequently within the same session, several sessions without hypnosis may be devoted to this part of the therapy (Brown & Fromm, 1986). After all, hypnosis is only one tool in a more comprehensive treatment.

Metaphoric Imagery. Patients regularly express something related, or referring, to their traumatic memories via a metaphoric expression or metaphoric images, among them dreams. The therapist may help patients to have a more distant involvement initially with the processing of their traumata by focusing the therapy first of all on these metaphors or symbols (van der Hart, 1985b; Witztum, van der Hart, & Friedman, 1988). Patients are asked initially to imagine in hypnosis the metaphor in question and to strive toward a solution within the metaphoric domain. If necessary, direct attention then may be given to the real memories. This approach assumes that a solution within the metaphoric domain facilitates the finding of a solution within the concrete domain, in this case the processing of traumatic memories (van der Hart, 1985). Besides using a dream reported by the patient, which has a symbolic connection to a trauma, the therapist may also suggest such a dream in the hypnosis session. In both cases the therapist can link into it by asking the patient to dream the dream again (in hypnosis), but now with a different cast, maybe in different surroundings, yet with the same meaning; and then once again; and so forth, until the original traumatic memory is dealt with directly (Erickson, 1952).

Perceiving From a Distance Versus Emotionally Experiencing. Patients may observe from a distance the images of their past experiences or they may re-experience them emotionally. Fromm (1965) spoke in this connection of the dissociation of the observing part from the experiencing part of the ego:

> The observing part of ego is asked to remain calm and attentive, while the experiencing part relives certain aspects of the traumatic situation. The hypnotherapist can carefully regulate the degree of dissociation in the service of uncovering and integration. He may suggest greater dissociation when the material has the potential of becoming overwhelming. As the patient demonstrates ability to cope with the material, the therapist may suggest re-merging of these two facets of the ego to facilitate integration. (Brown & Fromm, 1986, p. 281)

Erickson and Rossi (1979) described the so-called *sandwich-approach* that also seems grounded in this principle. First, the patient is given the suggestion to observe one aspect of the trauma from a distance, without feelings. Then the suggestion is given to forget these images and to only experience the feeling that goes with them. Then a combination of both is suggested. In the next round another aspect of the trauma is tackled. This continues until every aspect has been reviewed separately. Finally, the same procedure is executed with reference to the entire trauma.

Substitution. The so-called *substitution technique* was developed by Janet (1889, 1898) and interest in it is recently renewed (cf. Lamb, 1985; Miller,

1986a; van der Hart 1986). In essence, it assists the patient to imagine a more positive course of the traumatic event than was the case in reality. This leads to the integration of these images in personal consciousness and thus probably also to acceptance of the original happening. Its memories will then no longer interfere. Naturally, this procedure may also cause even stronger dissociation of the original traumatic memories. Janet, who resorted to this procedure after other attempts at integration of relevant memories had failed, as a rule determined himself the content of substituent images for the patient. In modern approaches patients are usually asked to do this for themselves.

Although the substitution technique is a useful instrument to reduce the complaints that are logically connected by the patient to the past, there are situations in our opinion where the technique is contraindicated. This is the case with traumata connected with experiences of physical and sexual violence about which the patient was never able or allowed to talk as a child (Kluft, personal communication, May 1987b). Patients with such a past have often experienced disbelief or denial of facts earlier in life. Using the substitution technique may easily be perceived as an extension of this collusion of silence. In the following example the patient indicated herself when this technique was useful in her case and when it was not.

Ms. L was a 43-year-old single woman who 4 years prior to her intake had a "complete breakdown" and had not since returned to work. She lived a very isolated life, was depressed and very anxious, and she seriously doubted the use of her continued existence. She had been in treatment before, but did not get much out of it. If anything, treatment had increased her anxiety. As she was growing up, she had been a very shy girl. Her parents' marriage was troubled, with many quarrels between husband and wife, and regular wife-beating. The parents divorced when she was 6 and since then she and her younger sister had not seen their father. The mother's contact with her family of origin was very poor, so that the children did not have any contact with it either. When Ms. L was 11, her mother died in an accident. She and her sister were placed in an old-fashioned, strict orphanage, where they were put in different sections. They seldom saw each other and the patient started to feel extremely lonely.

The substitution technique seemed to form a necessary part in the processing of the period after her mother's death. In hypnosis she really liked to imagine for instance how during that time there was someone after all who took her aside, gave her attention and a little bit of warmth, and who allowed her during breaks to play in a room together with her sister. In this case it was not one or the other "February Man" whom the patient imagined (cf. Dormaar, 1987; Erickson & Rossi, 1979), but one of the female counselors whom the patient considered capable of caring, but to whom she never dared reach out at that time in her life. Ms. L got consolation out of these experiences, and started to feel somewhat calmer. When in a later stage of the treatment, however, the fights between her parents came up for discussion (which she had witnessed when she was 4 or 5), she indicated herself that substitution did not work. No matter how difficult, she had to re-experience these events, and to share her feelings about them with the therapist.

As a matter of record, Erickson introduced his February Man in such a way that his patient did not realize at all that this was an imaginary figure. Our application of this technique has always been deliberately overt with the patient's consent.

Further Exploration. Traumatic events do not occur in a vacuum. Especially in cases of traumatic memories of physical and sexual violence in the family, it is important to also pay attention to the context in which the violence took place, and to the family history. Hypnosis may be called for to help elaborate this context.

The treatment of Maya offers an example. Maya was a 37-year-old woman with complaints of dissociation based on an incest past. Within as well as outside of the hypnosis sessions the loaded situation with her stepfather had been a regular topic of discussion, including her persistent sense of guilt about the sexual contact that lasted from ages 10 to 14. It was not until while in hypnosis her jealousy toward her mother was uncovered that Maya gained more insight into her feelings and their background. This led to acceptance of her own role in the drama and thus allowed her to continue working through her incest past.

HYPNOSIS AND WRITING ASSIGNMENTS

In our opinion, hypnotherapy is the treatment of choice when the therapist suspects that the patient has been exposed to extremely traumatic events, or when the patient shows strong dissociative symptoms. Hypnotherapy offers a wider range of possibilities than writing assignments for the exploration and processing of dissociated traumatic memories, the gradual elimination, and, if necessary, the reinstatement of amnestic barriers.

Often, however, a combination of hypnosis and writing assignments is possible even with such patients. In the processing and integration of traumatic memories, after or during the hypnotic exploration, writing is then a logical next step, sometimes even one of the last steps. When writing is mentioned as a possibility at some point, many patients indicate they find this a heavy assignment. "When I write it down, then it is there in black and white and it suddenly becomes real," as one patient said who found it still too difficult to do. Others mentioned that writing things down was threatening, because others could then read about their "secret." There are also patients who after a few hypnosis sessions start writing spontaneously about whatever came up in the session.

Agnes was a 30-year-old patient who was bothered by dissociative complaints (blackouts), which were connected with a traumatic incest past. She could talk about that past in general terms and without any emotion. All emotions and physical sensations remained dissociated. In hypnosis closer attention was paid to the traumatic events. When she was viewing the images on an imaginary monitor, she did experience the associated feelings, emotions and sensations. When in hypnosis, however, she could not describe what she was going through. Later, feelings of shame and guilt appeared to be responsible for the dissociation, and at that point Agnes took the initiative to write to the therapist. She wrote detailed stories about the experiences and feelings of "a little girl" as if it all concerned someone else. By temporarily maintaining the dissociation between herself as the adult and as the little girl, for the first time in her life she could express in words what had been done to her. The next step, not at all an easy one, was to tell the therapist outside of hypnosis that these events concerned herself; what she herself had felt while undergoing them; what influence they had had on her life, and how she now looked back upon them. Thus, the traumata received their place in Agnes' personal life history.

DISCUSSION

When Are Exploration and Integration of Traumatic Memories Indicated?

Psychotherapy has to be aimed at the reduction of suffering. The approaches described here are, however, far from painless. An essential question is whether it is always necessary, or desirable, to explore dissociated traumatic memories and to help patients integrate these in their personal consciousness. Is "covering" and forgetting not much more indicated, if treatment involves risks of decompensation, serious self-mutilation, or suicide (Bezemer, 1986)?

If people have hidden or encapsulated their traumatic memories via dissociation or repression, and manage to not personally be bothered by them, they probably do not develop overt psychiatric symptoms. More importantly, they probably do not come into therapy, unless their intimate relationships are affected to a degree that makes their partners or family members insist on their getting help. Some patients with serious dissociative disorders and a very traumatic past could thus be "in hiding" for years. But a new trauma, a period with much stress, or other triggering event may lead to eruption of the original traumata into the personal consciousness via nightmares or flashbacks, and to reactivation of earlier dissociative phenomena. Then these people may come into treatment presenting problems of blackouts, panic attacks, depression, suicide attempts, self-mutilation, and so forth. As a matter of interest, most patients we know with such problems have been treated for years by other methods without success.

As described earlier, the first phase of the treatment needs to be aimed at ego strengthening and stabilization. There are patients who consider this sufficient improvement and terminate therapy. In our experience this is especially true for survivors of World War II who are now bothered by nightmares and flashbacks to their traumatic war experiences, but not all that much by other dissociative phenomena. When they again function relatively well, they gladly take it for granted that they will be bothered by nightmares only from time to time. In such cases we as therapists will not insist on a more exploratory therapy either. Lange (1982) quite rightly pointed out in this context that with some victims of war the complaints tend to be ascribed too quickly to an unprocessed war past whereas at closer scrutiny they have more to do with the manner in which the family functions right now in the present. To focus the treatment exclusively on the individual's past is then incorrect.

However, when reliving of traumatic experiences in nightmares and flashbacks continues, and there continue to be other dissociative phenomena as well, in our opinion some form of treatment is indicated that is also directed at the processing of that past. There are indications that the prognosis of such treatment is favorable, and that as a rule the patients in question are not expected to spontaneously improve very much in their functioning (Kluft, 1986, 1987a). If such treatment is being considered by the therapist, it is extremely important to inform the patient thoroughly about its nature, which by the way comprises more than just exploration and integration of traumatic memories, as well as its long duration, and the difficulties that may be expected during its course. In our experience most patients with a past of physical and sexual violence choose in favor of such treatment.

In short, we suspect that the *measure* in which patients continue to be bothered by complaints, directly connected with unprocessed traumatic experiences, and the *intensity* of their effects, are the determining factors in the choice for exploratory and integrative treatment. Of course, the competence of the therapist in this area is a decisive factor in this choice also.

An Eclectic Use of Writing Assignments and Hypnosis

We have tried to give an indication when (and how) writing assignments and hypnosis fit into the exploration, processing, and integration of traumatic memories.

It is argued that there are a number of situations in which the choice for one or the other technique or for a combination of the two may be dependent on the preference of the therapist. However, directive therapy owes its reputation to the fact that it tries as much as possible to establish what is the best approach for *this* patient with *this* problem in *this* situation. Accumulating experience with the application of this type of technique with patients harboring a variety of problems leads us to believe that sometimes it is a writing assignment, sometimes hypnosis, and sometimes a combination of both. We argued that writing assignments are useful, if the patient experiences a clear link with past events, their memories are not too extremely traumatic, and the patient's reaction to them was not dissociative. Exploratory hypnotherapy is indicated if there is as yet no clear link, if the memories in question are too traumatic in nature, and if the patient dissociated them. Further, when the patient shows low ego strength, the initial aim of treatment should be to reinforce ego mastery, before exploration and processing of the past is to be initiated.

Possible Misunderstandings About Hypnosis

The application of the techniques discussed here, according to the principle of what fits this patient with this problem, may be obstructed by misunderstandings about, or even prejudices against, either one of these techniques. This is especially the case with exploratory hypnotic techniques.

For example, one argument sometimes heard against hypnosis is that patients consider it a therapist's lollipop rather than hard work (Lange, 1987). This may indeed be a patient's expectation. But the therapist, who knows better, can in those cases give explanation and information to the patient to set matters straight. Especially with regard to the use of hypnosis in the exploration and processing of traumatic memories, experience teaches us that it is an effective tool. The problem is rather that threatening memories may be uncovered too quickly for either the patient or therapist to manage. We have tried to indicate how this problem may be prevented.

Another argument heard against the use of hypnosis is that some patients have low hypnotizability. This is possible. However, patients with more or less dissociated traumatic memories, with which this writing is mainly concerned, have as a rule a good capability for trance. Both phenomena, traumatic memory and trance, are probably based on the same underlying phenomenon of dissociation (cf. Bliss, 1983; Hilgard, 1977; Janet, 1889; Putnam, 1985a). If such patients initially do not allow themselves to undergo hypnosis or only to light degree, they may have their own good reasons for that (van der Hart, 1986).

With patients who are bothered by an unpleasant feeling, which seems linked to the past, the affect bridge often leads quickly to the possibility of exploring the original situation to which that feeling can be linked. Whatever their score may be on a scale of hypnotizability, if patients are able to concentrate on the pertinent feeling and to reinforce it, they usually can also realize the suggestion that the feeling functions as a bridge back into time, and bring themselves back to the original event. This exemplifies the thesis of Beahrs that persons with a low score on the hypnotizability scale are able to go into hypnosis if a link is made with what they already experience, and is then reinforced (Beahrs, 1982; cf. van der Hart, 1982).

In addition, we pointed out that the use of the affect bridge is not recommended when the therapist suspects the existence of serious traumatic memories.

The Relationship Between Patient and Therapist

It is not customary in directive therapy to write much about the nature of the relationship between patient and therapist. The concepts of *transference* and *countertransference* are seldom used. An important principle is that the therapist treats the patient with respect and also in other ways exerts every effort to develop a positive rapport with the patient. It is exactly through such rapport that the therapist is able, for example, to give homework assignments, for which the patient might not feel easily motivated otherwise.

Especially in directive therapies, where the processing of traumatic memories is central to the treatment, it is important to realize that transference and countertransference also exist, often of a negative quality. Patients with a traumatic past are quickly inclined to perceive traits in the therapist that he or she seems to share with the person who interrogated, abused, or raped them in the past.

The reverse may happen too: Some attitude or behavior on the part of the patient may call forth feelings in the therapist, which are not appropriate. This sometimes happens when patients have gruesome stories to tell about their past.

The *inclination* to react with countertransference to traumatized patients is probably sometimes inevitable. What is needed is the therapist's awareness of the presence of such feelings and, if they start to interfere, a willingness to discuss them with a colleague who is experienced in this area. It is especially important to realize that not every therapist has to be able and willing to treat people with a gruesome past, whether concentration camp, or extreme sexual abuse, or other life tragedies. To provide such treatment should be a free choice (Sachs, personal communication, June 1987).

The most important positive element in the relationship between patient and therapist is probably the measure of trust the patient has developed toward the therapist (cf. Braun, 1986). We already indicated within the context of the preparatory phase of the treatment, how much proceeding at a slow speed is a condition for the establishment of trust. "To have a warm, caring, but nonseductive person available with whom the adult patient, *here and now*, can form a mature, real relationship is paramount in therapy" (Brown & Fromm, 1986, p. 20). This is especially true for patients with a severely traumatic past, and particularly for those who have been (sexually) abused by a parent: They have the greatest difficulty with trusting the therapist. Their life has been marked by the fact that no one person could be trusted, especially not those they were dependent upon. The trust such a patient may give a therapist means, at the most, that a next step in the treatment may be taken (Kluft, personal communication, May 1987), and, we may add, carefully.

If we tell our patients they can call us at any time, they may take this literally, call us out of bed at 4 a.m. because of a crisis, and feel very betrayed when it is made clear to them that this is not what was meant. Therapists have to tell patients exactly how and when they can be reached, and to whom else they can turn at other times. The integrity of therapists is, among other ways, expressed in the fact that they remain available once the therapy is set in motion, and they do not skip town when it gets difficult. Patients are able to accomplish difficult writing assignments, or exploratory activities in hypnosis, when they can count on their therapist being right alongside them on the painful road to recovery.

Chapter 18

EGO-STATE TRANSFERENCES IN THE HYPNOANALYTIC TREATMENT OF DISSOCIATIVE REACTIONS

JOHN G. WATKINS
HELEN H. WATKINS
The University of Montana

TRANSFERENCE REACTIONS IN PSYCHOANALYTIC THERAPY

The analysis of transference reactions is considered to be the most potent tool in psychoanalytic therapy. By experiencing simultaneously a past relationship as externalized onto a present inappropriate object, the patient is enabled to distinguish reality from past memory, achieve a genuine insight, and alter basic character structure. Unfortunately, in the classic psychoanalytic situation the arousal of such reactions may require many months to reach full fruition before interpretation can be effective. Hypnoanalytic treatment (e.g., analysis within the hypnotic modality) sometimes offers the opportunity to evoke transferences in a shorter period of time, even if more working through in the conscious state may be required (Brown & Fromm, 1986; Fromm, 1968b).

The psychoanalytic contributions of Federn (1952) and Weiss (1952) provide a theoretical framework for understanding transference manifestations in patients suffering from dissociative disorders when treated with hypnotic techniques. These techniques can shorten the period for evocation of transference reactions. We have modified and expanded ego-state theory and described its application to treatment recognizing a continuum of permeability and flexibility of ego-state boundaries within each patient (J.G. Watkins, 1978a, 1978b; J.G. Watkins, & H.H. Watkins, 1981, 1984). We also differentiate transference and countertransference reactions according to the particular ego state activated at particular times and in particular contexts. These concepts are explained here and two case histories are offered to illustrate their application.

THE EGO PSYCHOLOGY OF PAUL FEDERN

Paul Federn, a close associate of Freud's and his *protégé* Eduardo Weiss (1952), made several significant contributions to the understanding and treatment of these reactions that have not received the attention and recognition they deserve. However, to explain the procedures we use in treating dissociative reactions it is necessary to review the major concepts of ego-state theory and therapy.

Federn discarded Freud's "libido" and posited instead *two* basic energies: ego or self-cathexis, hence, an "I" or "me" energy, and object cathexis, an "it" or "not-me" energy. He held that whether a behavior, experience, or part of the body, was felt as "self" depended on whether it was invested with ego cathexis or object cathexis. If I move my hand up and down, the hand and its movement are innervated with ego cathexis, and I experience both as a part of my own self. If the hand is hypnotically anesthetized, rendered devoid of consciously controlled movement, and made to wag up and down by hypnotic suggestion, then its ego cathexis has been removed. It is now invested with object energy. I experience both the hand and its movement as ego-alien and no longer "mine." "It" is happening, but "I" am not doing it.

Likewise, if a thought of my dead father reaches conscious awareness, but is object cathected, then I no longer recognize it as "my" thought. I *see* my father and am diagnosed as hallucinating. The various dispositions of ego and object energy determine what is experienced as self and what not. When something conscious is ego-cathected I *experience* it; when object cathected, I *perceive* it.

THE CONCEPT OF EGO STATES

Federn's second significant contribution was that human personality is not necessarily a unity but is divided into segments or "ego states" by separating boundaries whose permeability lie on a continuum. At one end of the continuum are different attitudes and roles, like going to a party Saturday or working at the office on Monday. These situations represent normal, adaptive differentiation.

If the ego-state boundaries become more rigid and impermeable, the states move from adaptive differentiation, through covert status (like Hilgard's,

1977; "hidden observers"), toward maladaptive dissociation. At the other end of the continuum we find true multiple personalities, where the ego states alternate in being cathected with ego energy and emerging overtly. The covert alters, if at all energized, are at that time invested with object cathexis. If the executive state is aware of them, it perceives them as "he," "she," or "it." If the ego cathexis moves to an alter, that alter becomes the executive state, hence, the self of the moment. It is now experienced as "me."

EGO AND OBJECT ENERGIES

When significant figures are first introjected, they are invested with object or nonself -cathexis. If the introject is then ego-cathected, it becomes an identification. Federn, unlike object-relation theorists, did not put the concepts "self" and "object" together. If a pattern of behavior and experience is object-cathected, it is an "object" and perceived as outside the self. If it becomes ego-cathected, it is experienced as part of the self and is no longer "an object." The term *self-object* would be contradictory.

An abused child who internalizes his or her perceptions of a brutal parent may invest these with object energy. The child then suffers depression as the introjected object continues internally to abuse his or her "self." If the child invests this entity with ego cathexis, it becomes a segment of his or her self. He or she now identifies with the parent and no longer suffers the depression, but instead abuses his or her own children. In Federn's theory, "self" is simply an energy, not a collection of behaviors and experiences. This energy is characterized by having within it the *feeling* of selfness. Behaviors and experiences energized by this cathexis are felt as being within "my" self.

The concepts of object and ego cathexis and of ego states have important implications for understanding hypnosis and for dealing with transferences. Through hypnosis we can initiate anesthesia and undo it in parts of the body. Through hypnosis we can also change subject experiences to object perceptions, and vice versa. For example, we can suggest change in a dream so that the little girl who is seen running from a monster becomes "me" running from the monster, or vice versa. Accordingly, hypnosis is a modality for changing subject and object by manipulating ego and object cathexes in various areas of the soma and psyche (J.G. Watkins, 1977).

The concept of ego states is also very important in understanding and dealing with transferences. These reactions are not simply a matter of the relationship of "the whole patient" with some early parental figure being projected onto the analyst. If a person is not simply a unity but a complex organism differentiated into many different ego states, then we must consider how each segment perceived the original parent to evaluate its unrealistic projection onto the figure of the analyst.

TRANSFERENCE AND COUNTERTRANSFERENCE TO VARIOUS EGO STATES

Increasingly, we came to the realization that in dissociated patients it is not enough to perceive an obvious transference and then to interpret it, "You are reacting to me as if I were your father (mother), etc." We have to determine just which alter is dominant at the moment and relate *its* affect to *its* unique relation with the early parent. The current transference manifested may be quite different from that of another alter.

Because transferences are prone to initiate counter transferences we also need to know much about the needs, feelings, motivations and conflicts of each state if we are to understand the widely varying feelings each may generate in our own selves as therapists.

Finally, if such complexities of transference displacements can occur in true, overt multiple personalities, we should be cognizant that similar reactions may occur in the treatment of many more normal neurotic, psychosomatic and behavioral problems. Research with the hidden observer phenomena (Hilgard, 1977), hypnotically activated ego states in normal research subjects (J.G. Watkins & H.H. Watkins, 1979–1980, 1980), and with ego-state therapy itself (H.H. Watkins, 1978) suggest that transference reactions may stem from the displacement of feelings and perceptions onto the analyst by *covert* personality segments (e.g., ego states or "part-persons").

EGO-STATE TRANSFERENCES IN THE CASE OF MULTIPLE PERSONALITY

Multiple personality is a kind of controlled laboratory in that ego states are more clearly separated (Watkins & Johnson, 1982). Dissociated entities may transfer their contents onto the analyst differently from one another. Let us first consider this in relation to a clear, overt case of multiple personality.

During a 2-year period of intensive treatment some 18 different alters appeared in Sharon. She was a highly intelligent, professional woman, wife, and mother. She was talented in many areas. Like most multiples, she was the product of child abuse. However, I (JGW) found myself confused by the ever-changing fluctuations in her transference reactions. These would move from positive to negative and back again depending on which alter was executive during the various stages in the recall, re-experiencing, and working through of early traumas.

Gradually it was possible to sort these out and to make appropriate interpretations. When she manifested strong fear of me and huddled in the corner I came to recognize "Mary," who not only endured many beatings by Father, but was at the bottom of the hierarchy of alters (e.g., the one to whom the others displaced their pain). Mary suffered more than the others, and when "executive" might explode into fits of ungovernable anger that endangered her family.

Father was not always brutal toward the patient, but he sexually abused her in various ways. The alter "Christine" was often the object of his sexual play, whereas "Ghiselle" learned to please him with seductive behavior. As a consequence, Christine participated in sex with him but only endured it, but Ghiselle became promiscuous. When Christine was executive, and I was perceived as the "sexual" father, her reaction was anger and avoidance. If Ghiselle was out, I might be viewed similarly, but her behavior would be smiling and seductive. Both perceived the "father" in transference as sexually approaching her, but each behaved differently toward him.

Father was apparently bi-sexual, because at times he took the patient to gay bars and initiated oral and anal intercourse with her. Accordingly, a male alter, "Alex," who was a 9 to 12 year-old boy, had been created to deal with this situation. Alex was both an athlete and a musician. He, and he alone could play classical piano. When erotic transference toward a father figure was being manifested, my understanding of what was going on and my manner of response had to be different depending on whether Christine, Ghiselle, or Alex was executive at the time.

These same variations in the nature of the transferences onto current family members by different alters were quite confusing to the patient's children. "Tiger Mommy" and "Diana" were very nurturing and loving toward them. "Danny," "Karl," and "Megan" were jealous of "the little brats," perceiving them as the patient's siblings whom her parents had preferred. Alex enjoyed taking them skiing whereas "Alexandra" liked to dress the patient's daughters in artistic and feminine ways. The patient, in reporting to therapeutic sessions, would wear clothes that indicated which alter was present. If she appeared wearing pants, I expected to be addressed initially by the alter, Alex. Ghiselle and Christine wore dresses, but Ghiselle dressed more seductively. To illustrate the unique self-identity of each alter, Alex was disgusted if he emerged when the patient was wearing dresses and horrified if she was menstruating.

The displacement of affect from one state to another was especially evident in the alter's handling of pain. Diana had a cheerful and sociable disposition, which was maintained by repressing memories of the early child abuse, and by displacing all pain to other states. She was quite proud of her ability to turn off pain. Once when she reported having a headache I asked her to turn it off, which she did in a few seconds. I then asked to contact whoever had just noticed some recent pain. Mary stormed out, bitterly complaining of the sudden new headache.

On another occasion when Mary complained of pain in her hand, I suggested that she "give it back" to Diana. When Diana was contacted later she kept stroking her hand, stating that it seemed to have a sharp pain in it. By an "affect bridge" (J.G Watkins, 1971) I was able to regress Diana back to a situation at the family dinner when as a child she had put her elbows on the table, a taboo in that household. Father had stuck her hand with a fork, twisted her arm behind her back, took her to a bedroom and then beat her. This reaction enabled us to recover both a traumatic memory and its emotional experience—a step further along the road toward integration.

EGO-STATE TRANSFERENCES IN A NONMULTIPLE PATIENT

Techniques of ego-state hypnotherapy can be applied as successfully in the treatment of other serious psychopathologies as well as in multiple personalities. The treatment of "Little Roddy" illustrates this best. A young man in a pre-medical course at the university was deeply distressed, suicidal, homicidal, and schizoid in his relations with others. A child state emerged under hypnosis that related well to me (JGW—"Jack"). It would write letters to its "good Daddy," saying, "You stay with me." However, it was very afraid of Helen, who was a co-therapist on this case. Cowering and stuttering when hypnotically activated, Roddy would exclaim, "Helen has knife." At that time we did not understand the origin or meaning of Helen's "having knife."

In order that Helen could work with this patient during my absence, we first desensitized the "little Roddy" ego state by a behavior modification technique. While I stayed beside the patient Helen would come progressively down the hallway toward our study a bit closer each day, until his fear of her had apparently subsided. She (HHW) then treated him for some 2 months while I was at another university.

The "little Roddy" ego state was very spontaneous and emotional in contrast with the flat, depressed, and schizoid external manner of the patient. It became obvious that some traumas (probably related to mother) had caused a dissociation during which "Little Roddy" had split off from the main personality, taking with it all the spontaneity and joy of living and leaving only the schizoid ego state. However, the patient was not a multiple personality. The dissociated Roddy ego state existed in covert form and emerged only under hypnosis.

We embarked on a series of projective exploratory technique (J.G. Watkins, in press) designed to search out the traumatic sources, and if possible relieve them through controlled abreactions (J. Watkins & H. Watkins, 1978). One violent fear abreaction helped to reveal the origin of Roddy's transference anxiety that "Helen has knife." At about the age of 4 he had come into the house to ask whether he could go visit his grandmother, whom he dearly loved. His mother, who was in the kitchen paring potatoes, said, "No!" Under his breath Roddy muttered, "Son-of-a-bitch." His mother came running into the livingroom waving the knife and shouting at him. She then took off his belt and beat him into a state of unconsciousness.

This was apparently the moment at which the Little Roddy state dissociated and went into repression. During abreaction he screamed violently until he lapsed into unconsciousness. Through a series of similar re-living experiences, the fear was released and the origin of the knife phobia as transferred onto Helen explained.

Because the patient had released and overcome the unconscious fear of his mother and of Helen (his current mother-imago), the Roddy ego state was no longer needed. It was therefore desirable that its spontaneity, emotionality, and *joi de vivre* be integrated back into the main personality. This need was discussed with the little Roddy, and he tearfully volunteered that, "because I love you both, I am willing to die." With much sadness we parted from our little friend. Roddy was psychologically "put to death" through hypnotic suggestion. His "contents" returned to the patient, who then ceased to be a depressed and schizoid shell.

Much more working-through time was spent, but in the end the patient not only completed his undergraduate studies with distinction, but then went to medical school, graduated and completed an internship plus a residency at a prominent institution. We have had frequent contact now with him for over 10 years. He is an excellent doctor, enjoying life, creative, and able to give and receive love.

Perhaps the important point in this case was the procedure of working through the transferences all with "part-persons," or individual ego states, and not the whole personality. We had undone the dissociating traumas and moved ego cathexis back into the Roddy ego state. This made it possible for the qualities of the child state to be integrated back into the whole personality. Lest we be accused of trying to report a miracle, let us add that this result was achieved only after several years of intensive therapy, which involved supportive, directive, behavioral, cognitive, abreactive, and analytic techniques applied hypnoanalytically, but within the model of ego-state theory.

SUMMARY

Hypnoanalytic ego-state therapy, with its concepts of ego and object energies, which can be displaced through various segments of the soma and psyche, is not yet widely known in psychoanalytic circles. However, the findings of the hidden observer studies, plus the therapeutic experiences reported to us by many students and colleagues indicate that treating not only multiple personalities, but also normal and neurotic individuals as multiplicities, opens up new vistas for psychoanalytic and hypnoanalytic treatment (Beahrs, 1982).

Chapter 19

ON SILENCE AND THE HOLOCAUST: A CONTRIBUTION TO CLINICAL THEORY*

ARNOLD WILSON
New School for Social Research, New York

I am concerned in this chapter with the capacity of children of holocaust survivors to tolerate affects and the construction, in collaboration with a therapist, of a narrative account of data from the remembered, fantasized, and hitherto unexplored past. I suggest that tolerance for certain affects that are Holocaust sequelae is enhanced by the commitment to historical explanation and that such a narrative commitment, when supported by a therapeutic holding environment, constitutes a facilitative element of the treatment process.

I also examine a particular aspect of how trauma is perpetuated from one generation to the next. Several clinicians have examined this issue. Auerhahn and Prelinger (1983) cited the principle of repetition, in which the parent induces a re-creation of Holocaust images, fantasies, and experiences in his or her child in order to work through conflicts relating to meaninglessness and self-fragmentation originating in the death camps. The child, in turn, promotes the re-created images, fantasies, and experiences in order to make sense out of a turbulent parental biography shrouded in pain and ambiguity. Wilson and Fromm (1982) described the way the survivor parent may use his or her child as a "restitutive self-object," in which the child may simultaneously represent both a recapitulation of searing dissociated memories as

*Reprinted from Wilson, A. (1985). On silence and the holocaust: A contribution to clinical theory. *Psychoanalytic Inquiry* (pp. 63–84). Hillsdale, NJ: The Analytic Press.

well as the symbol for the parent to undo the trauma associated with those memories. In this day, sequestered Holocaust themes in the parent emerge and become enacted within the context of the parent–child relationship. The child, the object of identification with prior figures, may be overprotected or expelled, may be delegated to succeed or fail, or may fulfill the thwarted ego-ideal ambitions of the parent or be the object of their thwarted ego-ideal conflicts. Others have spoken of the parents' inability to absorb their children's aggression (Barocas & Barocas, 1973); the transmission of global mistrustfulness and fear that is part of a "survival complex" (Kestenberg, 1980); the necessity of a "parentogenic alliance" in which parents must forge a safe place between them, which contains their own development failures, fixations, and fantasies lest these forces overflow and envelop the vulnerable child (Herzog, 1982); and the intrafamilial vectors arising from the parental attempt to reverse their encounter with death and destruction (Klein, 1974; Lipkowitz, 1973; Sigal, Silver, Rukoff, & Ellin, 1973; Trossman, 1968).

There are many children of survivors whose parents have empathically and with appropriate concern prompted them to know the past and to creatively integrate it. I am concerned here primarily with individuals who either do not know, avoid knowing, or defend against knowing. The concepts contained here, however, have implications for those survivor families in which the parents could not help but dwell and obsess on the Holocaust and thus violated generational boundaries, which led to the children's needs to seek refuge in isolation, away from the overwhelming intrusiveness of the parents' innermost secrets.

AFFECTS AND AFFECT TOLERANCE

Affect was originally viewed largely within the economic point of view, as a means of drive representation that corresponded with discharge process (Rapaport, 1953b). Both affect and ideation were associated with memory traces—affects were the unstructuralized response of the ego to a cathexis of a memory trace, whereas ideation was the structuralized response. Both Schur (1953) and Rapaport (1953b) argued that affects themselves constitute structures and thus undergo a structuralization process. Their contributions set the stage for development theorists to study early mental life and the genesis of affective life. Issues such as the role of early object relations, the intertwining of cognition with specified affects, and the relationship of affects to psychobiological life became the focus of scrutiny. As a result, affects began to be viewed as ego states independent of complex metapsychological considerations. The work of Bibring (1953), Sandler and Joffe (1965), and Bemporad and Wilson (1978) in conceptualizing depression as a basic psychobiological affect are examples. Although affects have thus been scrutinized, the notion of affect tolerance has received relatively scant attention in the clinical psychoanalytic literature. Joffe (1969), Zetzel (1970), and Kernberg (1975) have addressed the notion of affect tolerance in some way, but Krystal's (1975) paper remains the most comprehensive evaluation of this concept.

Affect tolerance is the comfort, established incrementally through gradual familiarity and recognition, of a particular feeling state within the context of the self. This construct implies that we pay attention not to the absence or presence of an affect, but rather to the manner by which we experience, handle, or defend against an affective state. What clinically often looks like the absence of an affect may be a condition wherein a patient cannot control, master, or bear the affect; the intolerable affect therefore becomes repressed or dissociated and fails to be integrated into an expanding affect array. At other times, an affect may be accessible to conscious self-observation but minimized because it signals overwhelming tensions over which the patient possesses inadequate controls. Self-regulation of one's own affective experiences occurs through a gradual characteristic patterning of modes of action and defense, which usually are internalized functions of the self inherited from an early parent–child attunement.

In early development the good-enough mother allows her child a tolerable affective experience, intuitively knowing her child's capacities and how a child's affect array expands. She empathically organizes and filters through doses of increasingly strong and varied affective states until the experience approaches a traumatic level of overload, at which time she intervenes and frees the child from the unpleasure that has developed. This is part of the theory of the mother as an external or auxiliary stimulus barrier. The mother's specific influences on her child's developmental acquisition of affective states are complex and varied, as discussed in detail by Benedek (1956), Winnicott (1965b), and Mahler (1966). Jacobson (1964), too, has described affects not as unpleasurable tensions but as the discharge of psychic energies along preferred pathways that develop through the experiences of early object relationships. These object-relations views of affect formation are complemented by the work of theorists such as Tomkins (1962), Schmale (1964), Basch (1976), and Pine (1980), who noted the interaction of innate constitutional, biological, and instinctual factors with the role the mother plays.

What is generally agreed is that it is the caretaking experience that is essential to the form of affect development, the parent's ability to sense and organize the child's affective experience. When the child reaches higher levels of developmental maturity, the patterning of affective experiences becomes further fixed by age-specific internalization and self-regulatory processes. The dreading of emotions and characteristic ways of warding off emotions are further elaborated through the lifespan. As Zetzel (1970) emphasized, ways of dealing with affect are an ever-evolving lifelong developmental phenomena.

Of particular importance to my thesis is the intertwining of affect with unconsious and conscious ideation. Brenner (1974), among others, emphasized that affects occur in the presence of associated ideas, which are internalized reflections of early social experiences. In particular, he believed, anxiety and depression function in this way. In Brenner's view, anxiety is associated with the idea that something bad is about to happen, whereas depression is associated with the idea that something bad has already happened. Depression and anxiety perform a signaling function and act as a motive for defense or action. Jacobson (1964) has asserted that, depending on individual social experiences, many affects can perform a similar signaling function.

Tolerance for an affect is established developmentally through increasingly intensive and varied exposure to an affective state under conditions of security. The mother intuitively understands her infant's and toddler's threshold, above which the affective experience becomes unmanageable and potentially traumatic. The mother's regulatory function is eventually internalized by the child. The signal of traumatic overload represents a failure of the self-regulatory function during conditions of affect intolerance.

For children of Holocaust survivors, the affects cited by Brenner (1974), depression and anxiety, as well as rage, often serve this signaling function and are particular adult manifestations of ideation resulting from early experiences with their parents. The survivor parent who communicates to his or her child the idea that bad things will happen may thus promote a lack of anxiety tolerance. If the parent conveys to the child the idea that he or she has done bad things, a lack of depression tolerance may be the result. The survivor parent who communicates the idea that the child's aggression is overwhelming or destructive may promote a lack of rage tolerance. When children of survivors enter treatment as adults, affect tolerance can be enhanced through the therapeutic investigation of these ideas, with the result that the affects no longer serve as signals for action or defense; they can then be integrated into the group of affective experiences that are safe and tolerable.

Clinically, it is relatively easy to overlook affect tolerance as a goal of treatment. It is difficult to empathically perceive another person's regressed affective states because these are frequently lacking in obvious behavioral manifestations. Additionally, state-dependent primitive mental conditions are difficult to discern in patients because of the clinician's repression of the memories of his or her own infantile affects. This limitation is especially germane when the clinician is faced with the recognition of another's severe emotional pain. In the absence of his or her ability to recognize another's affect, a clinician may tend to assume that it is one in his or her own repertoire (Krystal, 1974). Thus, to the extent that affects are subject to regression (i.e., when state-conditions lead to regressions that result in primitive mental affective conditions) a clinician is vulnerable to projecting his or her own feeling state or mistakenly identifying a feeling state with which he or she can experience comfort or familiarity.

HOLOCAUST AFFECT TOLERANCE

The clinical observations in this chapter derive from psychoanalytic psychotherapy with children of survivors. One patient, Mr. A, was a 31-year-old man whose rage and lust for revenge against persecutors and victimizers often spilled over into many sectors of his life. He was unusually intelligent and articulate but could not stabilize himself in a career and eventually allied himself with an escapist cult group. His treatment was unusually difficult and was intermittently punctuated by fierce diatribes against mental health professionals, whom he perceived as representing a parasitical element that survived by passive reflection rather than active opposition to various social injustices. His parents, both survivors, had met in a deportation camp shortly before coming to the United States in 1946. Mr. A noted that the only time his father willingly talked about the camps was in recollecting the time he secretly pasted a picture of Hitler on the wall of a latrine, thereby risking death. Mr. A's mother was hypochondriacal and overprotective. Mr. A suffered from severe depression, which at times was defended against by overideational impulsivity. It was not until the first half of the second year of treatment that he was able to begin to examine the effects upon him of his parents' concentration camp experiences without retreating into rage and invective. The therapist attempted to remain interpretive and analytically neutral through the storms; gradually, as the patient's rage abated, he began to speak more and more of the hardships his parents had undergone. He initiated a deeper relation with his parents and coaxed them into telling him more about their camp experiences. At around the same time, he became capable of reflecting on his turbulent moods and depressive states with an increased capacity for self-observation, and joined the therapist in constructing a plausible history to explain their origins. As the Holocaust material unfolded, Mr. A was able to stabilize himself in treatment with a newly emerging positive transference and was able to reevaluate his relation with his parents. As he developed insight, his ongoing relation with them changed. His rage toward his father for the latter's emotional unavailability and refusal to be pleased by any of Mr. A's accomplishments abated. His rage against helpers was understood to derive, in part, from his mother's attempt in times of panic attacks to identify him with her own father (killed during the war), who had protected and soothed her and whom he idealized. After these panic episodes, she belittled Mr. A's attempt to perform this same soothing function and made him feel "toxic" to others and ashamed of himself. His parents also seemed to have a great deal of difficulty handling and absorbing his aggression, and often responded either counteraggressively or by withdrawing when he asserted himself against their wishes. The gradual introduction of Holocaust-related data brought about a new level of insight into his parents' lives, as well as a sense of how the Holocaust had entered into his life through his parents. When termination prematurely occurred (the therapist was moving to a different city), he was still symptomatic, but began work with a new therapist and continued to improve. His affective life was far more buoyant, and he no longer experienced his rage or depression with such overwhelming intensity. During the termination phase, he asserted that, in part, it had been the therapist's willingness to withstand his affective states without recoiling that had contributed to his ability to integrate them and not to feel as if he were "out of control" all the time. Depression, rage, and severe anxiety no longer signaled the onset of an ego-alien mental state that made him feel strange and isolated, compounding his lack of affect tolerance.

Mr. A's development of self-regulation through the expression and exploration of aggressive wishes in the transference is reminiscent of Winnicott's (1971) discussion of the value of the therapist who survives while he simultaneously allows himself to be destroyed as the patient wishes, so that the patient can be reassured that the therapist has the capacity to survive his unbridled psychic destructiveness. To Winnicott, such aggressive wishes represent an unresolved residue of the infant's normal unintentional destructive urges, arising from the natural vigor of his primary needs. What I draw attention to is how the analyst's holding function exemplifies the therapeutic provision of affect tolerance, of holding and containing the vicissitudes of aggression (however it manifests itself in feeling states) so that aggression is no longer dreaded and the patient no longer experiences him or herself as out of control.

After liberation from the death camps, many survivors presented an ominous clinical picture (although, to be sure, many did not). Manifold sequelae were directly traceable to the appalling camp experience.[1] Various clinicians described states of chronic reactive aggression, distorted identification with the dead, severe "survivor's guilt," and massive dependency conflicts with unresolved mourning. The turning of aggression against the self was seen to potentiate depression that was triggered by guilt. Chronic anxiety and tension states were seen to lead to disturbed family ties.

In survivor families, certain of the children's feeling states are frequently proscribed because they evoke Holocaust-related memories, identifications, and fantasies in the parents. Krystal (1978) remarked that in severely trauma

[1]Anthologies edited by Krystal (1968) and Dimsdale (1980) provide detailed descriptions of psychiatric symptomology and treatment of survivors.

tized adults "the fear of affects frequently represents the dread of the return of... trauma" (p.92). As with Mr. A, parental explosiveness often becomes associated with the evocation of certain feeling states; at other times, parental withdrawal results when dreaded or overwhelming affect states emerge into felt experience. What occurs may be understood as an intergenerational transmission of trauma: One generation's trauma leads to the next generation's lack of affect tolerance. Certain affects in the children become intolerable, split off, and their emergence into awareness is difficult and painful. The affects are feared and avoided by parents because the reawakening, remembering, and reliving in themselves is too immense and painful an ordeal. In much the same protective way, and for a variety of reasons (e.g., avoiding parental withdrawal or sensing severely conflictual and painful affective states), the children may collaborate with their parents' aim of forgetting by splitting off or dissociating affects that trigger horrible memories in their parents. The threshold of tolerance for these particular affects consequently becomes lowered and the affect is not integrated within the normal developing affect array. Discomfort with these affects may lead the child to avoid situations outside of the family in which they might be experienced, resulting in poor peer relations (Sigal, Silver, Rakoff,& Ellin, 1973), a sense of the world as hostile and malevolent (Barocas & Barocas, 1981), and the sense of the family as the sole source of pleasure, gratification, and protection (H. Klein, 1974).

When the child experiences difficulties in mastering and expressing such affects as anxiety, rage, or depression,[2] it may be due not so much to overt traumatization as to the child's failure to be helped to experience necessary increments of these affects when the affect in normal development had to be mastered, made familiar and comfortable, and then modulated. It is not gross trauma that lead to most difficulties with such individuals, it is the subphase inadequacies that began with uneven and ineffective modulation and then extended into other sectors of the personality.

Case reports of offspring of Holocaust survivors are sometimes described in which these affective states are not linked to sequelae of their parents' experience in the death camps. Quite often the survivor's child does not know this is the case and misidentifies the roots of his or her affectivity as ahistorical, his or hers alone. The survivor child, preferring to view the parent as a hero rather than a victim, is bereft of a historical perspective while experiencing the repetition of psychodynamics issuing from the amorphous

[2]Anxiety, rage, and depression intolerance does not characterize every child of survivors, just as not every parent presented a characteristic survivor syndrome. These descriptions originate from a "normative" rather than "privileged" competence (Spence, 1982), implying a description based upon the tendencies depicted in broad psychoanalytic research descriptions rather than the web of specific meanings unique to a particular case.

past. The pathway to insight, through comprehending that his or her affective difficulties represent the perpetuation of an ongoing intergenerational tragedy, is often not open to him or her.

Children of survivors, seen in psychoanalysis or psychotherapy, may characterologically have grown to dread and avoid Holocaust-generated emotions. They may settle into a style of object relations in which a multitude of events that might trigger them, such as nuances of intimacy or interpersonal conflict, are avoided. One rather schizoid and anhedonic patient, who strove to avoid expression of affects that might make him feel "attached" to another person, had never had a relationship outside his family in which he felt a reasonable amount of comfort and intimacy. He fantasized that this could only be possible were he to move to Israel. He described Israel as both a Jewish and a highly aggressive country. The relocation fantasy was understood to symbolize an unconscious idea that attachment to another person was possible only if he could truly understand himself as a Jew, but this required a surrounding millieu in which aggressivity could be tolerated, unlike the situation in his family. Like their parents, children of survivors tend to live with the dread that split-off, painful, maladaptive affective states will reach consciousness and overwhelm them. Thus, the therapeutic context may provide a basis for a creative reintegration, a concept similar to but more than what Zetzel (1970) called "bearing it." At issue here is the acquisition of Holocaust-affect tolerance—establishing comfort and constraints in the therapeutic relationship around anxiety, rage, and depression.

During the treatment of individuals with lowered Holocaust-affect tolerance, the clinician must be wary of the facile appeal of the hydraulic metaphor, which equates expression with riddance. Should the clinician find him or herself thinking in such abreactive terms, he or she might identify this thought as a specific countertransference response—his or her wish that the patient rid him or herself of an aversive mental state so that the clinician too may be rid of the problem of treating it. In such cases, the hydraulic concept is an antiquated anal metaphor that can only confuse one's therapeutic vision. This countertransference reaction may lead to severe acting out or the often-seen clinical phenomenon of the affect storm. One also runs the risk of losing patients who are naturally suspicious of psychotherapeutic help by encouraging cathartic release when the tolerance that would enable a patient to withstand such a release is absent.[3]One of the outcomes of countertransference-generated acting out might be the heightening of paranoid ideation and suspiciousness regarding the therapist's motives, perhaps

[3]A second generation patient who leaves treatment in this way may experience a need to emphasize his or her parents' heroism while denying their suffering; or he or she may develop a mistrust of the clinician with the underlying belief that the clinician is a persecutor; or the patient may deny conflict with an accompanying sense that he or she does not require assistance.

resulting in the abrupt termination of the treatment. Because affect tolerance is the problem, the articulation and experience of these affects is frightening, and character structure is likely to be organized around their minimization. It should also be stressed that the other extreme—when the therapist is frightened of the patient's mental states and blocks the expression of affects—results in an upsurge in the patient's dread of his or her feelings. This error also fails to address the therapeutic goal of tolerating previously intolerable affective states.

The effect on the child of experiencing the repercussions of the Holocaust while not knowing about the event may be paralyzing. What is in the air must be put into words, if not at home, then in the therapist's office. It is in the therapist's office that the silent parent can safely be heard, albeit through the imaginative discourse of the child and the interpretative reconstructive commitment of the therapist. It is precisely at this point in the treatment that it becomes important for the therapist to be acutely sensitive to what, in the patient's recounting, is constituted of fantasy and what of factually derived evidence. This is because fantasy has deeper meaning, but discourse of what was true of the Holocaust is at times beyond conflict and thus beyond formations arising from motives versus countermotives. Images of what occurred are not necessarily compromise formations. There might be no more rational way of viewing them. Psychoanalytic theory and practice, dating back to Freud's 1897 famous and fateful 69th letter to Fliess (Freud, 1954), with its emphasis on dreamwork, early memories, screen memories, and the necessity for free association, has never sharply defined a consistent distinction between what actually transpired in the object field of the patient and what meanings the patient has superimposed onto his experiences.

It has been argued that many factors prevent the accurate retelling of early experiences, although analogic correspondences are most frequently discerned through the transference. Such issues as the defensive function of memories (G. Klein, 1966; Loewald, 1976), one's position on the lifespan (Schafer, 1978), the context of time (Loewald, 1973), and the inherent subjectivity of the analytic process itself (Schimek, 1975) cast doubt on the objectivity of the process of recollection. And what of the survivor? Do his or her recollections become subject to these principles of regulation? Wiesel (1969) described how in his camp "flames were leaping up from a ditch, gigantic flames. They were burning something . . . little children. Babies? Yes I saw it—saw it with my own eyes . . . was I awake? I could not believe it . . . no, none of this could be true. It was a nightmare" (p.42). If only we could treat this as dreamlife, the product of primary-process condensation and displacement, the royal road that points us to unconscious infantile wishes, a symbolization of current conflicts. But this incredible madness was real, it occurred in this world and must be dealt with as such.

When a child of survivors discusses the Holocaust, dreams about it, fantasizes about it, we may be faced with the psychological representation of a rendition of the past upon which the bizarre logic of the nightmare reflects real events rather than the intrusion of unconscious processes. Comfort in this case is established through trust in the containing therapeutic holding action, not through the discovery of deeper meaning. Through this reliance on the therapeutic holding action, these data can be apprehended with clarity, and the child of survivors can appreciate the implications for his or her and his or her parents' lives, weaving past, present, and future into a meaningful continuum. Schafer (1979) made the point that in the course of a useful analysis a sense of multiple histories is usually created. As one looks backward from the present and forward from the past, past and present interact in a circular development of interpretations. As the life history continuum becomes established through the explication of memory, fact, and fantasy, the past, too, will evolve and assume an increasingly intelligible coherence. Loftus and Loftus (1980), from the perspective of experimental psychology, have shown that the manner in which we talk about a memory and the questions we ask of it tend to become part of the original memory. Thus, for the survivor's child, speaking of the past to a therapist serves the purposes of rewriting what is already known, as well as discovering what is new. The past that is constructed through such a recounting fills in the gaps and clarifies the distortions induced by the vicissitudes of silence.

Holocaust-affect tolerance is most likely to be developed gradually and indirectly, through two concurrent processes. The first is through the establishment of a narrative competence—a construction of the past, composed of fantasies, memories, and information that is organized textually, possesses verisimilitude (the appearance of truthfulness), and offers a historical framework for containing, explaining, and understanding. At the same time, in the therapeutic relationship, the comfort and modulation around affects that the good-enough mother intuitively provides becomes reenacted in the holding environment. Thus, what is unknown, unspoken, but pervasive enters into verbal discourse and becomes consciously negotiable therapeutic data. Here, the applicable formula is not only the topographic model of making conscious what was unconscious—and the structural model of creating ego where id had been—it is also the narrative model of rendering sayable what was unsayable.

TO KNOW OR NOT TO KNOW: NARRATIVE COMMITMENT AND AFFECT TOLERANCE

A notion of narrative commitment as an aspect of psychoanalytic explanation was initially formulated by Sherwood (1969), who stated that "psychoanalytic explanation begins with an individual case history, and the real job of explanation occurs through ordering the mass of biographical material and attempting to organize it into a coherent whole. This is accomplished by constructing some sort of narrative account containing as much of the material as possible" (p. 281).

Sherwood discussed narrative commitment within the context of psychoanalytic epistemology, asserting that much of what is considered to be explanation and generalization is really a commitment to present case history data in a coherent and consistent form.

By contrast, narrative commitment in this chapter may be understood as the willingness, despite discomfort, to create in the therapeutic context a coherent and meaningful verbal account of the personal past out of whatever shreds of information (whether in fantasy or reality) are available. its truth claim (Ricoeur, 1977) is to be evaluated, not in terms of reliance on the actual occurrences of events, but in terms of consistency, narrative intelligibility, and success in integrating meaningful information. The question of the explanatory potential of the narration is at first detectable by the therapist rather than the patient, because of the inherent nature of the listening process (G. Klein, 1965). The patient "feels" a particular affective configuration, which is the outcome of the situation whereby vital information has failed to be consciously represented in a way that spurs insight, self-regulation, and fosters the therapeutic alliance.

Des Pres (1976) warned:

> The concentration-camp experience represents an evil so appalling that we too, when we turn to face it, suffer psychic unbalance. Some hideous impression of Auschwitz is in every mind, far removed from conscious thought but *there*; . . . and anything connected with it, anything which starts it into consciousness, brings with it a horror too large and intensely personal to confront safely. (p. 170)

This, then, is a dilemma of the child of survivors— how to confront the appalling realities safely, how to transcend self and parental injunctions against knowing, how to counterbalance the psychic unbalance, how to tolerate the affective experiences whose origins and genesis are shrouded in mystery and cloaked with fantasy. In the treatment office, this dilemma becomes the therapist's as well. Because of the danger of both knowing as well as not knowing, the relationship between interpretation and the construction of the narrative subtly changes. Usually, in therapy, the construction of a narrative occurs through the interpretive work of the analytic process (Schafer, 1980; Spence, 1982). In the case of patients of the second generation, narrative commitment is constructed parallel to the narrative itself.[4] The patient provides bits of information that, in essence, are symbols that serve as preliminary interpretations of the past. The therapist then reinterprets the patient's symbolic or incomplete interpretation in the service of narrativity, conflict and defense, and verisimilitude. Narrative commitment is forged between therapist and patient; together they construct meanings and intentions that are an integral aspect of the therapeutic transaction. Thus narrative commitment is a dialectical process; it is present in the therapist, in the patient, and is synthesized between patient and therapist.

I have already stressed the value of the holding environment that the therapist provides for the child of survivors. The issue of what "holds" a patient in treatment and motivates a patient to keep coming back and to strive for health is controversial and dates back to Freud's (1910b, 1912b, 1915) papers on transference. In these papers he puzzled on a major paradox of psychoanalytic technique: The transference is simultaneously the major form of both attachment and resistance. How can the therapist rely on something in the patient that must be resolved? How is a therapist to evoke in the patient the interest and energy necessary for treatment while curbing the impulses from which this interest and energy are powered? Loewald (1960) has suggested that a particular childhood need sought in therapy is the need to identify with one's potential for growth as seen in the eyes of a parent. This type of therapeutic response provides hope and also structures one's vision of reality in a promising, optimistic way. The therapist thus holds the patient by being experienced as a guide to the riches the world offers. In essential agreement with this position, Friedman (1969), discussing the therapeutic alliance, asserted that the therapist

> must convey to the patient not only the direction he wants the patient to move in, but also the confidence that the movement in inherent in the patient, which means that what the uncured patient wants is indeed a representation, however, distorted, of what the cured patient will get. To the extent that the analyst fails to do the latter he will naturally lose significance to the patient. (p. 150)

For children of survivors, this direction of movement that the therapist conveys "holds" the patient when it takes the form of encouraging the encounter with Holocaust-derived memories and fantasies, narrativizing them, and promotes tolerance of their affective repercussions. Thus, beyond the patient's recognition that an alternative and better life is possible, an identification with the therapist's resoluteness in facing Holocaust themes constitutes an essential element of the holding environment. Although em-

[4]The construction of a narrative and the collaboration around narrative commitment has been written about and recommended by clinicians who treat children of survivors as a technique that appears to have the status of a parameter (Eissler, 1953). Gampel (1982) offered a poignant example of this process in a case she called "A Daughter of Silence."

pathically acknowledging a despairing world view, which follows from confrontations with the past, the therapist must also represent to the patient a direction out of the despair. The therapist's communication of confidence that the patient can withstand the confrontation with the past and that such a confrontation will lead to increased mental health provides a security as well as a motive for the patient to persevere. The patient may then identify with the therapist's conviction that affects associated with Holocaust material need not be dreaded or avoided but can be mastered.

The enhancement of affect tolerance is thus facilitated by construction of a historical narrative, which includes the Holocaust legacy, by support of such a remembered and discovered past in the holding context of the therapy and through the typical concerns of the transference. These processes are not mutually exclusive; clinically, they comprise complementary aspects of the therapeutic interaction. Certain affects express basic parental identifications, and these identifications need to be experienced affectively in the course of a successful treatment (Schafer, 1964). Information that is organized in the therapy according to narrative principles will simultaneously be played out in the dynamics of the transference as well as experienced according to one's tolerance for affective expression.

The defenses and resistances mobilized when the Holocaust survivor's child commits him or herself to the explication of Holocaust material are different from those a therapist finds when analyzing the analytic transference. The former arise from diverse sources: the patient's reluctance to assess his or her parents' victimization; the wish to cleanse him or herself of the repugnance of the death traces of the past; the dissonance with positive idealized transference elements; fear of destabilizing the balance of the present relation with the parents; or hesitance to abandon a seething hatefulness of certain aspects of the past in favor of an understanding tempered by forgiving and understanding. An important difference is that the therapist does not always attempt to dissolve them or bring them into awareness through interpretations from a position of technical neutrality. This is because they may serve a restraining function due to a lack of affect tolerance. The technique of interpreting defenses before impulses holds when the patient can tolerate the analysis of the defenses. It is for this reason that the therapist who treats these patients may, when the patient begins to assess the Holocaust-related material, have to assert an inordinate amount of control over the treatment and allow him or herself to be a receptacle for hostile or paranoid projections; the therapist may have to actively struggle with the patient through confrontation and clarification. Then, too, the therapist may have to abandon the technique of following the patient's associations and instead be prepared to lead the patient into the aversive material. Through evoking this material and then tolerating it without relegating it to the realm of a disguising fantasy to be interpreted, the therapist may serve a stimulus-regulating function parallel to the one the survivor's parent may have failed to serve many years earlier.

An example of this type of therapeutic action is the case of Mr. B. Mr. B was an energetic, at times hypomanic man, who lived a fairly frantic life, which left him little time for relaxation or recreation. He had a long series of unsuccessful heterosexual relationships, which tended to end because he became bored and irritated with his partners. Action-oriented, he felt restless and anxious when his girlfriends demanded intimacy and closeness. Mr. B spoke of his past as if it were unreal or an illusion that could be brushed aside and had no impact on his present life. His parents were both survivors. His father, a prominent European intellectual before the war, received compensation payments from the government of West Germany. The father maintained a tie with the past in part through an abstract philosophical preoccupation with the freedom of the human individual, a message with which he constantly harangued his son. Much of this preoccupation concerned his own experience of survival and the freedom of choices open to him after the utter tyranny of incarceration. Mr. B's mother, on the other hand, refused to speak about her life before coming to America and giving birth to Mr. B. It was understood in his family that she was not to be upset, and father and son protected her through a conspiracy of silence. In therapy, it gradually became clear that, like his mother, Mr. B was striving not to have a past. Like his father, he sought freedom by pitting himself against oppression, which in his case he contrived. Comments linking this dynamic with his parents' lives were well received, but made Mr. B quite anxious. Part of the therapeutic task at this juncture became to provide him with a history that could be experienced as alive. I led him into this material, despite the increasing level of his discomfort. As Mr. B spoke of his past, we both also came to understand that love and nurturance were not provided in his family when a member dwelled on the past. He was, however loved at other times, and both parents took pride in his intellectual and athletic prowess. However, the dread of the past had passed into his life and profoundly influenced his intimate relationships. He unconsciously expected that a sharing of personal history jeopardized relationships, introducing stresses that would overwhelm the love and care in the relationship.

Children of survivors can construct a multitude of bridges to the past. Perhaps the most taxing and fantasy-laden is through initiating a new level of dialogue with their parents. Mr. A, described earlier, insisted for over a year that he could not speak with his parents about the Holocaust experience, because such communication would provoke his father to murderous rage. When he did initiate this dialogue, he found that he did indeed rekindle rage in his father, but it was not directed at him. Although the exchanges were filled with stress, he also discovered pleasure in experiencing his father as an assertive and powerful figure, and proudly produced a series of fantasies and dreams concerning what his father had been like before imprisonment.

CONCLUSION

I have examined the importance of narrative commitment and the therapeutic holding environment in the treatment of children of survivors in mastering Holocaust imagery, unconscious fantasies, and defective affect tolerance that have been generated by intergenerational transmission of death camp trauma. I am suggesting that affect tolerance is enhanced by the commitment to historical explanation and that such a narrative commitment constitutes a facilitative element of the therapeutic holding environment and the treatment process. Insofar as the survivor's child experiences unknown incomprehensible repetitions of the parental past, the establishment in therapy of a narrative that spans the boundary of the generations permits the child to overcome destructive forces, to make integrative use of the parent's induction of Holocaust repetitions and of the child's reception of such repetitions. The resolution of concentration camp sequelae may be viewed as necessitating symbolic restoration of obliterated or disguised meanings, as the individual organizes and assimilates overwhelming messages and disguised images whose origins lie in the distant past. Therapist and patient collaborate on the interpretation of hidden or obscure themes and allusions, translating into words various forms of meaningful silence that conceal important personal history.

The affects cited (anxiety, rage, depression) may remain split-off and intolerable until the second generation individual can juxtapose them against the backdrop of the Holocaust as an organizing experience for his or her parents and for him or herself. Each new bit of historical information will change the narrative, which continually evolves in order to accommodate new findings and make sense out of the inchoate amorphous past. As these affects become less fearful, less aversive, fact and fiction become increasingly extricated from each other, and the process of affect tolerance gets under way. The patient increasingly becomes immersed in the psychoanalytic and psychotherapeutic process. The clinician provides the holding environment that promotes comfort with these affects and wherein they can be safely experienced, tolerated, explored, and explained. It is a fundamental psychoanalytic tenet that human memory retrieves information selectively in the service of current fears and conflicts. As a result, the exploration and differentiation of affects hitherto dreaded or inaccessible will also lead to the reevaluation of memories and ongoing experience.

The word "silence" has emerged into prominence largely in the context of ethics and morals in Holocaust-informed studies. It has been argued that much of what reaches public discourse either fails to capture the essence of the event or cheapens it through misrepresentation. Some prefer the alternative to such public discourse—silence—to an image tarnished and trivialized. For those concerned with the ethical aftermath, the preservation of the values and the moral indignation the Holocaust demands, such a position is fully understandable and perhaps laudable. But for clinicians charged with the health of the patients they talk to, discourse is different; it is not trivial; the event is not lost or explained away. Therefore, I am led to the conclusion that individuals touched by the horror of the Holocaust must define their personal involvement with its reverberations through the generations, rather than submit to the invisible forces of a pathogenic silence that perpetuates the destructiveness.

Chapter 20

HYPNOANALYSIS FOR STRUCTURAL PATHOLOGY: IMPAIRMENTS OF SELF-REPRESENTATION AND CAPACITY FOR OBJECT INVOLVEMENT

ELGAN L. BAKER
The Indiana Center for Psychoanalysis and
The Indiana University School of Medicine

AN HISTORICAL SHIFT IN PSYCHOANALYTIC THEORY AND PRACTICE

Traditional psychoanalytic conceptualizations of psychopathology have tended to emphasize dynamic propositions regarding disrupted homeostasis, frustrated or inhibited instinctual strivings and anxiety associated with the topographic compromise of the psyche (Baker, 1985a). These notions were central to Freud's classic theory of neurosis and were derived primarily from his clinical work with hysterical patients and his psychodynamic model of personality. Traditional psychoanalytic ideas about the therapeutic action of psychotherapy reflect this emphasis on the dynamic flex of libidinal energy in psychological functioning and relate improvement in treatment to the discharge of tension, the abreaction of traumatic experience, and the restoration of intrapsychic balance and stability (Loewald, 1960). For this reason, classic psychoanalytic technique has tended to focus on catharsis, transference-based regression for uncovering, interpretation with its potential to facilitate insight, and working through. Each of these technical processes is predicated on the core issues of "discharging" conflictual tensions and "freeing-up" psychic energy for adaption and growth.

In his later writings on metapsychology and the clinical technique of psychoanalysis, Freud (1923, 1926, 1933a) began to shift his focus to an increasing concern with structural issues in psychopathology: the organization of maturation of the ego, the formation of identity, and interpersonal variables in development. These ideas formed the foundation for the evolution of contemporary ego psychology and object relations theories that have contributed to a fundamental shift from primary concern with the management of instincts and their vicissitudes to primary concern with the maturity, stability, and structural integrity of the ego. This shift in metapsychological construction has also produced changes in the practice of psychoanalytic technique. These changes include an increased emphasis on the nontransferential aspects of the relationship between patient and therapist and the contemporary experience of these to potentiate more adaptive interpersonal involvement; the use of the therapeutic process to support adaptation and mastery rather than primarily being focused for regression and uncovering; an emphasis on affective containment, modulation, and neutralization rather than abreaction and catharsis; and increased technical attention to the facilitation of identification and introjective processes during treatment.

These conceptual and technical shifts have largely derived from psychoanalytic research relating to normal and deviant development (Jacobson, 1964; Mahler, 1968; Mahler, Pine, & Bergman, 1975) and from clinical experience in treating narcissistic, borderline, and psychotic patients (Kernberg, 1975). Problems with boundary stabilization, differentiation of self from other, identity integration and cohesion, and the inconsistent management of intense un-neutralized impulses and affects are frequently encountered in the treatment of pre-neurotic forms of psychopathology and require attention to defects in the organizational stability of the self. Attention to structural integrity expands the technical concentration on interpretation and resolution of dynamic conflicts central to the treatment of neurotic patients (Kernberg, 1975, 1976; Volkan, 1976). The emphasis on structural variables is derived from the conceptual premise that the internal organization of the self evolves from the intrapsychic representation of experience in the world.

PSYCHOANALYTIC TECHNIQUE AND STRUCTURAL REPAIR

Stable, consistent, and benevolent experience contributes to the development of mature, integrated psychic structure and to a positive, cohesive, and functional sense of self (Volkan, 1976). The lack of a consistent and responsive environment precludes adequate psychic maturation and prevents the integration of an appropriate sense of identity. From this perspective, the therapeutic action of psychoanalytic treatment vis-a-vis structural pathology results from the development of a consistent, gratifying interpersonal environment, the focused *experiencing* of this environment in a stable fashion across time, and the directed internal representation of this experience that is then integrated for identity cohesion and psychic maturation. This clinical approach is as much a product of the "being functions" of the therapist as it is the result of what he or she does (Winnicott, 1965a). It involves an approach to being with the patient and empathically sharing the experience of being together that has broadened our traditional understanding of "neutrality" in the psychoanalytic situation. Such a stance typically requires a greater degree of active intervention and processing of experience by the therapist than in the treatment of neurotic patients. It is precisely this active sharing and processing of experience that is crucial to this work and that is analogous to the interaction between mother and infant described by Winnicott (1965a) in his explication of the facilitative effects of a "holding environment" on the early processes of maturation.

This conceptualization of technique to address structural pathology emphasizes the contemporary experiential features of treatment as well as the interpretation of historical antecedents to psychopathology, and attempts to construct therapeutic experiences that will remediate specific structural defects. These experiences typically recapitulate the normal course of development and facilitate the adaptive resolution of specific developmental tasks that remain unfinished and that account for arrests and defects in structural integrity (Kernberg, 1975; Kohut, 1971). Such a maturational sequence of experiential involvement moves from a concern with symbiosis and attachment processes to separation and individuation processes (Mahler et al., 1975). At each point, these processes are explored and related to specific structural sequelae such as boundary definition and management, object permanence and object constancy, and identity differentiation and integration. The goal is not simply to explicate and to interpret the developmental roots of failures in the epigenesis of structural maturity but also to create an interpersonal environment in treatment which facilitates compensatory restructuralization and allows a second chance at maturational resolution and growth.

HYPNOANALYTIC TECHNIQUE AND STRUCTURAL REPAIR

A number of hypnoanalytic writers have attempted to extend the paradigm shifts of ego psychology and object-relations theory to the practice of hypnosis (Baker, 1981, 1983a, 1983b, 1983c, 1985b, 1986, in press; Brown & Fromm, 1986; Copeland, 1986; Fromm & Gardner, 1979; Gruenewald, Fromm, & Oberlander, 1972). Traditional hypnoanalytic technique, parallel to the technical *zeitgeist* of psychoanalysis proper, emphasized the regressive aspects of hypnosis and its importance for uncovering and abreaction. The more contemporary approach emphasizes the integrative potential of hypnosis and its importance for structural maturation and mastery.

Hypnosis is uniquely well-suited as a technique to address structural pathology, for it is intrinsically experiential as well as interactive (i.e., shared).

Hypnosis enhances the sensory-perceptual and ideomotor phenomenology of the patient and structures, directs, interprets, or reframes these phenomena for symptom resolution and enhanced general adaptation. Hypnotic technique allows for the direction of a specific experience in external sensory reality or mediated via internal imagery that can then be focused, elaborated, given meaning and internally integrated to facilitate the resolution of unfinished developmental work. The experience of hypnosis involves repeated experience with the boundaries of reality and of the self through the unfolding of regression and dissociative processes. The management of these with the support of the therapist helps to stabilize the demarcations and functions of boundaries and reinforces the patient's sense of efficacy and security in their autonomous control. The experience of hypnosis also involves a series of experiences of "being with the other," with varying degrees of intensity in object relatedness. The interpersonal essence of trance induction and utilization and the interactive essence of trance containment and modulation demonstrate that interpersonal connections can be tolerable, safe, and even gratifying, while providing secure opportunities to intensify or to dilute the degree of interpersonal interaction.

Hypnosis, like other altered states of consciousness, varies across the continuum from relatively autistic to externally anchored and interactive. In experiencing these phenomenological shifts, the patient also experiences an emerging capacity to manage connections with the external world. The experience of hypnosis also allows for a directed symbolization of experience through imagery and via the evocative use of linguistic symbols and metaphors. The language of hypnotherapy is frequently figurative and linked to less-defended affects than experienced in typical waking consciousness. In this sense, symbolization in trance may well occur on the threshold between primary and secondary process functioning, with unique opportunities to facilitate maturational transitions to more adaptive internal organizers of experience, in much the way that Piaget (1954) described the evolution of consensually validated schemata for the organization of thought. With this emphasis on the personal and internal elaboration of external and/or shared experience, hypnosis also reinforces the connections between inner and outer; intrapsychic and interpersonal connections often defensively blocked by the security needs of the patient but crucial to flexible adaptation in the world. When established, such connections also facilitate the introjective processes that are seen as crucial to structural maturation (Cameron, 1961; Giovacchini, 1967; Hendrick, 1951; Knight, 1940; Volkan, 1968) and the mechanisms of identification that support integrated individuation (Brody & Mahoney, 1964; Erikson, 1956; Greenson, 1954; Kramer, 1955; Miller, Pollock, Bernstein, & Robbins, 1968; Schafer, 1968; Volkan, 1982).

Baker (1981, 1982, 1983a, 1983c, 1985a, 1985b, in press) has attempted to explore specific applications of hypnosis in the intensive treatment of borderline and psychotic patients. Meaningful psychotherapy with these patients is frequently very difficult because of problems in establishing a consistent and valid therapeutic alliance. These patients resist interpersonal involvement due to fears of merger, rejection, or malevolent destruction. Further, attempts at alliance are disrupted by labile shifts in affect, with the intrusion of primitive aggression; shifts in the experience of self and other due to the absence of an integrated internal representation world; and erratic and transient regressions with increases in autistic involvement and the use of primitive defenses such as splitting, denial, and projective identification (Volkan, 1976). The lack of structural integrity is a core aspect of these patients' psychopathology and becomes a crucial focus in any intervention.

Experience with a consistent and facilitative environment is a cornerstone of meaningful psychotherapy. However, consistent experience with the environment is limited by the fragmentation, disorganization, lability, and regressive propensity of these patients. Therefore, therapeutic intervention must be able to establish clear and reliable boundaries; to provide a consistent and secure experiential environment within those boundaries; to develop a capacity to titrate engagement with that environment at a level tolerable to the patient; to establish avenues to internally represent, process and integrate that experience; and to contain episodic disengagement and regression without disruption, abandonment or retaliation. The unique capacity of hypnosis to differentially delineate experience, to modultate the intensity and locus of experiential involvement, and to process this experience in an interactive/interpersonal fashion offers a useful technical adjunct to the strategic management of these parameters in intensive treatment. The therapeutic relationship and the therapeutic process then can evolve in a form conducive to structural mutation and psychological maturation.

TECHNICAL MODIFICATIONS OF HYPNOANALYTIC TECHNIQUE

A number of technical alterations are important in applying hypnosis to patients organized at this primitive level of development. A clear demarcation of the boundaries of trance with specific cues and sensory referents helps to contain the experience of altered consiousness without undue regression and to anchor this experience to a dependable external reality. The clarity of these boundaries also serves to stabilize the patient's own ego boundaries and to demonstrate the patient's capacity to form and to maintain the boundaries of the self. Formal and structured inductions, the comparison of experience in and out of trance, "open-eyed" trance to episodically check the permanence and continuity of external reality, limits on undirected association during trance, and specific ideomotor signals to alter trance involvement and to maintain interactive connectedness with the therapist are useful and important technical considerations in structuring hypnosis. The touch of the therapist's hand, focused sensory awareness of the weight of the feet on the floor, or the clenching or unclenching of a fist can provide sensory anchors for images, suggestion, or interpretations that can than be reliably replicated to establish the consistency and mutuality of the experience or to recall the experience for further elaboration. This "grounding" of intervention in sensory experience parallels the way in which internal concepts are grounded in sensoriperceptual exploration and experience across the course of development (Jacobson, 1964) and supports the evolution of a consistent internal organizing structure for experience. As the patient learns to enhance body awareness or to use body experiences to control tension, to recapture a soothing image, to restore a sense of security rooted in the relaxation of trance or to access attention or problem-solving processes, he or she also develops a sense of mastery and a sense of self as master. This emerging sense of self as one with the physical reality of the body, comfortable with awareness of the body, and in control of body experience is fundamental to the development of a stable self-concept fueled by a sense of self-efficacy and self-esteem.

It is generally accepted that the development of a sense of self allows for the full and stable integration of historical and contemporary experience and makes possible far more flexible adaptation (Fairbairn, 1963; Kernberg, 1976; Volkan, 1976). The experience of self parallels the experience of other and reciprocally determines the quality of interactions with external objects. Hypnosis provides opportunities to direct specific experiences with and of the external world including the therapist and to elaborate these as building blocks of the internal self-structure. The relaxation of trance, the soothing and gratifying attention of the therapist and the calm serenity of the office provide an experiential referent for the perception of self as comfortable (and comforted), safe (and securable), and gratified (and therefore deserving of gratification). Simultaneously, such experience can be utilized to demonstrate the security and goodness of involvement with the world. Altered attention in trance, muscle tension discharge, and motor control during hypnosis can enhance awareness of the integrity of the body (and self as strong) and control over motor and sensory processes (and self as efficacious and/or autonomous). Such experiences can be elaborated with internal symbols and structured fantasies to expand the certainty and integrity of identity and the consistency and safety of others in the external world.

Hypnotic images are often useful for these patients in creating a sense of self as whole, as attractive, or as lovable. Problems with object permanence—the continuity of object and self across time and space—can be addressed by images that evoke a single consistency of the self or object representation elaborated or focused across imagined situations. One patient I treated had a favorite yellow scarf that we regularly included in images of self in varying situations and temporal frames. Another focused on a characteristic birthmark to assure himself that he was able to exist unchanged across time. Difficulties with object constancy—the integrity of self and object across situations with changing affective valences—can also be treated with hypnotic imagery and sensorimotor experience. Images of blending and mixing can support the working through of splitting defenses without overwhelming anxiety. Images that emphasize the integration of parts, the uniqueness of parts that remain securely anchored to a whole, and fantasies about the ability of relationships to continue despite changes in self and other are all evocative of emerging representational constancy and structural stability. With one patient, I would often ask him to imagine that one hand was becoming very, very heavy while the other hand became very, very light and then to focus these sensations while simultaneously experiencing that both hands were part of his body, that both sensations were a part of his experience of himself, and that he could move both hands together or apart. We then reversed the sensory experience so that the light hand became heavy and the heavy hand began to feel light. This experience became a sensory focus for work on the constancy of his identity across varying feeling states and for his ability to tolerate and manage opposing feelings simultaneously in anticipation of an emerging capacity for neurotic ambivalence rather than primitive and discontinuous affective lability.

Just as the integrity and stability of the self-structure emerge from secure and gratifying experiences of the other and the world, the increased maturity of the self makes possible an expanded capacity for object involvement. Hypnotic images of the therapist can be used as a representation of his or her permanence and constancy. Recall of these images with sensory cues can serve a transitional object function for self-soothing in the face of separation anxiety or for conflict resolution in the absence of external structure and support. Such hypnotically elaborated images can move from partial representations to whole pictures (part objects to whole objects) to support structural cohesion, much as Giovacchini (1967) described the action of the "analytic introject" in work with severely disturbed patients. Experiences with being "together but apart" can be developed through hypnotic interactions involving alternating sharing/not sharing of experience such as dreams retold or kept private during trance, sensory alterations that involve hearing the therapist's voice as coming from near or far away, or alternately feeling and being anesthetic to pressure on the back of a hand. Such experiences reinforce the patient's ability to maintain a secure sense of self in interaction with others and to control the privacy of internal experience and the regulation of stimulus barriers requisite for social involvement. Hypnotic fantasy may also be utilized to help the patient imagine an expanding world of parallel and interactive object involvement and to profit from the gratification and rehearsal functions such fantasy can serve.

A DEVELOPMENTAL CONTINUUM OF EXPERIENCES

Experiences are developed for patients along a developmental continuum as they can tolerate involvement with them, and then repeated across several sessions until patients can access them autonomously and comfortably. Technically, such experiences typically move from sensorimotor anchoring, to internal representation via images, to linguistic and symbolic elaboration, because this sequence roughly parallels the developmental acquisition of the structural organization of experience. Attention to the stability and integrity of identity proceeds from self-awareness and self-definition; to self-permanence and self-control; to self-agency and self-cohesion; to self-esteem and unique and flexible self-expression. Attention to object involvement parallels this sequence and moves from object awareness and functional object definition; to parallel object involvement and object identification (whole object definition); to expanded and differentiated object relatedness and whole object representation; to a capacity for interpersonal mutuality and reciprocal intimacy. These sequences emphasize the phenomenological aspects of structural maturation and the parallel dynamic movement from concerns with attachment to concerns with separation to concerns with individuation.

CONCLUSION

It is important to emphasize that hypnotic images do not change psychic structure. The experience of involvement with the therapeutic process across time and the eventual conscious understanding and integration of the process potentiates structural changes in intensive psychoanalytic treatment. However, hypnosis can help to direct experience, to contain and to modulate the process, and to facilitate its internal representation and integration in a fairly direct fashion not typically available in waking, verbal psychotherapy. This unique aspect of hypnosis is especially helpful in addressing structural pathology with preneurotic patients who otherwise demonstrate significant problems in engaging and tolerating the process central to the work of psychotherapy.

The integration of hypnosis with the parameters of psychoanalytic technique offers unique opportunities for the creative facilitation of the therapeutic process, especially for those patients who lack a consistent capacity to engage and to modulate that process via verbal and introspective activity alone. The application of psychoanalytic constructs to inform our understanding of hypnotic phenomena and to direct our formulation of the hypnotherapeutic process offers an enriched foundation for our treatment of complicated patients and helps to ensure the integrity of our technique.

REFERENCES

Abrams, S. (1964). The use of hypnotic technique with psychotics: A critical review. *American Journal of Psychotherapy, 18*, 79-94.

Achterberg, J. (1985). *Imagery in healing: Shamanism and modern medicine*. Boston: New Science Library.

Adams-Tucker, C. (1982). Proximate effects of sexual abuse in childhood. *American Journal of Psychiatry, 139*, 1252-1258.

Alexander, F, & French, T.M. (1946). *Psychoanalytic therapy: Principals and application*. New York: Ronald Press.

Allen, S.A. (1985). *Hypnotic responsiveness in children: Imaginative and creative correlates*. Unpublished doctoral dissertation, University of Wyoming, Laramie, WY.

Allison, R.B. (1947). A new treatment approach for mutiple personalities. *American Journal of clinical Hypnosis, 17*, 15-32.

Alman, B.M., & Carney, R.E. (1980). Consequences of direct and indirect suggestions on success of posthypnotic behavior. *American Journal of Clinical Hypnosis, 23*, 112-118.

American Medical Association. (1985). Council report: Scientific status of refereshing recollection by the use of hypnosis. *Journal of the American Medical Association, 253*, 1918-1923.

Andersen, M.S. (1985). Hypnotizability as a factor in the hypnotic treatment of obesity. *International Journal of Clincial and Experimental Hypnosis, 33*, 150-159.

Apfel, R.J., Kelly, S.F., & Frankel, F.H. (1986). The role of hypnotizability in the pathogenesis and treatment of nausea and vomiting of pregnancy. *Journal of Psychosomatic obstetrics and Gynecology, 5*, 179-186.

Araoz, D.L. (1984). Hypnosis in management training and development. In W.C. Wester & A.H. Smith (Eds.), *Clinical hypnosis: A multidisciplinary approach* (pp 558-573). Philadelphia: Lippincott.

Araoz, D.L. (1989a,July) Thinking for success. *Human resources forum*. New York: American Management Association.

Araoz, D.L. (1989b, September). Right brain management. *Human resources forum*. New York: American Management Association.

Araoz, D.L., & Negley-Parker, E. (1988). *The new hypnosis in family therapy*. New York: Brunner/Mazel.

Armstrong, L. (1978). *Kiss daddy good-night: A speak-out on incest*. New York: Hawthorne Books.

Armstrong, S. (1980). Dual focus in brief psychodynamic psychotherapy. *Psychotherapy and Psychosomatics, 33,* 147-154.

Armsworth, M.W. (1984). *Post-traumatic stress responses in women who experienced incest as children or adolescents*. Unpublished doctoral dissertation, University of Cincinnati, Cincinnati, OH.

Arroyo, W., & Eth, S. (1985). Children traumatized by Central American warfare. In S. Eth & R.S. Pynoos (Eds.), *Posttraumatic stress disorder in children* (pp 101-120). Washington, DC: American Psychiatric Press.

Auerhahn, N., Prelinger, E. (1983). Repetition in the concentration camp survivor and her child. *International Reveiw of Psychoanalysis, 10,* 31-46.

Avery-Clark, C., O'Neil, J., & Laws, D.R. (1981). A comparison of intrafamilial sexual and physical child abuse. In M. Cook & K. Howells (Eds.), *Adult sexual interest in children* (pp. 3-40). London: Academic Press.

Bach, S. (1985). *Narcissistic states and the therapeutic process*. New York: Jason Aronson.

Baker, E. (1981). An hypnotherapeutic approach to enhance object relatedness in psychotic patients. *The International Journal of Clinical and Experimental Hypnosis. 29,* 136-147.

Baker, E. (1982).The management of tranference phenomena in the treatment of primitive states. *Psychotherapy: Theory, Research and Practice, 19,* 194-197.

Baker, E. (1983a). The use of hypnotic dreaming in the treatment of the borderline patient: Some thoughts on resistance and transitional phenomena. *International Journal of Clinical and Experimental Hypnosis, 31,* 19-27.

Baker, E. (1983b). Resistance in the hypnotherapy of primitive states: It's meaning and management. *International Journal of Clinical and Experimental Hypnosis, 31,* 82-89.

Baker, E. (1983c). The use of hypnotic techniques with psychotics. *American Journal of Clinical Hypnosis, 25,* 283-288.

Baker, E. (1985a.) Psychoanalysis and psychoanalytic psychotherapy. In S. Lynn & J. Garske (Eds.) *Contemporary psychotherapies: Models and methods* (pp. 19-68). Columbus, OH: Charles E. Merrill.

Baker, E. (1985b). Ego psychology and hypnosis: Contemporary theory and practice. *Psychotherapy in Private Practice, 3,* 115-122.

Baker, E. (1986). Developmental aspects of the hypnotherapy relationship. *Contemporary Psychoanalysis,* 7, 114-137.

Baker, E. (1987). The state of the art of clinical hypnosis. *International Journal of Clinical and Experimental Hypnosis, 35,* 203-214.

Baker, E. (in press). Hypnotherapy with borderline spectrum disorders: A developmental approach. *Contemporary Psychoanalysis*.

Baker, E.L., & Levitt, E.E. (1989). The hypnotic relationship: An investigation of compliance and resistance. *International Journal of Clinical & Experimental Hypnosis, 37,* 145-153.

Balson, P.M., & Dempster, C.R. (1980). Treatment of war neurosis from Victnam. *Comprehensive Psychiatry, 21,* 167-175.

Bandura, A. (1977). Self-efficacy: Toward a unifying theory of behavior change. *Psychological Review, 84,* 191-215.

Banquet, J.P. (1973). Spectral analysis of the EEG in meditation. *Electroencephalography and Clinical Neurophysiology, 35,* 143-151.

Banyai, E. (1985, August). *On the interactional nature of hypnosis: A social psychophysiological approach.* Paper presented at the International Congress of Hypnosis and Psychosomatic Medicine, Toronto, Canada.

Banyai, E., & Hilgard, E.R. (1976). A comparison of active-alert hypnotic induction with traditional relaxation induction. *Journal of Abnormal Psychology, 85,* 218-224

Bányai, E., Mészáros, I., & Csokay, L. (1985). Interaction between hypnotist and subject:A social psychophysiological approach (preliminary report). In D. Waxman, P.C. Mizra, M. Gibson, & M.A. Baker (Eds.), *Modern trends in hypnosis* (pp. 97-108). New York & London: Plenum Press.

Barber, J. (1977). Rapid induction analgesia: A clinical report. *American Journal of Clinical Hypnosis, 19,* 138-147.

Barber, J. (1980a). Hypnosis and the unhypnotizable. *American Journal of Clinical Hypnosis, 23,* 4-9.

Barber, J. (1980b). Utilizing hypnosis in the treatment of pain. In D.J. Oborne, M.M. Grueberg, & J.R. Eiser (Eds.), *Research in psychology and medicine* (Vol.1, pp. 35-40). London: Academic Press.

Barber, T.X. (1969). *Hypnosis: A scientific approach.* New York: Van Norstrand.

Barber, T.X. (1978). "Hypnosis," suggestions, and psychosomatic phenomena: A new look from the standpoint of recent experimental studies. *American Journal of Clinical Hypnosis, 21,* 13-27.

Barber, T.X. (1985). Preface. In D.L. Araoz *The new hypnosis.* New York: Brunner/Mazel.

Barber, T.X., & Calverley, D.S. (1966). Toward a theory of "hypnotic" behavior: Experimental analysis of suggested amnesia. *Journal of Abnormal Psychology, 71,* 95-107.

Barber, T.X., & Wilson, S.C. (1978). The Barber Suggestibility Scale and the Creative Imagination Scale: Experimental and clinical applications. *American Journal of Clinical Hypnosis, 21,* 84-108.

Barocas,J.,& Barocas, C. (1973). Manifestations of concentration camp effects on the second generation. *American Journal of Psychiatry, 130,* 820-821.

Barocas, J.& Barocas, C. (1981). Wounds of the fathers: The next generation of holocaust victims. *International Review of Psychoanalysis, 6,* 331-341.

Barrucand, D.(1967). *Histoire de l'hypnose en France [A history of hypnosis in France].* Paris: PUF.

Basch, M.F. (1976). The concept of affect: A re-examination. *Journal of American Psychological Association, 24,* 759-777.

Bass, E.,& Davis,L. (1988). *Healing the incest wound: Adult survivors in therapy.* New York: Norton.

Bass,E.,& Thornton, L. (Eds.). (1983). *I never told anyone: Writing by women survivors of child sexual abuse.* New York: Harper & Row.

Bates, B.L., Miller,J., Cross, H.J., & Brigham, T.A. (1988). Modifying Hypnotic suggestibility with the Carleton Skills Training program. *Journal of Personality and Social Psychology, 55,* 120-127.

Baum,L.F. (1960). *The wonderful Wizard of Oz.* New York: Dover. (Original work published 1900)

Beahrs, J.O. (1982). *Unity and multiplicity: Multilevel consciousness of self in hypnosis, psychiatric disorder and mental health.* New York: Brunner/Mazel.

Beaumont, J.G., Young, A.W., & McManus, I.C. (1984). Hemisphericity: A critical review. *Cognitive Neuropsychology, 1,* 191-212.

Beck, J., & van der Kolk B. (1987). *Women with a history of incest in the mental hospital.* Manuscript submitted for publication.

Belicki, D., & Belicki, K. (1982). Nightmares in a university population. *Sleep Research, 11,* 116.

Belicki, K., & Belicki, D. (1984). Frequent nightmares and hypnotic ability: An extended replication. *Sleep Research, 13,*110.

Bellak, L., Faithorn, P., & Plishka, P.C. (1981). *Crisis and special problems in psychoanalysis and psychotherapy.* New York: Brunner/Mazel.

Bellak, L., Hurvich, M., & Gediman, H. (1973).*Ego functions in schizophrenics, neurotics and normals.* New York: Wiley.

Bemporad, J.R., & Wilson, A. (1978). A developmental approach to depression in childhood and adolescence. *Journal of American Academy of Psychoanalysis, 6,* 325-352.

Benaron, H.B.W.,Tucker, B.E., Andrews, J.P., Boshes, B., Cohen, J., Fromm, E., & Yacorzynski, G.K. (1960). Effect of anoxia during labor and immediately after birth on the subsequent development of the child. *American Journal of Obstetrics and Gynecology, 80,* 1129-1142.

Bender, L., & Blau, A. (1937). The reaction of children to sexual relations with adults. *American Journal of Orthopsychiatry, 7,* 500-518.

Benedek, E.P. (1985). Children and psychic trauma: A brief review of contemporary thinking. In S. Eth & R.S. Pynoos (Eds.), *Post-traumatic stress disorder in children* (pp. 1-16). Washington, DC: American Psychiatric Press.

Benedek, T. (1956). Psychobiological aspects of mothering. *American Journal of Orthopsychiatry, 26,* 272-278.

Benward, J., & Densen-Gerber, J. (1975). Incest as a causative factor in anti-social behavior: An exploratory study. *Contemporary Drug Problems, 4*(3), 323-340.

Bergeret, J. (1974). La depression ct les etas limites [*Depression and borderline disorders.*]. Paris: Dayot.

Bernstein, E.M., & Putnam, F.W. (1986). Development, reliability, and validity of a dissociation scale. *Journal of Nervous and Mental Disease, 174,* 727-735.

Beutler, L.E, (1979). Toward specific psychological therapies for specific conditions. *Journal of Consulting and Clinical Psychology, 47,* 882-897.

Bezemer, W. (1986). Behandelen of niet bahandelen: Een mistig gebied [To treat or not to treat: A foggy territory]. In C. van Lichtenburcht, W. Bezemer, & W. Gianotten (Eds.), *Verder na incest: Hulpverlening bij het verwerken van incestervaringen* [Life after incest: Processing the incest experience] (pp.63-69). Baarn, The Netherlands: Ambo.

Bibring, E. (1953). The mechanism of depression. In P. Greenacre (Ed.), *Affective disorders.* (pp. 13-48).New York: International University Press.

Biddle, W.E. (1967). *Hypnosis in the psychoses.* Springfield, IL: Charles C. Thomas.

Birdwhistell, R.L. (1970). *Kinesics and context: Essays on body motion communication.* Philadelphia: University of Pennsylvania Press.

Black, S. (1969). *Mind and body.* London: Wm. Kimber.

Bleich, A., Garb, R., & Kotler, M. (1986). Treatment of prolonged combat reaction. *British Journal of Psychiatry, 148,* 493-496.

Bliss, E.L. (1983). Multiple personalities, related disorders and hyponosis. *American Journal of Clinical Hypnosis, 26,* 114-123.

Bliss, E.L. (1984). Hysteria and hypnosis. *Journal of Nervous and Mental Disease, 172,* 203-206.

Bliss, E.L., & Jeppsen, E.A. (1985). Prevalence of multiple personality among inpatients and out patients. *American Journal of Psychiatry, 142,* 250-251.

Bliss, E.L., & Larson, E.M. (1985). Sexual criminality and hypnotizability. *Journal of Nervous and Mental Disease, 173,* 522-526.

Blum, G.S. (1979). Hypnotic programming techniques in psychological experiments. In E. Fromm & R.E. Shor (Eds.), *Hypnosis: Developments in research and new perspectives* (pp.457-481). New York: Aldine.

Bourgeois, P. (1981). L'approche hypnotique dans les psychotherapies breves [Hypnotic method in brief psychotherapy]. *L'evolution psychiatrique* [The evolution of psychiatry], 56, 106-127.

Bower, G.H. (1981). Mood and memory. *American Psychologist, 36,* 129-148.

Bowers, K.S. (1976). *Hypnosis for the seriously curious.* New York: Jason Aronson.

Bowers, K.S. (1979). Stress, disease, and hypnosis. *Journal of Abnormal Psychology, 88,* 490-505.

Bowers, K.S. (1981). Has the sun set on the Stanford Scales? *American Journal of Clinical Hypnosis, 24,* 79-88.

Bowers, K.S. (1982). The relevance of hypnosis for cognitive behavioral therapy. *Clinical Psychology Review, 2,* 67-78.

Bowers, K.S., & Kelly, P. (1979). Stress, disease, psychotherapy, and hypnosis. *Journal of*

Abnormal Psychology, 88, 490–505.

Bowers, P. (1982). The classic suggestion effect: Relationships with scales of hypnotizability, effortless experiencing, and imagery vividness. *International Journal of Clinical and Experimental Hypnosis, 30,* 270–279.

Bowers, P., & Bowers, K. (1979). Hypnosis and creativity: A theoretical and empirical rapprochement. In E. Fromm & R.E. Shor (Eds.), *Hypnosis: Developments in research and new perspectives* (pp.351-379). New York: Aldine.

Braber, B. (1987). *Passage naar vrijheid: Joods verzet in Nederland 1940-1945* [Passage to freedom: Jewish resistance in The Netherlands 1940–1945]. Amsterdam: Balans Publishers.

Brant, R., & Tisza, V. (1977). The sexually misused child. *American Journal of Orthopsychiatry, 47*(1), 80–90.

Braun, B.G. (1984). Uses of hypnosis with multiple personality. *Psychiatric Annals, 14,* 34–40.

Braun, B.G. (Ed.). (1986). *Treatment of multiple personality disorder.* Washington, DC: American Psychiatric Press.

Brende, J.O. (1984). An educational-therapeutic group for drug and alcohol abusing combat veterans. *Journal of Contemporary Psychotherapy, 14,* 122–136.

Brende, J.O., & Benedict, B.D. (1980). The Vietnam combat delayed stress syndrome: Hypnotherapy of "dissociative symptoms." *American Journal of Clinical Hypnosis, 23,* 34–40.

Brenner, C. (1974). On the nature and development of affects: A unified theory. *Psychoanalytic Quarterly, 43,* 532–556.

Breuer, J., & Freud, S. (1955). Studies of hysteria. I: On physical mechanisms of hysterical phenomena: Preliminary communication. In J. Strachey (Ed.), *Standard Edition* (Vol-2,pp.1-335). London: Hogarth Press. (Original work published 1895)

Briere, J.,& Runtz, M. (1986). Suicidal thoughts and behaviours in former sexual abuse victims. *Canadian Journal of Behavioral Science, 18,* 413–423.

Brody, M., & Mahoney, V. (1964). Introjectin, identification and incorporation. *International Journal of Psychoanalysis, 45,* 57–63.

Brooks, B. (1983). Preoedipal issues in a postincest daughter. *American Journal of Psychotherapy, 37,* 129–136.

Brown, D. (1977). A model for the levels of concentrative meditation, *International Journal of Clinical and Experimental Hypnosis, 25,* 236–273.

Brown, D. (195). Hypnosis as an adjunct to the psychotherapy of the severely disturbed patient: An affective development approach. *International Journal of Clinical and Experimental Hypnosis, 33,* 281-301.

Brown, D.,& Fromm, E. (1986). *Hypnotherapy and hypnoanalysis.* Hillsdale, NJ: Lawrence Erlbaum Associates.

Brown, D.,& Fromm, E. (1987). *Hypnosis and behavioral medicine.* Hillsdale, NJ: Lawrence Erlbaum Associates.

Browne, A., & Finkelhor, D. (1986). Impact of child sexual abuse: A review of the literature. *Psychological Bulletin, 99,* 66–77.

Browning, D., & Boatman, B. (1977). Incest: Children at risk. *American Journal of Psychiatry, 134,* 69–72.

Brownmiller, S. (1975). *Against our will: Men, women and rape.* New York: Simon & Schuster.

Bruch, H. (1974). *Learning psychotherapy: Rationale and ground rules.* Cambridge, MA: Harvard University Press.

Bryer, J.B., Nelson, B.A., Miller, J.B., & Krol, P.A. (1987). Childhood sexual and physical abuse as factors in adult psychiatric illness. *American Journal of Psychiatry, 144*(11), 1426–1430.

Buchenholz, B., & Frank, R. (1949). The "concept of the self" in acute traumatic neurosis of war. *Journal of Nervous and Mental Disease, 107,* 55–60.

Burgess, A.W., Hartman, C.R., & McCormack, A. (1987). Abused to Abuser: Antecedents of Socially Deviant Behaviors. *American Journal of Psychiatry, 144*(11), 1431–1436.

Burgess, A.W., Holmstrom, L.L. (1974). Sexual trauma of children and adolescents: Pressure, sex and secrecy. *Nursing Clinics of North America, 10,* 554-563.

Burrows, G.D, & Dennerstein, L. (1980). *Handbook of hypnosis and psychosomatic medicine.* Hillsdale, NJ: Lawrence Erlbaum Associates.

Butler, S. (1978). *Conspiracy of silence: The trauma of incest.* New York: Bantam Books.

Cameron, N. (1961). Introjection, reprojection and hallucination in the interaction between schizophrenic patients and the therapist. *International Journal of Psychoanalysis, 42,* 86-96.

Campbell, D.T., & Fiske, D.W. (1959). Convergent and discriminant validation by the multitrait-multimethod matrix. *Psychological Bulletin, 56,* 81-105.

Campbell, J., & Moyers, B. (1988). *The power of the myth.* New York: Doubleday.

Castaneda, C. (1972). *Ixtlan.* New York: Simon & Schuster.

Castaneda, C. (1985). *The fire from within.* New York: Simon & Schuster.

Cedercreutz, C. (1972). The big mistake: A note. *International Journal of Clinical and Experimental Hypnosis, 20,* 15-16.

Cedercreutz, C. (1978). Hypnotic treatment of 100 cases of migraine. In F.H. Frankel & H.S. Zamansky (Eds.), *Hypnosis at its bicentennial: Selected papers* (pp. 225-259). New York: Plenum Press.

Cheek, D., & LeCron, L. (1968). *Clinical hypnotherapy.* New York: Grune & Stratton.

Chen, A.C.N., Dworkin, S.F., & Bloomquist, D.S. (1981). Cortical power spectrum analysis of hypnotic pain control in surgery. *International Journal of Neuroscience, 13,* 127-136.

Chertok, L. (1982). The unconscious and hypnosis. *International Journal of Clinical and Experimental Hypnosis, 30,* 95-107.

Chertok, L. (1983). Psychoanalysis and hypnosis theory: Comments on five case histories. *American Journal of Clinical Hypnosis, 25,* 209-224.

Chertok, L.,& Borch-Jacobsen, M. (1987). *Hypnose et psychanalyse* [Hypnosis and psychoanalysis]. Paris: Dunod.

Chertok, L., & De Saussure, R. (1973). *Naissance du psychanalyse* [Beginnings of psychoanlysis]. Paris: Payot.

Cladder, J.M., & lens, J.W.M. (1985). *Moderne hypnotherapie* [Modern hypnotherapy]. Lisse, The Netherlands: Swets & Zeitlinger.

Clarke, C.J., & Jackson, A.J. (1983). *Hypnosis and behavior therapy: The treatment of anxiety and phobias.* New York: Springer.

Cleaver, E. (1968). *Soul on ice* New York: Del.

Coe, W.C.,& Ryken, K. (1979). Hypnosis and risks to human subjects. *American Psychologist Association, 34,* 673-681.

Coe, W.C., St. Jean, R.L., & Burger, J.M. (1980). Hypnosis and enhancement of visual imagery. *International Journal of Clinical and Experimental Hypnosis, 28,* 225-243.

Cohen, J.A. (1981). Theories of narcissism and trauma. *American Journal of Psychotherapy, 35,* 93-100.

Cohen, N.L., & Alpert, M. (1978). Locus of control as a predictor of outcome in treatment of obesity. *Psychological Reports, 42,* 805-806.

Cole, E. (1982). Sibling incest: The myth of benign sibling incest. *Women and therapy, 5,* 79-89.

Conn, J.H. (1972). Is hypnosis really dangerous? *International Journal of Clinical and Experimental Hypnosis, 20,* 61-79.

Constantine, L.L. (1980). Effects of early sexual experiences: A review and synthesis of research. In L.L. Constantine & F.M. Martinson (Eds.), *Children and sex: New findings,new perspectives* (pp. 217-244). Boston: Little, Brown.

Conte, J.R., & Schuerman, J.R. (1987). Factors associated with an increased impact of child sexual abuse. *Child Abuse & Neglect, 2,* 210-211.

Coons, P.M. (1980). Multiple personality: Diagnostic considerations. *Journal of Clinical Psychiatry, 41,* 330-336.

Cooper, I., & Cormier, M. (1982). Inter-generational transmition of incest. *Canadian Journal of Psychiatry, 278,* 231-235.

Copeland, D. (1986). The application of object relations theory to the hypnotherapy of developmental arrests. *International Journal of Clinical and Experimental Hypnosis, 34,* 157-168.

Corby, J.C. Roth, W.T., Zarcone, V.P., & Kopell, B.S. (1978). Psychophysiological correlates of the practice of Tantric Yoga meditation. *Archives of General Psychiatry, 35,* 571-577.

Council, J.R., Kirsch, I., & Hafner, L.P. (1986). Expectancy versus absorption in the prediction of hypnotic responding. *Journal of Personality and Social Psychology, 50,* 182-189.

Courtois, C.A. (1979). Characteristics of a volunteer sample of adult women who experienced incest in childhood and adolescence. *Dissertation Abstracts International, 40A,* 3194-A.

Courtois, C.A. (1988). *Healing the incest wound: Adult survivors in therapy.* New York: Norton.

Courtois, C.A., & Hinckley, J.A. (1981). Grandfather-granddaughter incest. *Journal of Sex Education and Therapy, 7,* 37-42.

Crasilneck, H.B. (1980). Clinical assessment and preparation of the patient. In G.D. Burrows & L. Dennerstein (Eds.), *Handbook of hypnosis and psychosomatic medicine* (pp. 105-116). Amsterdam: Elsevier/North-Holland Biomedical Press.

Crasilneck, H.B., & Hall, J.A. (1959). Physiological changes associated with hypnosis: A review of the literature since 1948. *International Journal of Clinical and Experimental Hypnosis. 7,* 9-50.

Crasilneck, H.B., & Hall, J.A. (1985). *Clinical hypnosis: Principles and applications* (2nd ed.). New York: Grune & Stratton.

Crawford, H.J. (1982). Hypnotizability, daydreaming styles, imagery vividness, and absorption: A Multidimensional study. *Journal of Personality and Social Psychology, 42,* 915-926.

Crawford, H.J. (1989). Cognitive and psychological flexibility: Multiple pathways to hypnotic responsiveness. In V. Ghorghui, P. Netter, H. Eysenck, & R. Rosenthal (Eds.), *Suggestion and suggestibility: Theory and research* (pp. 155-168). Heidelberg & New York: Springer.

Crawford, H.J. (1990,July). *Cold pressor pain with and without suggested analgesis: EEG correlates as moderated by hypnotic susceptibility level.* Paper presented at the fifth International Conference of Psychophysiology, Budapest, Hungary.

Crawford, H.J., & Allen, S.N. (1983). Enhanced visual memory during hypnosis as mediated by hypnotic responsiveness and cognitive strategies. *Journal of Experimental Psychology: General, 112,* 662-685.

Crawford, H.J., & Brown, A. (1989). *Intensity of emotions: Differences between low and high hypnotizables.* Unpublished manuscript.

Crawford, H.J., Clarke, S.N., Kitner-Triolo, M., & Olesko, B. (1989,August). *EEG correlates of emotions: Moderated by hypnosis and hypnotic level.* Paper presented at the American Psychological Association Annual meeting, New Orleans, LA.

Crawford, H.J., Gur, R., Skolnick, B., Gur, R., & Benson, D. (1986,July). *Regional cerebral blood flow and hypnosis: Differences between low and high hypnotizables.* Paper presented at third International Conferences of the International Organization of Psychophysiology, Vienna, Austria.

Crawford, H.J., Hilgard, J.R., & MacDonald, H. (1982). Transient experiences following hypnotic testing and special termination procedures. *International Journal of Clinical and Experimental Hypnosis, 30,* 117-126.

Crawford, H.J., Nomura, K., & Slater, H. (1983). Spatial memory processing: Enhancement during hypnosis. In J.E. Shorr, J. Comella, G. Sobel, & L. Robin (Eds.), *Imagery: Theoretical aspects and applications* (pp. 209-216). New York: Plenum.

Crawford, H.J., Wallace, B., Nomura, K., & Slater, H. (1986). Eidetic-like imagery in hypnosis: Rare but there. *American Journal of Psychology, 99,* 527-546.

Cronin, D.M., Spanos, N.P., & Barber, T.X. (1971). Augmenting hypnotic suggestibility by providing favorable information about hypnosis. *American Journal of Clinical Hypnosis, 13,* 159-264.

Dahlstrom, W.G., Welsh, G.S., & Dahlstrom, L. (1972). *An MMPI handbook. Vol.1. Clinical interpretation.* Minneapolis: University of Minnesota Press.

Dahlstrom, W.G., Welsh, G.S., & Dahlstrom, L. (1975). *An MMPI handbook. Vol.2. Research applications.* Minneapolis: University of Minnesota Press.

Davanloo, H. (Ed.). (1978). *Basic principles and techniques in short-term dynamic psychotherapy.* New York: Spectrum.

Davanloo, H. (1980). *Short-term dynamic psychotherapy.* New York: Jason Aronson.

Davanloo, H. (1986). Intensive short-term dynamic psychotherapy with highly resistant patients. I. Handling resistance. *International Journal of Short-term Psychotherapy, 1,* 107-133.

Dave, R. (1979). Effects of hypnotically induced dreams on creative problem-solving. *Journal of Abnormal Psychology, 88,* 293-302.

Davis, L.W., Husband, R.W. (1931). A study of hypnotic susceptibility in relation to personality traits, *Journal of Abnormal and Social Psychology, 26,* 175-182.

Deikman, A.J. (1971). Bimodal consciousness. *Archives of General Psychiatry, 25,* 481-489.

De Moor, W. de. (1987). *De psychotherapeutische interventie. II. De behandelingsstrategische fase.* [Psychotherapeutic interventions: Behavioral strategies. Stage II.] Deventer: Van Loghum Slaterus.

Dengrove, E. (Ed.). (1976). *Hypnosis and behavior therapy.* Springfield, IL: Charles C. Thomas.

DePascalis, V., & Imperiali, M.G. (1984). Personality, hypnotic susceptibility and EEG responses: Preliminary study. *Perceptual and Motor Skills, 59,* 371-378.

DePascalis, V., & Palumbo, G. (1986). EEG alpha asymmetry: Task difficulty and hypnotizability. *Perceptual and Motor Skills, 62,* 139-150.

DePascalis, V., Silveri, A., & Palumbo, G. (1988). EEG asymmetry during covert mental activity and its relationship with hypnotizability. *International Journal of Clinical and Experimental Hypnosis, 36,* 38-52.

Des Pres, T. (1976). *The survivor: An anatomy of life in the death camps.* New York: Oxford University Press.

Devens, M., & Strauss, B.S. (1989). *The hypnosis experiment and stress related effects.* Paper presented to 40th Annual Scientific meeting of Society for Clinical and Experimental Hypnosis, St. Louis, MO.

Deyoub, P.L. (1979a). Hypnotizability and obesity. *Psychological Reports, 45,* 974.

Deyoub, P.L. (1979b). Hypnosis in the treatment of obesity and the relationship of suggestibility to outcome. *Journal of the American Society of Psychosomatic Dentistry and Medicine, 26,* 137-149.

De Young, M. (1981). Siblings of Oedipus: Brothers and sisters of incest victims. *Child Welfare, 60,* 561-568.

De Young M. (1982). Self-injurious behavior in incest victims: A research note. *Child Welfare, 61,* 577-584.

Diamond, M.J. (1972). The use of observationally presented information to modify hypnotic susceptibility. *Journal of Abnormal Psychology, 79,* 174-180.

Diamond, M.J. (1974). Modification of hypnotizability: A review. *Psychological Bulletin, 81,* 180-199.

Diamond, M.J. (1988). Accessing archaic involvement: Toward unraveling the mystery of Erickson's hypnosis. *International Journal of Clinical and Experimental Hypnosis, 36,* 141-155.

Diamond, M.J. (1987). The interactional basis of hypnotic experience: On the relational dimensions of hypnosis. *International Journal of Clinical and Experimental Hypnosis, 35,* 95- 115.

Diener, E., Larsen, R.J., Levine, S., & Emmons, R.A. (1985). Frequency and intensity: The underlying dimensions of affect. *Journal of Personality and Social Psychology, 48,* 1253-1265.

Dimsdale, J. (Ed.). (1980). *Survivors, victims, and perpetrators: Essays on the Nazi holocaust.* New York: Hemisphere.

Di Piano, F.A., & Salzberg, H.C. (1979). Clinical applications of hypnosis to three psychosomatic disorders. *Psychological Bulletin, 86,* 1223-1235.

Dixon, K.N., Arnold, L.E., & Calestro, K. (1978). Father-son incest: Underreported psychiatric problem? *American Journal of Psychiatry, 135,* 835-838.

Donaldson, M.A., & Gardner, R. (1985). Diagnosis and treatment of traumatic stress among women after childhood incest. In C.R. Figley (Ed.), *Trauma and its wake: The study and treatment of post-traumatic stress disorder* (pp. 356-377). New York: Brunner/Mazel.

Dormaar, J.J.M. (1987). February man revisited. *American Journal of Clinical Hypnosis, 30*(1), 28-35.

Doron, J.B. (1982, July). *Multiple victimizations: Those who suffer more than once.* Paper presented at the National Research Conference of Family Violence, Durham,NH.

Draijer, N. (1988). *Seksuell misbruik van door verwanten: Een landelijk onderzoek naar de omvang, de aard, de gezinsachtergronded, de emotionele betekenis en de psychische en psychosomatische gevolgen* [Sexual abuse of girls by relatives: A nation-wide survey of the nature, emotional signs and psychological and psychosomatic sequelae.] Den Haag: Ministerie van Sociale Zaken en Verkgelegenheid.

Dyckman, J.M., Cowan, P.A. (1978). Imaging vividness and the outcome of in vivo and imagined scene desensitization. *Journal of Consulting and Clinical Psychology, 46,* 1155-1156.

Ebbers, J. (1988). The role of family members in leave-taking rituals. In O. van der Hart (Ed.), *Coping with loss: The therapertic use of leave-taking rituals* (pp. 97-111). New York: Irvington.

Edelstien, M.G. (1982). *Trauma, trance, and transformation.* New York: Brunner/Mazel.

Eisen, M., & Fromm, E. (1983). The clinical use of self-hypnosis in hypnotherapy: Tapping the functions of imagery and adaptive regression. *International Journal of Clinical and Experimental Hypnosis, 31,* 243-255.

Eissler, K. (1953). The effect of the structure of the ego on psychoanalytic technique. *Journal of American Psychological Association, 1,* 104-143.

Ellenberger, H.(1970). *The discovery of the unconscious.* New York: Basic Books.

Ellenson, G.S. (1986). Disturbances of perception in adult female incest survivors. *Social Casework, 67,* 149-159.

Elsenga, S., & Emmelkamp, P.(1989). Een gedragstherapie bij een cliente met agorafobie en incestervaringen [A behavioral therapy in a client with agoraphobia and incest]. *Directieve Therapie., 9,* 4-17.

Elson, B.D., Hauri, P., & Cunis, D. (1977). Physiological changes in Yoga meditation. *Psychophysiology, 14,* 52-57.

Erikson, E. (1956). The problem of ego identity. *Journal of the American Psychoanalytic Association, 4,* 56-121.

Erickson, M.E. (1952). Deep hypnosis and its induction. In L.M. LeCron (Ed.), *Experimental hypnosis* (pp. 70-114). New York: Macmillan.

Erickson, M.E., & Rossi, E.L. (1979). *Hypnotherapy: An exploratory casebook.* New York: Irvington.

Erickson, M.E., Rossi, E.L., & Rossi, S.I. (1976). *Hypnotic realities: The induction of clinical hypnosis and forms of indirect suggestion.* New York: Irvington.

Eth, S., & Pynoos, R.S.(Eds.). (1985). *Post-traumatic stress disorder in children.* Washington, DC: American Psychiatric Press.

Fairbairn, W.R. (1963). Synopsis of an object-relations theory of the personality. *International Journal of Psychoanalysis, 44,* 224-255.

Farah, M.J. (1988). The neuropsychology of mental imagery: Converging evidence from brain-damaged and normal subjects. In J. Stiles-Davis, M. Kritchevsky, & U. Bellugi (Eds.), *Spatial cognition: Brain bases and development* (pp. 33-56). Hillsdale, NJ: Lawrence Erlbaum Associates.

Faw, V., Sellers, D.J., & Wilcox, W.W. (1968). Psychopathological effects of hypnosis. *International Journal of Clinical and Experimental Hypnosis, 22,* 281-298.

Federn, P. (1952). *Ego psychology and the psychoses* (E. Weiss,Ed.). New York: Basic Books.

Fenichel, O. (1945). *The psychoanalytic theory of neurosis.* New York: Norton.

Ferenczi, S. (1949). Confusion of tongues between the adult and the child. *International Journal of Psychoanalysis, 30,* 225-231.

Ferenczi, S. (1950). *Introjection and transference. Sex in psychoanalysis.* New York: Brunner. (Original work published 1909)

Ferenczi, S., & Rank, O. (1925). *Development of psychoanalysis* (C. Newton, Trans.). New York: Nervous and Mental Disease Publishing.

Finkelhor, D. (1978). Psychological, cultural and family factors in incest and family sexual abuse. *Journal of Marriage and Family Counseling, 4,* 41-49.

Finkelhor, D. (1979). *Sexually victimized children.* New York: The Free Press.

Finkelhor, D. (1980). Risk factors in the sexual victimization of children. *Child Abuse & Neglect, 4,* 265-273.

Finkelhor, D.(1984). *Child sexual abuse: New theory and research.* New York: The Free Press.

Finkelhor, D.,& Browne, A. (1985). The traumatic impact of child sexual abuse: A Conceptualization. *American Journal of Orthopsychiatry, 55,* 530-541.

Fish-Murray, C.C., Koby E.V., & van der Kolk, B.A. (1987). Evolving ideas: The effect of abuse on children's thought. In B.A. van der Kolk (Ed.), *Psychological trauma* (pp. 89-110). Washington, DC: American Psychiatric Press.

Fisher, C. (1943). Hypnosis in treatment of neuroses due to war and to other causes. *War Medicine, 4,* 565-576.

Flannery, R.B., Jr. (1987). From victim to survivor: A stress management approach to the treatment of learned helplessness. In B. van der Kolk (Ed.), *Psychological trauma* (pp. 217-232). Washington, DC: American Psychiatric Press.

Forward, S., & Buck, C. (1978). *Betrayal of innocence: Incest and its devastation.* Los Angeles: J.P. Tarcher.

Fossum, M.A., & Mason, M.J. (1986). *Facing shame.* New York: Norton.

Fourie, D.P., & Lifschitz, S. (1988). Not seeing the wood for the trees: Implications of susceptibility testing. *American Journal of Clinical Hypnosis, 30,* 166-177.

Frankel, F.H. (1976). *Hypnosis: Trance as a coping mechanism.* New York: Plenum Press.

Frankel, F.H. (1978a). Scales measuring hypnotic responsivity: A clinical perspective. *American Journal of Clinical Hypnosis, 21,* 208-218.

Frankel, F.H. (1978b). Hypnosis and altered states of consciousness in treatment of patients with medical disorders. In T.B. Karasu & R.I. Steinmuller (Eds.), *Psychotherapeutics in medicine* (pp. 181-201). New York: Grune & Stratton.

Frankel, F.H. (1981). Reporting hypnosis in the medical context. *International Journal of Clinical & Experimental Hypnosis, 29,* 10-14.

Frankel, F.H. (1982). Hypnosis and hypnotizability scales: A reply. *International Journal of Clinical & Experimental Hypnosis, 30,* 377-392.

Frankel, F.H. (1987). Significant developments in medical hypnosis during the past 25 years. *International Journal of Clinical and Experimental Hypnosis, 35,* 215-230.

Frankel, F.H., Apfel, R.J., Kelly, S.F., Benson, H., Quinn, T., Newmark, J., & Malmaud, R. (1979). The use of hypnotizability scales in the clinic: A review after six years. *International Journal of Clinical & Experimental Hypnosis, 27,* 63-73.

Frankel, F.H., Apfel-Savitz, R., Nemiah, J.C., & Sifneos, P.E. (1977). The relationship between hypnotizability and alexithymia. *Psychotherapy and Psychosomatics, 28,* 172-178.

Frankel, F.H., & Orne, M.T. (1976). Hynotizability and phobic behavior. *Archives of General Psychiatry, 33,* 1259-1261

Fraser, B.G.(1981). Sexual child abuse: The legislation and the law in the United States. In P.B. Mrazek & C.H. Kempe (Eds.), *Sexually abused children and their families* (pp. 55-74). New York: Pergamon Press.

Frederick, C. (1985). Children traumatized by catastrophic situations. In S. Eth & R.S. Pynoos (Eds.), *Post-traumatic stress disorder in children* (pp.71-99). Washington, DC: American Psychiatric Press.

French, T.M. (1952-1958). *The integration of behavior* (3 vol.). Chicago: The University of Chicago Press.

French, T.M. (1954). The integrative process in dreams. In T.M. French (Ed.), *The integration of behavior* (Vol. 2). Chicago: The University of Chicago Press.

French, T.M., & Fromm, E. (1964). *Dream interpretation: A dynamic approach.* New York: Basic Books.

Freud, A. (1936/1946). The ego and mechanisms of defense. In A. Freud, *The writings of Anna Freud;* (Vol. 2, pp.3-91), (C. Baines Trans.), New York: International Universities Press.

Freud, S. (1900). The interpretation of dreams. In J Strachey (Ed. & Trans.), *The standard edition of the complete psychological works of Sigmund Freud* (4-5). London: Hogarth Press.

Freud, S. (1910a). Five lectures on psychoanalysis. *Standard Edition, 11,* 3-58.

Freud, S. (1910b). The future prospects of psychoanalytic therapy. *Standard Edition, 11,* 139-152.

Freud, S. (1912a). Totem and taboo, *Standard Edition, 13,* 1-164.

Freud, S (1912b). The dynamics of transference. *Standard Edition,* 12, 97-108.

Freud, S (1915). Observations on transference-love. *Standard Edition, 12,* 157-174.

Freud, S. (1917). Introductory lectures on psychoanalysis. *Standard Edition, 15-16,* 3-481.

Freud, S (1918). Lines of advance in psycho-analytic therapy. *Standard Edition, 17,* 157-168.

Freud, S (1919). The uncanny. *Standard Edition, 17,* 219-252

Freud, S (1921). Group psychology and the analysis of the ego. *Standard Edition, 18,* 69-145

Freud, S. (1923). The ego and the id. *Standard Edition, 19,* 3-66.

Freud, S. (1926). Inhibitions, symptoms and anxiety. *Standard Edition, 20, 20-178.*

Freud, S. (1933a). New introductory lectures on psychoanalysis *Standard Edition, 22,* 3-184.

Freud, S (1933b). The question of a "Weltanschaung." *Standard Edition, 22,* 158-184.

Freud, S (1934). Moses and monotheism. *Standard Edition, 23,* 6-137

Freud, S. (1940). Splitting of the ego in the process of defence. *Standard Edition, 23,* 271-278.

Freud, S (1954). *Origins of psychoanalysis.* New York: Basic Books. (Original work published 1887-1902)

Freud, S (1966). *The complete introductory lectures on psychoanalysis* (J. Strachey, Trans.). New York: Norton. (Original work published 1917, 1933)

Fricton, J.R., & Roth, P. (1985). The effects of direct and indirect hypnotic suggestions for analgesia and high and low susceptible subjects. *American Journal of Clinical Hypnosis, 27,* 226-231.

Friedman, L. (1969). The therapeutic alliance. *International Journal of Psychoanalysis, 50,* 129-136.

Friedrich, W.N., & Boriskin, J.A. (1976). The role of the child in abuse: A review of the literature. *American Journal of Orthopsychiatry, 46*(4), 580-590.

Frishcholz, E.J., Spiegel, H., & Spiegel, D. (1981). Hypnosis and the unhypnotizable: A reply to Barber. *American Journal of Clinical Hypnosis, 24,* 55-58.

Frischholz, E.J., Spiegel, D., Spiegel, H., Balma, D.L., & Markell, C.S.(1982). Differential hypnotic responsivity of smokers, phobics and chronic pain control patients: A failure to confirm. *Journal of Abnormal Psychology, 91,* 269-272.

Frischholz, E.J., Tryon, W.W., Fisher, S., Maruffi, B.L., Vellios, A.T., & Spiegel, H. (1980). The relationship between the Hypnotic Induction Profile and the Standford Hypnotic Susceptibility Scale, Form C: A replication. *American Journal of Clinical Hypnosis, 22,* 185-196.

Fritz, G.S., Stoll, K., & Wagner, N.N. (1981). A comparison of males and females who were sexually molested as children. *Journal of Sex and Marital Therapy,* 7, 159-164.

Fromm, E. (1946). Study of a case of pseudo deaf-muteness—Psychic deafness. *Journal of Nervous and Mental Disease, 103,* 37-59.

Fromm, E. (1958). The psychoanalytic interpretation of dreams and projective techniques. *American Journal of Orthopsychiatry, 28,* 67-72

Fromm, E. (1960). Projective aspects of intelligence testing. In A. I. Rabin & M. Haworth (Eds.), *Projective techniques with children* (pp. 225-236). New York: Grune & Stratton.

Fromm, E. (1965). Hypnoanalysis: Theory and two case excerpts. *Psychotherapy: Theory, Research, and Practice, 2,* 127-133.

Fromm, E. (1968a). Dissociative and integrative processes in hypnoanalysis, *American Journal of Clinical Hypnosis, 10,* 174-177.

Fromm, E. (1968b). Transference and counter-transference in hypnosis. *International Journal of*

Clinical and Experimental Hypnosis, 16, 77-84.

Fromm, E. (1969). The manifest and the latent content of two paintings by Hieronymus Bosch: A psychoanalytic contribution to the study of creativity. *American Imago, 26,* 145-166.

Fromm,E. (1970). Age regression with unexpected reappearance of a repressed childhood language. *International Journal of Clinical and Experimental Hypnosis, 18,* 79-88.

Fromm, E. (1972a). Ego activity and ego passivity in hypnosis. *International Journal of Clinical and Experimental Hypnosis, 20,* 238-251.

Fromm, E. (1972b). Quo vadis hypnosis? Predictions of future trends in hypnosis research. In E Fromm & R. E. Shor (Eds.), *Hypnosis: Research developments and perspective* (pp. 575-586). Chicago: Aldine-Atherton.

Fromm, E. (1975). Self-hypnosis: A new area of research. *Psychotherapy: Theory, Research and Practice, 12,* 295-301.

Fromm, E. (1976). Altered states of consciousness and ego psychology. *Social Service Review, 50,* 557-569.

Fromm, E. (1977a). Altered states of consciousness and hypnosis: A discussion. *International Journal of Clinical and Experimental Hypnosis, 25,* 325-334.

Fromm, E. (1977b). An ego-psychological theory for altered states of consciousness. *International Journal of Clinical and Experimental Hypnosis, 25,* 373-387.

Fromm, E. (1978/1979). Primary and secondary process in waking and in altered states of consciousness. *Journal of Altered States of Consciousness, 4,* 115-128.

Fromm, E. (1979). The nature of hypnosis and other altered states of consciousness: An ego-psychological theory. In E. Fromm & R.E. Shor (Eds.), *Hypnosis: Developments in research and new perspectives* (pp. 81-103). New York: Aldine.

Fromm, E. (1980). Values in psychotherapy. *Psychotherapy: Theory, Research and Practice, 17,* 425-430.

Fromm, E. (1981). Ego-psychological parameters of hypnosis and their clinical applications. In H.J. Wain (Ed.), *Clinical and theoretical aspects of hypnosis* (pp. 33-53). Miami, FL: Symposia Specialists Medical Books.

Fromm, E. (1984a). Hypnoanalysis—with particular emphasis on the borderline patient. *Psychoanalytic Psychology, 1,* 61-76.

Fromm, E. (1984b). Theory and practice of hypnoanalysis. In W.C. Wester & A. Smith (Eds.), *Clinical hypnosis: A multidisciplinary approach* (pp.142-154). New York: J.B. Lippincott.

Fromm, E. (1987a). Psychoanalysis and hypnoanalysis: A professional history and a challenge. *Psychoanalytic Psychology, 4,* 207-218.

Fromm, E. (1987b). Significant developments in clinical hypnosis during the past 25 years. *International Journal of Clinical and Experimental Hypnosis, 35,* 215-230.

Fromm, E., Boxer, A.M., & Brown, D.P. (1985). Representations of self-hypnosis in personal narratives. In D. Waxman, P.C. Misra, M. Gibson, & M.A. Baker (Eds.), *Modern trends in hypnosis* (pp. 215-222). New York & London: Plenum Press.

Fromm, E., & Brown,D. (in press). The hypnoanalytic treatment of developmental deficit caused by early incest. In O.van der Hart (Ed.), *Trauma, dissociation and hypnosis.*

Fromm, E., Brown, D.P., Hurt, S.W., Oberlander, J.Z., Boxer, A.M., & Pfeifer, G. (1981). The phenomena and characteristics of self-hypnosis. *International Journal of Clinical and Experimental Hypnosis, 29,* 189-246.

Fromm, E., & Eisen, M. (1982). Self-hypnosis as a therapeutic aid in the mourning process. *American Journal of Clinical Hypnosis, 25,* 3-14.

Fromm, E., & French, T.M. (1962). Formation and evaluation of hypotheses in dream interpretation. *Journal of Psychology, 54,* 271-283.

Fromm, E., & Gardner, G. (1979). Ego psychology and hypnoanalysis: An integration of theory and technique. *Bulletin of the Menninger Clinic, 33,* 413-422.

Fromm, E., & Hartman, L.D. (1955). *Intelligence—A dynamic approach.* New York: Random House.

Fromm, E., Hartman, L.D., & Marschak, M.(1954). A contribution to a dynamic theory of intelligence testing in children. *Journal of Clinical and Experimental Psychopathology and Quarterly Review of Psychiatry and Neurology, 15,* 73-95.

Fromm, E., Hartman, L.D., & Marschak, M. (1957). Children's intelligence tests as a measure of dynamic personalty functioning. *American Journal of Orthopsychiatry, 27,* 134-144.

Fromm, E., & Hurt, S.W. (1980). Ego-psychological parameters of hypnosis and altered states of consciousness. In G.D. Burrows & L. Dennerstein (Eds.), *Handbook of hypnosis and psychosomatic medicine* (pp. 13-28). New York: Elsevier/North-Holland Biomedical Press.

Fromm, E., & Kahn, S. (1990) *Self hypnosis: The Chicago paradigm.* New York: Guilford.

Fromm, E., Oberlander, M.I., & Gruenewald, D. (1970). Perceptual and cognitive processes in different states of consciousness: The waking state and hypnosis. *Journal of Projective Techniques and Personality Assessment, 29,* 189-246.

Fromm, E., Sawyer, J., & Rosenthal, V. (1964). Hypnotic simulation of organic brain damage. *Journal of Abnormal and Social Psychology, 69,* 482-492.

Fromm, E., & Shor, R.E. (Ed.). (1972a). *Hypnosis: Research developments and perspectives.* Chicago: Aldine-Atherton.

Fromm, E., & Shor, R.E. (1972b). Hypnosis: Underlying theoretical issues. In E. Fromm & R.E. Shor (Eds.), *Hypnosis: Research developments and perspectives* (pp.495-509). Chicago: Aldine-Atherton.

Fromm, E., & Shor, R.E.(1979). *Hypnosis: Developments in research and new perspectives* (Rev. 2nd. ed.). New York: Aldine

Fromm, E., Skinner, S., Lombard, L., & Kahn, S. (1987/1988). The modes of the ego in self-hypnosis. *Imagination, Congnition and Personality, 7,* 335-349.

Fromuth, M.E. (1986). The relationship of childhood sexual abuse with later psychological adjustment in a sample of college women. *Child Abuse and Neglect, 10,* 5-15.

Gaddini, R. (1983). Incest as a developmental failure. *Child Abuse & Neglect, 7,* 357-358.

Gagnon, J.H. (1965). Female child victims of sex offeness. *Social Problems, 13,* 176-192.

Galbraith, G.D., London, P., Leibovitz, M.P., Cooper, L.M., & Hart, J.T. (1970). EEG and hypnotic susceptibility. *Journal of Comparative and Physiological Psychology, 72,* 125-131.

Gampel, Y. (1982). A daughter of silence. In M. Bergman & M. Jucovy (Eds.), *Generations of the Holocaust* (pp. 120-136). New York: Basic Books.

Ganzarain, R. & Buchele, B. (1986). Countertransference when incest is the problem. *International Journal of Group Psychotherapy, 36*(4), 549-566.

Gardner, G.G., & Olness, K. (1981). *Hypnosis and hypnotherapy with children.* New York: Grune & Stratton

Gartner, A., & Kelly, F. (1983). *Borderline pathology in post-incest female adolescents: Diagnostic and theoretical considerations.* Paper presented at the Annual Convention of the American Psychological Association, Anaheim, CA.

Gartner, A.F, & Gartner, J. (1988). Borderline pathology in post-incest female adolescents: Diagnostic and theoretical considerations. *Bulletin: The Menninger Clinic, 52*(2), 101-113.

Gedo, J.E., & Goldberg, A. (1973). *Models of the mind: A psycho-analytic theory.* Chicago: University of Chicago Press.

Geiser, R.L. (1981). Incest and psychological violence. *International Journal of Family Psychiatry, 2,* 291-300.

Gelinas, D.J. (1983). The persisting negative effects of incest. *Psychiatry, 46,* 313-332.

Gendlin, E.T. (1978). *Focusing.* New York: Everest House.

Gerschman, J., Burrows, G.D., Reade, P., & Foenander, G. (1979). Hypnotizability and the treatment of dental phobic behavior. In G.D. Burrows, D.R. Collison, & L. Dennerstein (Eds.), *Hypnosis* (pp. 33-39). New York: Elsevier.

Gersons, B.P.R. (1988). Afweermechanismen en afscheidsrituelen [Defense mechanisms and leave-taking rituals]. In O. van der Hart (Ed.), *Coping with loss: The therapretic use of leave-taking rituals* (pp.135-149). New York: Irvington.

Gfeller, J.D., Lynn, S.J., & Pribble, W.E. (1987). Enhancing hypnotic susceptibility: Interpersonal and rapport factors. *Journal of Personality and Social Psychology, 52,* 586-595.

Gill, M.M (1982). *Analysis of transference, volume 1: Theory and technique.* New York: International Universities Press.

Gill, M.M., & Brenman, M. (1959). *Hypnosis and related states: Psychoanalytic studies in regressison.* New York: International Universities Press.

Gillett, P.L., & Coe, W.C. (1984). The effects of rapid induction analgesia (RIA), hypnotic susceptibility and the severity of discomfort on reducing dental pain. *American Journal of Clinical Hypnosis, 27,* 81-91.

Giovacchini, P. (1967). The frozen introject. *International Journal of Psychoanalysis, 48,* 62-67.

Glick, B.S. (1970). Some limiting factors in reciprocal inhibition theory. *Psychiatric Quarterly, 44,* 223-230.

Gold, E.R. (1986). Long-term effects of sexual victimization in childhood: An attributional approach. *Journal of Consulting and Clinical Psychology, 54,* 471-475.

Goldstein, K. (1963). *The organism.* Boston: Beacon Press.

Gomes-Schwartz, B., Horowitz, J.M., & Sauzier, M. (1985). Severity of emotional distress among sexually abused preschool, school-age, and adolescent children. *Hospital and Community Psychiatry, 36,* 503-508.

Goodwin, J. (1985). Post-traumatic symptoms in incest victims. In S. Eth & R.S. Pynoos (Eds.), *Post-traumatic stress disorder in children* (pp. 155-168). Washington, DC: American Psychiatric Press

Goodwin, J. (1989). *Sexual abuse: Incest victims and their families.* Chicago: Year Book Medical Publishers.

Goodwin, J., Cormier,L., & Owen, J. (1983). Grandfather-granddaughter incest: A trigenerational view. *Child Abuse & Neglect, 7,* 163-170.

Goodwin, J., & DiVasto, P. (1979). Mother-daughter incest. *Child Abuse & Neglect, 3,* 953-957.

Goodwin, J., McCarthy, T., & DiVasto, P. (1981). Prior incest in mothers of abused children. *Child Abuse & Neglect, 5,* 87-95.

Gorassini, D.R., & Spanos, N. P. (1986). A social-cognitive skills approach to the successful modification of hypnotic susceptibility. *Journal of Personality and Social Psychology, 50,* 1004-1012.

Gordon, R. (1949). An investigation into some factors that favor the formation of stereotype images. *British Journal of Psychology, 39,* 156-167.

Gravitz, M.S. (1987). Two centuries of hypnosis specialty journals. *International Journal of Clinical and Experimental Hypnosis, 35,* 265-276.

Green, A.H. (1985). Children traumatized by physical abuse. In S. Eth & R.S. Pyoons (Eds.), *Post-traumatic stress disorder in children* (pp.133-152). Washington, DC: American Psychiatric Press.

Greenson, R. (1954). The struggle against identification. *Journal of the American Psychoanalytic Association, 2,* 200-217.

Grinder, J., & Bandler, R. (1981). *Trance-formations: Neuro-linguistic programming and the structure of hypnosis.* Moab, UT: Real People Press.

Grinker, R.R., & Spiegel, J.P. (1945). *Men under stress.* Philadelphia: Blakiston.

Groddeck, G.W. (1949). *The book of the It.* London: Vision Press Limited.

Gross, M. (1979). Incestuous rape: A cause for hysterical seizures in four adolescent girls. *American Journal of Psychiatry, 49,* 704-708.

Gross, R.J., Doerr, H., Caldirola, D., Guzinski, G.M., & Ripley, H.S. (1980-1981). Borderline syndrome and incest in chronic pelvic pain patients. *International Journal of Psychiatry in Medicine, 10,* 79-96.

Grossman, C.M., & Grossman, S. (1965). *The wild analyst, the life work of Georg Groddeck.* New York: George Baziller.

Groth, A.N. (1982). The incest offender. In S.M. Sgroi (Ed.), *Handbook of clinical intervention in child sexual abuse* (pp.215-239). Lexington, MA: D.C. Heath.

Gruber, K.J. (1981). The child victim's role in sexual assault by adults. *Child Welfare League of American, LX*(5), 305-311.

Gruenewald, D. (1971). Hypnotic techniques without hypnosis in the treatment of dual personality. *Journal of Nervous and Mental Disease, 153,* 41-46.

Gruenewald, D. (1977). Multiple personality and splitting phenomena: A reconsideration. *Journal of Nervous and Mental Disease, 164,* 385-393.

Gruenewald, D. (1978). Analogues of multiple personality in psychosis. *International Journal of Clinical and Experimental Hypnosis, 26,* 1-8.

Gruenewald, D. (1982a). Problems of relevance in the application of laboratory data to clinical situations. *International Journal of Clinical & Experimental Hypnosis, 30,* 345-353.

Gruenewald, D. (1982b). A psychoanalytic view of hypnosis. *American Journal of Clinical Hypnosis, 24,* 185-190.

Gruenewald, D. (1982c). Some thoughts on the distinction between the hypnotic situation and the hypnotic condition. *American Journal of Clinical Hypnosis, 25,* 46-51.

Gruenewald, D. (1984). On the nature of multiple personality: Comparisons with hypnosis. *International Journal of Clinical and Experimental Hypnosis, 32,* 170-190.

Gruenewald, D., & Fromm, E. (1967). Hypnosis, simulation and brain damage, *Journal of Abnormal Psychology, 72,* 191-192.

Gruenewald, D., Fromm, E., & Oberlander, M. (1972). Hypnosis and adaptive regression: An ego-psychological inquiry. In E. Fromm & R. Shor (Eds.), *Hypnosis: Developments in research and new perspectives* (pp 499-509). Chicago: Aldine-Atherton,

Gruzelier, J. (1987). The neuropsychology of hypnosis. In M. Heap (Eds.), *Experimental and clinical hypnosis: Current clinical, experimental and forensic practices* (pp 68-76). London: Croom Helm.

Gruzelier, J., Brown, T., Perry, A., Rhonder, J., & Thomas, M. (1984). Hypnotic susceptibility: A lateral predisposition and altered cerebral asymmetry under hypnosis. *International Journal of Psychophysiology, 2,* 131-139.

Gutheil, T.G., & Avery, N.C. (1977). Multiple overt incest as family defense against loss. *Family Process, 16,* 105-116.

Gwynn, M.I., Spanos, N.P., Gabora, N.J., & Jarrett, L.E. (1988), Long term and short term follow-up on the Harvard Group Scale of Hypnotic Susceptibility: Form A. *British Journal of Experimental & Clinical Hypnosis, 5,* 117-124.

Haley, J. (1967a). *Advanced techniques of hypnosis and therapy: Selected papers of M.H. Erickson, M.D.* New York: Grune & Stratton.

Haley, J.(Ed.). (1967b). *Medical hypnosis and therapy: the selected papers of Milton H. Erickson, M.D.* New York: Grune & Stratton.

Hall, H.R. (1983). Hypnosis and the immune system: A review with implications for cancer and the psychology of healing. *American Journal of Clinical Hypnosis, 25,* 92-103.

Harner, M.J. (1980). *The way of the Shaman: A guide to power and healing.* San Francisco: Harper & Row.

Harris, J.M. (1986, May). *Model training seminar for adult incest survivors.* Paper presented at the Fourth National Conference on the Sexual Victimization of Children, Children's Hospital National Medical Center, New Orleans, LA.

Hart, H.H. (1961). A review of the psychoanalytic literature on passivity. *Psychiatric Quarterly, 35,* 331-352.

Hart, B.B. (1985). Type of suggestion and hypnotizability in clinical work. *British Journal of Experimental & Clinical Hypnosis, 2,* 89-93.

Hartman, C.R., & Burgess, A.W. (1986). Child sexual abuse: Generic roots of the victim experience. *Treating Incest: A Multimodal Systems Perspective,* 83-92.

Hartmann, H. (1958). *Ego psychology and the problem of adaptation.* New York: International Universities Press.

Haugaard, J.J. (1987). *The consequences of child sexual abuse: A college survey.* Unpublished manuscript, Department of psychology, University of Virginia, Charlottesville , VA.

Haugaard, J.J., & Reppucci, N.C. (1988). *The sexual abuse of children: A comprehensive guide to current knowledge and intervention strategies.* San Francisco: Jossey-Bass.

Hebb, D.O. (1975). Science and the world of imagination, *Canadian Journal of Psychology, 16,* 4-11.

Hebb, D.O. (1980). *Essay on mind.* Hillsdale, NJ: Lawrence Erlbaum Associates.

Hebert, R., & Lehmann, D. (1979). Theta bursts: An EEG pattern in normal subjects practicing the transcendental meditational technique. *EEG and Clinical Neurophysiology, 42,* 397-405.

Henlin, H., Pollinger-Hass, A., Singer, P., Houghton, W., Schwartz, M.R., & Wallen, V. (1985). The reliving experience in Vietnam veterans with post-traumatic stress disorders. In W.E. Kelly (Ed.), *Post-traumatic stress disorder and the war veteran patient* (pp. 72-84). New York: Brunner/Mazel.

Hendrick, I. (1942). Instinct and the ego during infancy. *Psychoanalytic Quarterly, 11,* 33-58.

Hepps, R.B., & Brady, J.P. (1967). Hypnotically induced tachycardia: An experiment with simulating controls. *Journal of Nervous and Mental Disease, 145,* 131-137.

Herman, J. (1981). *Father-daughter incest.* Cambridge MA: Harvard University Press.

Herman, J., & Hirschman, L. (1981). Families at risk for father-daughter incest. *American Journal of Psychiatry, 138,* 967-970.

Herman, J., Perry, J.C., & van der Kolk, B (1989). Childhood trauma in borderline personality disorder. *American Journal of Psychiatry, 146,*(4), 490-495.

Herman, J., Russell, D., & Trocki, K. (1986). Long-term effects of incestuous abuse in childhood. *American Journal of Psychiatry, 143,*(10), 1293-1296.

Herzog, J. (1982). World beyond metaphor: Thoughts on the transmission of trauma. In M. Bergmann & M. Jucovy (Eds.), *Generations of the holocaust* (pp. 103-119). New York: Basic Books.

Hilgard, E.R. (1965). *Hypnotic susceptibility.* New York: Harcourt, Brace & World.

Hilgard, E.R. (1975). Hypnosis. *Annual Review of Psychology, 26,* 19-44.

Hilgard, E.R. (1977). *Divided consciousness. Multiple controls in human thought and action.* New York: John Wiley & Sons.

Hilgard, E.R. (1978). The Stanford Hypnotic Susceptibility Scales as related to other measures of hypnotic responsiveness. *American Journal of Clinical Hypnosis, 21,* 68-83.

Hilgard, E.R. (1979a). Divided consciousness in hypnosis: The implications of the hidden observer. In E. Fromm & R.E. Shor (Eds.), *Hypnosis: Developments in research and new perspectives* (pp. 45-80). New York: Aldine.

Hilgard, E.R. (1979b). The Stanford Hypnotic Susceptibility Scales as related to other measures of hypnotic responsiveness, *American Journal of Clinical Hypnosis, 30,* 194-403.

Hilgard, E.R. (1980). Hypnosis in the treatment of pain. In G.D. Burrows & L. Dennerstein (Eds.), *Handbook of hypnosis and psychosomatic medicine* (pp. 233-268). Amsterdam: Elsevier/ North-Holland Biomedical Press.

Hilgard, E.R. (1981a). Further discussion of the HIP and the Stanford Form C: A reply to a reply by Frischholz, Spiegel, Tryon, and Fisher. *American Journal of Clinical Hypnosis, 24,* 106-108.

Hilgard, E.R. (1981b). The eye roll sign and other scores of the Hypnotic Induction Profile (HIP) as related to the Stanford Hypnotic study by Frischholz and others. *American Journal of Clinical Hypnosis, 24,* 89-97.

Hilgard, E.R. (1982). Hypnotic susceptibility and implications for measurement. *International Journal of Clinical & Experimental Hypnosis, 30,* 394-403.

Hilgard, E.R. (1984). A book review of E. Rossi (Ed.), *"The collected papers of Milton H. Erickson on hypnosis"* (4 vol.). *International Journal of Clinical and Experimental Hypnosis, 32,* 257-265.

Hilgard, E.R. (1987). Research advances in hypnosis: Issues and methods. *International Journal of Clinical & Experimental Hypnosis, 25,* 248-264.

Hilgard, E.R., Crawford, H.J., & Wert, A. (1979). The Stanford Hypnotic Arm Levitation

Induction and Test (SHALIT): A six minute hypnotic induction and measurement scale. *International Journal of Clinical & Experimental Hypnosis, 27,* 111-124.

Hilgard, E.R., & Hilgard, J.R. (1975). *Hypnosis in the relief of pain.* Los Altos, CA: William Kaufman.

Hilgard, E.R., Sheehan, P.W., Monteiro, K.P., & MacDonald, H. (1981). Factorial structure of the Creative Imagination Scale as a measure of hypnotic responsiveness: An international comparative study. *International Journal of Clinical & Experimental Hypnosis, 29,* 66-76.

Hilgard, J.R. (1974a). Imaginative involvement: Some characteristics of the highly hypnotizable and the non-hypnotizable. *International Journal of Clinical & Experimental Hypnosis, 22,* 138-156.

Hilgard, J.R. (1974b). Sequelae to hypnosis. *International Journal of Clinical and Experimental Hypnosis, 22,* 281-298.

Hilgard, J.R. (1979). *Personality and hypnosis: A study of imaginative involvement* (2nd ed.) Chicago: University of Chicago Press.

Hilgard, J.R., Hilgard, E.R., & Newman, M.R. (1961). Sequelae to hypnotic induction with special reference to earlier chemical anesthesia. *Journal of Nervous and Mental Disease, 133,* 461-478.

Hilgard, J.R., & Hilgard, E.R. (1979) Assessing hypnotic responsiveness in a clinical setting: A multi-item clinical scale and its advantages over single item scales. *International Journal of Clinical & Experimental Hypnosis, 27,* 134-150.

Hilgard, J.R., & LeBaron, S. (1984). *Hypnotherapy of pain in children with cancer.* Los Altos, CA: William Kaufmann.

Hinshelwood, R.D. (1989). *A dictionary of Kleinian thought.* London: Free Association Books.

Holotyd, J. (1985-86). Hypnosis applications in psychological research. *Imagination, cognition and personality, 5,* 103-115.

Holroyd, J. (1986, August).*Hypnotizability and treatment outcome in psychiatric patients.* Paper presented to the International Congress of Hypnosis and Psychosomatic Medicine, Toronto, Canada.

Holt, R.R. (1963). *Manual for the scoring of primary process manifestations in Rorschach responses* (9th ed). Unpublished manuscript, Research Center for Mental Health, NY.

Holt, R.R. (1964). Imagery: The return of the ostracized, *American Psychologist, 19,* 254-264.

Hoogduin, K. (1980). De drie brieven [The three letters]. In K. van der Velden (Ed.), *Directieve Therapie* (Vol.2, pp 257-266). Deventer, The Netherlands: Van Loghum Slaterus.

Hoogduin, K., & De Jong, P.(1984). Hypnotiseerbaarheid en hypnotherpaie bij dwangneurose: Eerste bevindingen [Hypnotizability in clients with obsessive compulsive disorder: Initial findings]. *Directieve Therapie, 4,* 320-326.

Hoogduin, K., & De Jong, P. (1986). Hypnosis and hypnotizability in obsessive-compulsive disorders: Preliminary findings. *Hypnos, 13,* 3-7.

Horne, R.L. (1985, August). *Hypnotizability and treatment outcome in psychiatric patients,* Paper presented at the International Congress of Hypnosis and Psychosomatic Medicine, Toronto, Canada.

Horowitz, M.J. (1970). *Image formation and cognition.* New York: Appleton-Century-Crofts.

Horowitz, M.J. (1976). *Stress response syndromes.* New York: Jason Aronson.

Horowitz, M.J. (1986). *Stress response syndromes* (2nd ed.). Northvale, NJ: Jason Aronson.

Husain, A., & Chapel, J.L. (1983). History of Incest in Girls Admitted to a Psychiatric Hospital. *American Journal of Psychiatry, 140*(5), 591-593.

Ilfeld, F.W. (1976). Validation of the PSI. *Psychological Reports, 39,* 1215-1228.

Jackson, D.N. (1974). *The Personality Research Form Manual.* Goshan, NY: Research Psychology Press.

Jackson, J.A., & Merrington, H.N. (1980). Hypnosis in family medicine. In G.D. Burrows & L. Dennerstein (Eds.), *Handbook of hypnosis and psychosomatic medicine* (pp. 185-204). Amsterdam: Elsevier/North-Holland Biomedical Press.

Jackson, L.S. (1981). Current research in self-hypnotic phenomenology: The Chicago paradigm.

International Journal of Clinical and Experimental Hypnosis, 29, 247-258.

Jacobson, E. (1964). *The self and the object world.* New York: International Universities Press.

Jaffe, R. (1968). Dissociative phenomena in former concentration camp inmates. *International Journal of Psycho-Analysis, 49,* 310-312.

James, J., & Meyerding, J. (1977). Early Sexual Experience and Prostitution. *American Journal of Psychiatry, 134*(12), 1381-1385.

Janet, P. (1889). *L'Automatisme psychologique* [Psychological automatism]. Paris: Felix Alcan.

Janet, P. (1893). L'Amnesie continue [The amnesia continues]. *Revue Generale des Sciences, 4,* 167-179.

Janet, P. (1894). Histoire d'une idee fixe [History of a fixed idea]. *Revue Philosiphique, 37*(1), 121-168.

Janet, P. (1898). *Nevroses et idees fixes* (Vol.1) [Neuroses and fixed ideas]. Paris: Felix Alcan.

Janet, P. (1903). *Les obsessions et la psychasthenie* [Obsessions and psychasthenia]. Paris: Felix Alcan.

Janet, P. (1904). L'Amnesie et la dissociation des souvenirs par l'emotion [Amnesia and dissociation of memories by emotions]. *Journal de Psychologie Normale et Pathologique, 1,* 417-453.

Janet, P. (1909). Problemes psychologiques del'emotion [Psychological problems of emotion]. *Revue Neurologique, 17*(2), 1578-1687).

Janet, P. (1919). *Les medications psychologiques* [Psychological healing]. Paris: Felix Alcon.

Janet, P. (1935). Realisation et interpretation [Realization and interpretation]. *Annales Medico-Psychologiques, 93,* 329-366.

Janoff-Bulman, R., & Frieze, I. (1983). A theoretical perspective for understanding reactions to victimization, *Journal of Social Issues, 38,* 1-18.

Jehu, D., Gazan, M., & Klassen, C. (1985). Cognitive restructuring of distorted beliefs associated with childhood sexual abuse. *Journal of Social Work and Human Sexuality, 4,* 49-69.

Joffe, W.G. (1969). A critical review of the status of the ego concept. *International Journal of Psychoanalysis, 50,* 533-547.

John, R., Hollander, B., & Perry, C. (1983). Hypnotizability and phobic behavior: Further supporting data. *Journal of Abnormal Psychology, 92,* 390-392.

Johnson, L.S., (1981) Current research in self-hypnotic phenomenology: The Chicago paradigm. *International Journal of Clinical and Experimental Hypnosis, 29,* 247-258.

Johnson, L.S., Dawson, S.L., Clark, J.L., & Sikorsky, C. (1983). Self-hypnosis versus heterohypnosis: Order effects and sex differences in behavioral and experimental impact. *International Journal of Clinical and Experimental Hypnosis, 31,* 139-154.

Johnson, L.S., & Weight, D.G. (1976), Self-hypnosis versus hetero-hypnosis: Experiential and behavioral comparisons. *Journal of Abnormal Psychology, 85,* 523-526.

Josephson, G.A., & Fong-Beyette, M.L. (1987). Factors assisting female clients' disclosure of incest during counseling. *Journal of Counseling and Development, 65,* 475-478.

Judd, F.K., Burrows, G.D., & Dennerstein, L. (1986). Clinician's perceptions of the adverse effects of hypnosis: A preliminary survey. *Australian Journal of Clinical and Experimental Hypnosis, 13,* 49-60.

Justice, B., & Justice, R. (1979). *The broken taboo: Sex in the family.* New York: Human Sciences Press.

Kahn, S., Fromm, E., Lombard, L., & Sossi, M.S. (in press). The relation of self-reports of hypnotic depth in self-hypnosis to hypnotic susceptibility and imagery production. *International Journal of Clinical and Experimental Hypnosis.*

Kandel, E., (1983). From metapsychology to molecular biology: Explorations into the nature of anxiety. *American Journal of Psychiatry, 140,* 1277-1293.

Kandel, E., & Schwartz, R. (1985). *Principles of neural science* (2nd ed.). New York: Elsevier.

Karlin, R.A. (1979). Hypnotizability and attention. *Journal of Abnormal and Social Psychology, 88,* 92-95.

Karlin, R., Cohen, A., & Goldstein, L. (1982). *A shift to the right: Electroencephalo graphic changes from rest to hypnotic induction.* Unpublished manuscript.

Karlin, R., Goldstein, L., Cohen, A., & Morgan, D. (1980 Sept.). *Quantitated EEG, hypnosis and hypnotizability.* Paper presented at the annual meeting of the American Psychological Association, Montreal, Canada.

Kasamatsu, A., & Hirai, T. (1969). An EEG study on the Zen meditation (Zazen). In C.T. Tart (Ed.), *Altered states of consciousness* (pp. 489-501). New York: Wiley.

Kaufman, J., & Zigler, E. (1987). Do abused children become abusive parents? *American Journal of Orthopsychiatry, 57,* 186-192.

Kazdin, A.E. (1979). Imagery elaboration and self-efficacy in the covert modeling treatment of unassertive behavior. *Journal of Consulting and Clinical Psychology, 47,* 725-733.

Kazdin, A.E. (1986). The evaluation of psychotherapy: Research design and methodology. In S.L. Garfield & A.E. Bergin (Eds.), *Handbook of psychotherapy and behavior change* (3rd ed., pp. 23-68). New York: Wiley.

Keane, T.M., Fairbank, L.A., Caddell, J.M., Zimering, R.T., & Bender, M.E. (1985). A behavioral approach to assessing and treating post-traumatic stress disorder in Vietnam veterans. In C.R. Figley (Ed.), *Trauma and its wake* (pp. 257-294). New York: Brunner/Mazel.

Kelly, S.R. (1984). Measured hypnotic response and phobic behavior. *International Journal of Clinical & Experimental Hypnosis, 32,* 1-5.

Kempe, R., & Kempe, H. (1984). *The common secret.* New York: Freeman.

Kennedy, M., & Cormier, B. (1969). Father-daughter incest—Treatment of the family. *Laval Medical, 40,* 946-950.

Kernberg, O. (1975). *Borderline conditions and pathological narcissism.* New York: Jason Aronson.

Kernberg, O. (1976). *Object relations theory and clinical psychoanalysis.* New York: Jason Aronson.

Kernberg, O. (1977). The structural diagnosis of borderline personality organization. In P. Hartocollis (Ed.), *Borderline personality disorders: The concept, the syndrome, the patient* (pp. 87-121). New York: International Universities Press.

Kestenberg, J. (1980). Psychoanalyses of children of survivors from the holocaust: Case presentations and assessment. *Journal of American Psychoanalysis Association, 28,* 775-804.

Kihlstrom, J.F. (1985). Hypnosis. *Annual Review of Psychology, 36,* 385-417.

Kihlstrom, J.F., & Evans, F.J. (1979). *Functional disorders of memory.* Hillsdale, NJ: Lawrence Ealbaum Associates.

Kinney, J.M., & Sachs, L.B. (1974). Increasing hypnotic susceptibility. *Journal of Abnormal Psychology, 83,* 145-150.

Kinsey, A.C., Pomeroy, W.B., Martin, C.E., & Gebhard, P. (1953). *Sexual behavior in the human female.* Philadelphia: Saunders.

Kirmayer, L.J. (1988). Word magic and the rhetoric of common sense: Erickson's metaphor for mind. *International Journal of Clinical and Experimental Hypnosis, 36,* 157-172.

Klein, G. (1965). On hearing one's own voice: An aspect of cognitive control in spoken thought. In N.S. Greenfield & W.C. Lewis (Eds.), *Psychoanalysis and current biological thought* (pp.245-273). Madison,WI: University of Wisconsin Press.

Klein, G. (1966). The several grades of memory. In R.M. Lowenstein, L.M.Newman, M. Schur, & A.J. Solnit (Eds.), *Psychoanalysis-a general psychology: Essays in honor of Heinz Hartmann* (pp.337-389). New York: International University Press.

Klein, H. (1974). Children of the holocaust: Mourning and bereavement. In E. J. Anthony (Ed.), *Children of the Holocaust, International Yearbook of Child Psychiatry, 12,* 393-804.

Kleinhauz, M., & Eli, I. (1987). Potential deleterious effects of hypnosis in the clinical setting. *American Journal of Clinical Hypnosis, 29,* 155-159.

Kluft, R.P. (1984). Treatment of multiple personality disorder. *Psychiatric Clinics of North America, 7,* 9-30.

Kluft, R.P. (Ed.), (1985). *Childhood antecedents of multiple personality.* Washington, DC: American Psychiatric Press.

Kluft, R.P. (1986). Personality unification in multiple personality disorder: A follow-up study.

In B. G. Braun (Ed.), *Treatment of multiple personality disorder* (pp.29-60). Washington, DC: American Psychiatric Press.

Kluft, R.P. (1987a). An update of multiple personality disorder. *Hospital & Community Psychiatry, 38*(4), 363-373.

Knight, R. (1940). Introjection, projection and identification. *Psychoanalytic Quarterly, 9,* 334-341.

Koch, M. (1980). Sexual abuse in children. *Adolescence, 15*(59), 643-648.

Kohut, J. (1971). *The analysis of the self.* New York: International Universities Press.

Koss, M., & Harvey, M. (1987). *The rape victim: Clinical and community approaches to treatment.* Lexington, MA: The Stephen Greene Press.

Kramer, P. (1955). On discovering one's identity. *The Psychoanalytic Study of the Child, 10,* 47-74.

Krener, P. (1985). After incest: Secondary prevention? *Journal of the American Academy of Child Psychiatry, 24*(2), 231-234.

Kris, E. (1972). *Psychoanalytic expressions in art.* New York: International Universities Press. (Original work published, 1936)

Kroger, W.S. (1963). *Clinical and experimental hypnosis.* Philadelphia: Lippincott.

Kroger, W.S., & Fezler, W.D. (1976). *Hypnosis and behavior modification: Imagery conditioning.* Philadelphia: Lippincott.

Krystal, H. (Ed.). (1968). *Massive psychic trauma.* New York: International University Press.

Krystal, H. (1974). The genetic development of affects and affect regression. *Annals in Psychoanalysis, 2,* 98-126.

Krystal, H. (1975). Affect tolerance. *Annals in Psychoanalysis, 3,* 179-219.

Krystal, H. (1978). Trauma and affects. *Psychoanalytic Study of the Child, 33,* 81-116.

Kubie, L.S. (1943a). Manual of emergency treatment for acute war neuroses. *War Medicine, 4,* 582-599.

Kubie, L.S. (1943b). The use of induced hypnotic reveries in recovery of repressed anmesic data. *Bulletin of the Menninger Clinic, 7,* 172-182.

Kubie, L.S. & Margolin, S. (1944). The process of hypnotism and the nature of the hypnotic state. *American Journal of Psychiatry, 100,* 611-622.

Krystal, H. (1984). Psychoanalytic views on human emotional damage. In B.A. van der Kolk (Ed.), *Post-traumatic stress disorder: Psychological and biological sequelae* (pp. 1-28) Washington, DC: American Psychiatric Press.

LaBriola, F., Karlin, R., & Goldstein, L. (1987). EEG laterality changes from prehypnotic to hypnotic periods. In B. Taneli, C. Perris, & D. Kemali (Eds.), *Neurophysiological correlates of relaxation and psychopathology. Advances in Biological Psychiatry, 16,* 1-5.

Lagache, D. (1952). Le probleme du transfert [The problem of transference]. *Revue francaise de psychanalyse, 16,* 5-115.

Lamb, C.S. (1985). Hypnotically-inducing deconditioning: Reconstruction of memories in the treatment of phobias. *American Journal of Clinical Hypnosis, 24*(4), 266-271.

Lamb, S. (1986). Treating sexually abused children: Issues of blame and responsibility. *American Journal of Orthopsychiatry, 56,* 303-307.

Landis, J. (1956). Experiences of 500 children with adult sexual deviants. *Psychiatric Quarterly Supplement, 30,* 91-109.

Lang, P.J., Lazovik, A.D., & Reynolds, D.J. (1965). Desensitization, suggestibility and pseudotherapy. *Journal of Abnormal Psychology, 70,* 395-402.

Lange, A. (1977). Het gebruik van symbolen en het toepassen van de zelfperceptietheorie [The use of symbols and the application of self-perception theory]. In K. van der Velden (Ed.), *Directieve therapie* (Vol. 1, pp. 62-70). Deventer: Van Loghum Slaterus.

Lange, A. (1982). Re-attributie in de directieve gezinstherapie met een oorlogsslachtoffer [Re-attribution in directive family therapy with a war-victim]. *Directieve Therapie 2*(4), 288-303.

Lange, A. (1987). Leeftijdsregressie op papier [Age-regression on paper]. *Directieve Therapie* 7(1),

70-78.

Laredo, C. (1982). Sibling incest. In S.M. Sgroi (Ed.) *Handbook of clinical intervention in child sexual abuse* (pp. 177-189). Lexington, MA: D.C. Heath.

Laurence, J.R., & Nadon, R. (1986). Reports of hypnotic depth: Are they more than mere words? *International Journal of Clinical & Experimental Hypnosis, 34,* 215-233.

Laurence, J.R., & Perry, C.W. (1981). The "hidden observer" phenomena in hypnosis: Some additional findings. *Journal of Abnormal Psychology, 90,* 334-344.

Laurence, J.R., & Perry, C.W. (1988). *Hypnosis, will and memory: A psycholegal history.* New York: Guilford.

Lavoie, G. (1985a). The language of hypnosis: In quest of the hypnotic subject. In Guantieri (Ed.) *Hypnosis in psychotherapy and psychosomatic medicine* (pp. 17-30). Verona: I1 Signo. Editions post-universitaires.

Lavoie, G. (1985b). *Hypnosis and the unconscious.* Presidential address to the 10th International Congress of Hypnosis and Psychosomatic Medicine, Toronto, Canada.

Lavoie, G. (1988). Hypnose clinique [Clinical hypnosis]. In P. Lalonde & F. Grunberg (Eds.), *Psychiatrie clinique: Approche bio-psycho-sociale* (pp. 1216-1240) Montreal: Gaetan Morin.

Lavoie, G., & Elie, R. (1985). The clinical relevance of hypnotizability in psychosis: With reference to thinking processses and sample variances. In D. Waxman, P. Misra, M. Gibson, & M.A. Basker (Eds.), *Modern trends in hypnosis* (pp. 41-66). New York: Plenum Press.

Lavoie, G., Michaud, M., Elie, R., & Amar, V. (1987). Hypnotizability as a prognostic index in schizophrenia. II: The functional relationship between increasing mastery over autistic thinking disorders and improvement in hypnotic response over a 10-17 year period. *International Journal of Clinical and Experimental Hypnosis, 35,* 179.

Lavoie, G., & Sabourin, M. (1980). Hypnosis and schizophrenia: A review of experimental and clinical studies. In G.D. Burrows & L. Dennerstein (Ed.), *Handbook of hypnosis and psychosomatic medicine* (pp. 377-420). New York: Elsevier/North-Holland Biomedical Press.

Lavoie, G., Sabourin, M., Ally, G., & Langlois, J. (1976). Hypnotizability as a function of adaptive regression among chronic psychotic patients. *International Journal of Clinical Hypnosis, 24,* 238-257.

Lazar, B.S., & Dempster, C.R. (1981). Failures in hypnosis and hypnotherapy: A review. *American Journal of Clinical Hypnosis, 24,* 48-54.

Lazarus, A.A. (1973). "Hypnosis" as a facilitator in behavior therapy. *International Journal of Clinical & Experimental Hypnosis, 21,* 25-31.

Leahy, M.R., Martin, I.C.A. (1967). Successful hypnotic abreaction after 20 years. *British Journal of Psychiatry, 113,* 383-385.

Levitt, E.E., & Baker, E.L. (1983). The hypnotic relationship: another look at coercion, compliance and resistance. *International Journal of Clinical & Experimental Hypnosis, 31,* 115-131.

Levitt, E.E., & Baker, E., & Fish, R. (1990). Some conditions of compliance and resistance among hypnotic subjects, *American Journal of Clinical Hypnosis, 32,* 225–236

Levitt, E.E., Baker, E.L., Hacker, T., Klion, R., Krause, A.A., Lytle, R., & Vanderwater-Piercy, J. (in press). Compliance and resistance in the hypnotic state: The effect of a social and an academic counter-motivation. *Proceedings of the 11th International Congress of Hypnosis, & Psychosomatic Medicine,* The Hague, The Netherlands.

Levitt, E.E., & Hershman, S. (1963). The clinical practice of hypnosis in the United States: A preliminary survey. *International Journal of Clinical and Experimental Hypnosis, 11,* 55-65.

Lew, M. (1988). *Victims no longer.* New York: Nevraumont.

Lewis, M., & Rosenblum, L. (Eds.). (1978). *The development of affect.* New York: Plenum Press.

Lewis, M., & Sarrel, P. (1969). Some psychological aspects of seduction, incest, and rape in childhood. *Journal of the American Academy of Child Psychiatry, 8,* 609-619.

Lichtenberg, J.D. (1975). The development of a sense of self. *Journal of the American Psychoanalytic Association, 23,* 453-483.

Lindberg, F.H., & Distad, L.J. (1985a). Post-traumatic stress disorders in women who experienced childhood incest. *Child Abuse and Neglect, 9,* 329-334.

Lindberg, F.H., & Distad, L.J. (1985b). Survival responses to incest: Adolescents in crisis. *Child Abuse and Neglect, 9,* 521-526.

Lindholm, K.J. (1984). *Consequences of abuse on children's development and mental health: A conceptual model.* Unpublished manuscript, University of California, Los Angeles, CA.

Lipkowitz, M.H. (1973). The child of two survivors. A report of an unsuccessful therapy. *Israel Annals Psychiatry & Related Disciplines, 2,* 363-374.

Lister, E.D. (1982). Forced silence: A neglected dimension of trauma. *American Journal of Psychiatry, 139,* 862-876.

Loewald, H. (1960). On the therapeutic action of psychoanalysis. *International Journal of Psychoanalysis, 41,* 16-33.

Loewald, H. (1973). On internalization. *International Journal of Psychoanalysis, 54,* 9-17.

Loewald, H. (1976). Perspectives on memory. In M. Gill & P. Holzman (Eds.), *Psychology versus metapsychology: Psychoanalytic essays in honor of George Klein, Psychological Issues,* Mongraph 36, pp. 299-325.

Loftus, E.F. (1979). *Eyewitness testimony.* Cambridge: Harvard University Press.

Loftus, E.F., & Loftus, G.R. (1980). On the permanence of stored information in the brain. *American Psychology, 35,* 409-420.

Lombard., L., Fromm, E. & Kahn, S. (in press). The role of imagery in self-hypnosis: Its relationship to personality characteristics and gender. *International Journal of Clinical and Experimental Hypnosis.*

Luborsky, L. (1984). *Principles of psychoanlaytic psychotherapy: A manual for supportive-expressive treatment.* New York: Basic Books.

Lukianowicz, N. (1971). Incest. *British Journal of Psychiatry, 120,* 210-212.

Lustig, N., Dresser, J.W., Spellman, S.W., & Murray, T.B. (1966). Incest: A family group survival pattern. *Archives of General Psychology, 14,* 31-40.

Lynn, S.J., Neufeld, V., & Matyi, C.L. (1987). Inductions versus suggestions: Effects of direct and indirect working on hypnotic responding and experience. *Journal of Abnormal Psychology, 96,* 76-79.

Lynn, S.J., Weekes, J.R., Matyi, C.L., & Neufeld, V. (1988). Direct versus indirect suggestions, archaic involvement, and hypnotic experience. *Journal of Abnormal Psychology, 97,* 296-301.

MacFarlane, K., & Korbin, J. (1983). Confronting the incest secret long after the fact: A family study of multiple victimization with strategies for intervention. *Child Abuse & Neglect, 7,* 225-240.

MacFarlane, K., & Waterman, J. (with Conerly, S., Dramon, L., Durfee, M., & Long, S.). (1986). *Sexual abuse of young children.* New York: Guilford.

MacHovec, F. (1988). Hypnosis complications, risk factors and prevention. *American Journal of Clinical Hypnosis, 31,* 40-49.

MacLeod-Morgan, C. (1979). Hypnotic susceptibility, EEG theta and alpha waves, and hemispheric specificity. In G.D. Burrows, D.R. Collision, & L. Dennerstein (Eds.), *Hypnosis 1979* (pp. 181-188). Amsterdam: Elsevier-North Holland.

MacLeod-Morgan, C. (1982). EEG lateralization in hypnosis: A preliminary report. *Australian Journal of Clinical and Experimental Hypnosis, 10,* 99-102.

MacLeod-Morgan, C., & Lack, L. (1982). Hemispheric specificity: A physiological concomitant. *Psychophysiology, 19,* 687-690.

MacVicar, K., & Dillon, M. (1980). Childhood and adolescent development of ten female prostitutes. *Journal of the American Academy of Child Psychiatry, 19,* 145-159.

Machota, P., Pittman, F.S., & Flomenhoft, K. (1966). Incest as a family affair. *Family Process, 6,* 98-116.

Mahler, M. (1966). Notes on the development of basic moods: The depressive affect. In R.M. Loewenstein, L.M. Newman, M. Shur, & A.J. Solnit (Eds.), *Psychoanalysis—A general psychology* (pp. 152-168). New York: International University Press

Mahler, M. (1968). *On human symbiosis and the vicissitudes of individuation.* New York: International Universities Press.

Mahler, M., Pine, F., & Bergman, A. (1975). *The psychological birth of the human infant.* New York: Basic Books,

Malan, D.H. (1963). *A study of brief psychotherapy.* New York: Plenum Press.

Malan, D.H. (1976). *The frontier of brief psychotherapy: An example of the convergence of research and clinical practice.* New York: Plenum Press.

Malan, D.H. (1979). *Individual psychotherapy and the science of psychodynamics.* London: Butterworth.

Maltz, W., & Holman, B. (1987). *Incest and sexuality.* Lexington, MA: Lexington Books.

Mann, J. (1973). *Time limited psychotherapy.* Cambridge, MA: Harvard University Press.

Mann, J., & Goldman, R. (1982). *A casebook in time-limited psychotherapy.* New York: McGraw-Hill.

Margolis, C. (1983). Hypnotic imagery with cancer patients. *American Journal of Clinical Hypnosis, 25,* 128-135.

Margolis, M. (1984). A case of mother-adolescent son incest: A follow-up study. *Psychoanalytic Quarterly, 53,* 355-385.

Marks, I.M., Gelder, M.G., & Edwards, G. (1968). Hypnosis and desensitization for phobias: A controlled prospective trial. *British Journal of Psychiatry, 114,* 1263-1274.

Maslach, C., Zimbardo, P.G., & Marshall, G. (1979). Hypnosis as a means of studying cognitive and behavioral control. In E. Fromm & R.E. Shor (Eds.), *Hypnosis: Development in research and new perspectives* (pp. 649-683). New York: Aldine.

Masson, J.M. (1984). *The assault on truth: Freud's suppression of the seduction theory.* New York: Farrar, Straus & Giroux.

Matthews, W.J., Bennett, H., Bean, W., & Gallagher, M. (1985). Indirect versus direct hypnotic suggestions: An initial investigation. *International Journal of Clinical & Experimental Hypnosis 33,* 219-223.

Matthews, W.J., Kirsch, I., & Mosher, D. (1985). Double hypnotic induction: An initial empirical test. *Journal of Abnormal Psychology, 94,* 92-95.

Matthews, W.J., & Mosher, L. (1988). Direct and indirect hypnotic suggestion in the laboratory setting. *British Journal of Experimental & Clinical Hypnosis, 5,* 63-71.

McConkey, K.M., & Sheehan, P.W. (1982). Effect and experience on the Creative Imagination Scale (CIS). *International Journal of Clinical & Experimental Hypnosis, 30,* 280-288.

McConkey, K.M., Sheehan, P.W., & White, K.D., (1979). Camparison of the Creative Imagination Scale and the Harvard Scale of Hypnotic Susceptibility, Form A. *International Journal of Clinical & Experimental Hypnosis, 27,* 265-277.

McCormick, A., Janus, M.D., & Burgess, A.W. (1986). Runaway youths and sexual victimization: Gender differences in an adolescent runaway population. *Child Abuse and Neglect, 10,* 387-395.

McIntyre, K. (1981). Role of mothers in father-daughter incest: A feminist analysis. *Social Work, 81,* 462-466.

McLemore, C.W. (1972). Imagery in desensitization. *Behaviour, Research and Therapy, 10,* 51-57.

Meares, A. (1961). An evalution of the dangers of medical hypnosis. *American Journal of Clinical Hypnosis, 4,* 90-97.

Meiselman, K.C. (1978). *Incest: A psychological study of cause and effects with treatment recommendations.* San Francisco: Josey-Bass.

Meldman, M.J. (1960). Personality decompensations after hypnotic symptom suppression. *Journal of the American Medical Association, 173,* 359-361.

Mésázros, I., & Bányai, E.I.(1978). Electrophysiological characteristics of hypnosis. In K Lissak. (Ed.), *Neural and neurohumoral organization of motivated behavior* (pp. 173-187). Budapest: Akedemiai Kiado.

Mésázros, I., Bányai, E. I., & Greguss, A.C. (1985a). Evoked potential correlates of verbal versus imagery coding in hypnosis. In D. Waxman, P.C. Misra, M. Gibson, & M.A. Basker (Eds.), *Modern trends in hypnosis,* (pp. 161-168). New York and London: Plenum Press.

Mészáros, I., Bányai, E.I., & Greguss, A.C.(1985b). *Enhanced right hemisphere activation during hypnosis: EEG and behavioral task performance evidence.* Paper presented at the third international conference of the International Organization of Psychophysiology, Vienna, Austria.

Mészáros, I., Crawford, J.H., Szabó, C., Nagy-Kovács, A., & Révész, M.A. (1989). Hypnotic susceptibility and cerebral hemisphere preponderance; verbal-imaginal discrimination task. In V Ghorghui, R. Netter, H. Eysenck, R. Rosenthal (Eds.), *Suggestion and suggestibility: Theory and research,* (pp. 191-204). Heidelberg & New York: Springer.

Michaud, M., Lavoie, G., Elie, R., & Amar, V. (1987). Hypnotizability as prognostic index in schizophrenia I: Prediction of personality improvement and discharge rate over a 10-17 year period. *International Journal of Clinical and Experimental Hypnosis, 35,* 179.

Miller, A. (1986a). Brief reconstructive hypnotherapy for anxiety reactions: Three case reports. *American Journal of Clinical Hypnotherapy, 28*(3), 138-146.

Miller, A. (1986b). Hypnotherapy in a case of dissociated incest. *The International Journal of Clinical and Experimental Hypnosis, 34,* 13-28.

Miller, A., Pollock, G., Bernstein, H, & Robbins, F. (1968). An approach to the concept of identification. *Bulletin of the Menninger Clinic, 32,* 239-252.

Modell, A.H. (1968). *Object love and reality: An introduction to a psychoanalytic theory of object relations.* New York: International Universities Press.

Molnar, G., & Cameron, P. (1975). Incest syndromes: Observations in a general hospital psychiatric unit. *Canadian Psychiatric Association Journal, 20,* 373-377.

Moreno, J.L. (1934). *Who shall survive?* Washington, DC: Nervous and Mental Disease Publishing.

Morgan, A.H., & Hilgard, J.R. (1978-1979a). The Stanford Hypnotic Clinical Scale for Adults. *American Journal of Clinical Hypnosis, 21,* 134-147.

Morgan, A.H., & Hilgard, J.R. (1978-1979b). The Stanford Hypnotic Clinical Scale for Children. *American Journal of Clinical Hypnosis, 21,* 148-169.

Morgan, A.H., Johnson, D.J., & Hilgard, E.R, (1974). The stability of hypnotic susceptibility. *International Journal of Clinical & Experimental Hypnosis, 42,* 249-257.

Morgan, A.H., Macdonald, H., & Hilgard, E.R. (1974). EEG alpha and lateral asymmetry related to task and hypnotizability. *Psychophysiology, 11,* 275-282.

Moss C.S. (1967). *The hypnotic investigation of dreams.* New York: Wiley.

Mott, T. (1979). The clinical importance of hypnotizability. *American Journal of Clinical Hypnosis, 21,* 263-269.

Mott, T. (1982). The role of hypnosis in psychotherapy. *American Journal of Clinical Hypnosis, 24,* 241-248.

Mott, T. Jr. (1987). Editorial: Adverse reactions in the use of hypnosis. *American Journal of Clinical Hypnosis, 4,* 147-148.

Mrazek, P.B. (1981). The nature of incest: A review of contributing factors. In P.B. Mrazek & C.H. Kempe (Eds.) *Sexually abused children and their families,* (pp. 97-107). Elmsford, NY: Pergamon.

Mrazek, P.B., & Kempe, C.J. (Eds.). (1981). *Sexually abused children and their families.* Elmsford, NY: Pergamon.

Murphy, L.B. (1962). *The widening world of childhood.* New York: Basic Books.

Nash, M.R. (1987). What, if anything, is regressed about hypnotic age regression? A review of the empirical literature. *Psychological Bulletin, 102,* 42-52.

Nash, M.R. (1988). Hypnosis: A window on regression. *Bulletin of the Menninger Clinic, 52,* 383-403.

Nash, M.R., Johnson, L.S., & Tipton, R.D. (1979). Hypnotic age regression and the occurrence of transitional object relationships, *Journal of Abnormal Psychology, 88,* 547-555.

Nash, M.R., Lynn, S.J., & Givens, D.L. (1984). Adult hypnotic susceptibility, childhood punishment, and child abuse: A brief communication. *International Journal of Clinical & Experimental Hypnosis, 32,* 6–11.

Nash, M.R., & Spinler, D. (1989). Hypnosis and transference: a measure of archaic involvement. *International Journal of Clinical & Experimental Hypnosis, 37,* 129–144.

Nemiah, J.C. (1974). Conversion: Fact or chimera? *International Journal of Psychiatry in Medicine, 5,* 443–448.

Newton, B. (1983). The use of hypnosis in the treatment of cancer patients. *American Journal of Clinical Hypnosis, 25,* 104–133.

Oberlander, M.I. (1978, October). *What happens when you don't listen to your feelings.* Paper presented at 30th Annual Scientific Meeting of the Society for Clinical and Experimental Hypnosis, Asheville, NC.

Oberlander, M.I., Gruenewald, D., & Fromm, E. (1970). Content and structural characteristics of thought processes during hypnosis, *Proceedings of the 78th Annual Convention of the American Psychological Association.*

O'Connell, D.N., Orne, M.T., & Shor, R.E. (1966). A comparison of hypnotic susceptibility as assessed by diagnostic ratings and initial standardized test scores. *International Journal of Clinical & Experimental Hypnosis, 14,* 324-332.

Oppenheimer, E. (1936) On the correlation between intellect and motor development in mentally defective children and youths. *Psychiatrische en Neurologische Bladen,* 249-260.

Oppenheimer, E. & Speijer, N. (1937). Results of the Rorschach test in a case of dementia paralytica before and after malaria treatment, *Psychiatrische en Neurologische Bladen, 3.*

Orne, M.T. (1959). The nature of hypnosis: Artifact and essence. *Journal of Abnormal and Social Psychology, 58,* 277-299.

Orne, M.T. (1965). Undesirable effects of hypnosis: The determinants and management. *International Journal of Clinical and Experimental Hypnosis, 13,* 226-237.

Orne, M.T. (1977). The construct of hypnosis: Implications of the definition for research and practice. *Annals of the New York Academy of Science, 296,* 277–299.

Orne, M.T. (1979a). On the simulating subject as a quasicontrol group in hypnosis research: What, why, and how. In E. Fromm & R.E. Shor (Eds.), *Hypnosis: Developments in research and new perspectives* (pp. 519-566). New York: Aldine.

Orne, M.T. (1979b). The use and misuse of hypnosis in court. *International Journal of Clinical and Experimental Hypnosis, 27,* 311-341.

Orne, M.T. (1980). On the construct of hypnosis: How its definition affects research and its clinical application. In G. D. Burrows & L. Dennerstein (Eds.) *Handbook of hypnosis and psychosomatic medicine* (pp. 29-51). Amsterdam: Elsevier/North Holland Biomedical Press.

Orne, M.T., & Hammer, A.G. (1974). Hypnosis. *Encyclopedia Britannica* (15th ed., pp. 133–140). Chicago: William Benton.

Orne, M.T., Hilgard, E.R., Spiegel, H., Spiegel, D., Crawford, H.J., Evans, F.J., Orne, E.C., & Frischholz, E.J. (1979). The relationship between the Hypnotic Induction Profile and the Stanford Hypnotic Susceptibility Scales, Forms A and C. *International Journal of Clinical & Experimental Hypnosis, 27,* 85–102.

Orne, M.T., & McConkey, D.M. (1981). Toward convergent inquiry into self-hypnosis. *International Journal of Clinical and Experimental Hypnosis, 29,* 313-323.

Orne, M.T., & O'Connell, D.N. (1967). Diagnostic ratings of hypnotizability. *International Journal of Clinical & Experimental Hypnosis, 15,* 125–133.

Orne, M.T., Whitehouse, W.G., Dinges, D., & Orne, E.C. (1988). Reconstructing memory through hypnosis: Forensic and clinical implications. In H. Pettinati (Ed.), *Hypnosis and memory* (pp. 21-63). New York: Guilford.

Oyle, I. (1976). *Magic, mysticism and modern medicine.* Millbrae, CA: Celestial Arts.

Parker, H., & Parker, S. (1986). Father–daughter sexual abuse: An emerging perspective. *American Journal of Orthopsychiatry, 56,* 531–549.

Parson, E.R. (1984). The reparation of the self: Clinical and theoretical dimensions in the treatment of Vietnam combat veterans. *Journal of Contemporary Psychotherapy, 14,* 4-56.

Paulson, M.J. (1978). Incest and sexual molestation: Clinical and legal issues. *Journal of Clinical Child Psychology, 7,* 177-180.

Pelletier, G., & Handy, L.C. (1986). Family dysfunction and the psychological impact of child sexual abuse. *Canadian Journal of Psychiatry 31,* 407-412.

Perrault, M., & Montplaisir, J. (1984). Sleepwalking and hypnotic susceptibility. *Sleep Research, 13,* 111.

Perry, C. (1977). Is hypnotizability modifiable? *International Journal of Clinical & Experimental Hypnosis, 25,* 125-146.

Perry, C., Gelfand, R., & Marcovitch, Ph. (1979). The relevance of hypnotic susceptibility in the clinical context. *Journal of Abnormal Psychology, 88,* 592-603.

Perry, C., & Laurence, J.R. (1980). Hypnotic depth and hypnotic susceptibility: A replicated finding. *International Journal of Clinical and Experimental Hypnosis, 28,* 272-280.

Perry, C., & Mullen, G. (1975). The effect of hypnotic susceptibility on reducing smoking behavior treated by an hypnotic technique. *Journal of Clinical Psychology, 31,* 498-505.

Peters, J.J. (1976). Children who are victims of sexual assault and the psychology of offenders. *American Journal of Psychotherapy, 30,* 398-421.

Pettinati, H.M. (1982). Measuring hypnotizability in psychotic patients. *International Journal of Clinical & Experimental Hypnosis, 30,* 404-416.

Pettinati, H.M. (1988). *Hypnosis and memory.* New York: Guilford.

Pettinati, H.M., & Wade, J.H. (1986). Hypnosis in the treatment of anorexic and bulimic patients. *Seminars in Adolescent Medicine, 2,* 75-79.

Phelan, P. (1987). Incest: Socialization within a treatment program. *American Journal of Orthopsychiatry, 57*(1), 84-92.

Piaget, J. (1954). *The construction of reality in the child.* New York: Basic Books.

Pincus, H.A.,& Pardes, H. (Eds.). (1985). *The integration of neuroscience and psychiatry.* Washington, DC: American Psychiatric Press.

Pine, R. (1980). On the expansion of the affect array: A developmental description. In R. L. Lax, S. Bach, & J. A. Burland (Eds.), *Rapprochment: The critical subphase of separation-individuation,* pp. 217-233). New York: Aronson.

Price, D.D., & Barber, J. (1987). An analysis of factors that contribute to the efficacy of hypnotic analgesia. *Journal of Abnormal Psychology, 96,* 46-51.

Price, R. (1987). Dissociative disorders of the self: A continuum extending into multiple personality. *Psychotherapy, 24,* 387-391.

Putnam, F.W. (1985a). Dissociation as a response to extreme trauma. In R.P. Kluft (Ed.), *Childhood antecedents of multiple personality* (pp.65-97). Washington, DC: American Psychiatric Press.

Putnam, F.W. (1985b). Pieces of the mind: Recognizing the psychological effects of abuse. *Justice for Children, 1,* 1-7.

Rapaport, D. (1951). States of consciousness: A psychopathological and psychodynamic view. In M.M. Gill (Ed.), *The collected papers of David Rapaport* (pp. 385-404). New York: Basic Books.

Rapaport, D. (1953a). On the psychoanalytic theory of affects. In M.M. Gill (Ed.), *The collected papers of David Rapaport* (pp. 476-512). New York: Basic Books.

Rapaport, D. (1953b). Some metapsychological considerations concerning activity and passivity. In M.M. Gill (Ed.), *The collected papers of David Rapaport* (pp. 530-568). New York: Basic Books.

Rapaport, D. (1959). The theory of attention cathexis: An economic and structural attempt at the explanation of cognitive processes. In. M.M. Gill (Ed.), *The collected papers of David Rapaport* (pp.778-794). New York: Basic Books.

Rapaport, D., Gill, M.M. & Schafer, R. (1945-1946). *Diagnostic psychological testing* (2 vol.). Chicago: Yearbook Publishers.

Reeves, J.L., Redd, W.H., Strom, F.K., & Minagawa, R.Y. (1983). Hypnosis in the control of pain during hyperthermia treatment of cancer. In J.J. Bonica, U. Lindblom, & A. Iggo (Eds.), *Advances in pain research and therapy* (Vol. 5., pp. 857-861).New York: Raven Press.

Register, P.A., & Kihlstrom, J.F. (1986). Finding the hypnotic virtuoso. *International Journal of Clinical & Experimental Hypnosis, 34,* 84-97.

Reiff, R., & Scheerer, M. (1959). *Memory and hypnotic age regression: Developmental aspects of cognitive functioning explored through hypnosis.* New York: International Universities Press.

Reps, P. (N.D.). *Zen flesh, zen bones.* Garden City, NY: Anchor Press Doubleday.

Reyher, J. (1963). Free imagery: An uncovering procedure. *Journal of Clinical Psychology, 19,* 454-459.

Reyher, J., & Smeltzer, W. (1968). Uncovering properties of visual imagery and verbal association: A comparative study. *Journal of Abnormal Psychology Monograph, 78,* 218-222.

Ricoeur, P. (1977). The question of proof in Freud's psychoanalytic writing. *Journal of American Psychoanalytical Association, 25,* 835-871.

Rieker, P., & Carmen, E. (1986). The victim-to-patient process: The disconfirmation and transformation of abuse. *American Journal of Orthopsychiatry, 56,* 360-370.

Rist, K. (1979). Incest: Theoretical and clinical views. *American Journal of Orthopsychiatry, 49,* 680-691.

Rorschach, H. (1949). Psychodiagnostics (4th ed.). Berne: Verlack Hans Huber.

Rosenberg, S.W. (1983). Hypnosis in cancer care: Imagery to enhance the control of the psychological "side effects" of cancer therapy. *American Journal of Clinical Hypnosis, 25,* 122-127.

Rosenfeld, A.A. (1979). Incidence of a history of incest among 18 female psychiatric patients. *American Journal of Psychiatry, 136,* 791-796.

Rossi, E. (1980). *The collected papers of Milton H. Erickson* (4 vol.). New York: Irvington Press.

Rossi, E. (1986). *The psychobiology of mind-body healing: New concepts in therapeutic hypnosis.* New York: Norton.

Rossi, E., & Cheek, D. (1988). *Mind-body therapy: Methods of ideodynamic healing in hypnosis.* New York: Norton.

Ruch, J.C. (1975). Self-hypnosis: The result of heterohypnosis or vice versa? *International Journal of Clinical and Experimental Hypnosis, 23,* 228-304.

Rush, F. (1980). *The best kept secret: Sexual abuse of children.* Englewood Cliff, NJ: Prentice-Hall.

Russell, D.E.H. (1984). The prevalence and seriousness of incestuous abuse: Stepfathers vs. biological fathers. *Child Abuse & Neglect, 8,* 15-22.

Russell,D.E.H. (1986). *The secret trauma: Incest in the lives of girls and women.* New York: Basic Books.

Sabourin, M.E. (1982). Hypnosis and brain function: EEG correlates of state-trait differences. *Research Communications in Psychology, Psychiatry and Behavior, 7,* 149-168.

Sabourin, M.E., Cutcomb, S.D., Crawford, H.J., & Pribram, K. (in press). EEG correlates of hypnotic susceptibility and hypnotic trance; spectra analysis and coherence. *International Journal of Psychophysiology.*

Sacerdote, P. (1967). *Induced dreams.* New York: Vantage Press.

Sacerdote, P. (1982a). A non-statistical dissertation about hypnotizability scales and clinical goals: Comparison with individualized induction and deepening procedures. *International Journal of Clinical & Experimental Hypnosis, 30,* 354-376.

Sacerdote, P. (1982b). Further reflections on the hypnotizability scales: A comment. *International Journal of Clinical & Experimental Hypnosis, 30,* 393.

Sachs, L.B., & Anderson, W.L.(1967). Modification of hypnotic susceptibility. *International Journal of Clinical & Experimental Hypnosis, 15,* 172-180.

Sacks, O. (1984). *A leg to stand on.* New York: Harper & Row.

Said, T., & Worchel, J. (1986). *International Journal of Short-term Psychotherapy, 1,* 281-295.

Saletu, B. (1987). Brain function during hypnosis acupuncture and transcendental meditation. In

B. Taneli, C. Perris, & D. Kemali (Eds.), *Neurophysiological correlates of relaxation and psychopathology. Advances in Biological Psychiatry, 16,* 18-40.

Sanders, S. (1986). The Perceptual Alteration Scale: A scale measuring dissociation. *American Journal of Clinical Hypnosis, 29,* 95-102.

Sandler, J., & Joffe, W.G. (1965). Notes on childhood depression. *International Journal of Psychoanalysis, 46,* 88-96,

Sarbin, T.R., & Sable, R. (1979). Hypnosis and psychophysiological outcomes. In E. Fromm & R.E. Shor (Eds.), *Hypnosis: Developments in research and new perspectives.*(pp. 135-214). New York: Aldine.

Satir, V. (1972). *Peoplemaking.* Palo Alto, CA: Science & Behavior Books.

Scagnelli, J. (1980). Hypnotherapy with psychotic and borderline patients: The use of trance by patient and therapist. *American Journal of Clinical Hypnosis, 22,* 164-169.

Scagnelli-Jobsis, J. (1982). Hypnosis with psychotic patients: A review of the literature and presentation of a theoretical framework. *American Journal of Clinical Hypnosis, 25,* 33-45.

Scagnelli-Jobsis, J. (1983). Hypnosis with psychotic patients: Response to Spiegel. *American Journal of Clinical Hypnosis, 25,* 295-298.

Schacter, D.L. (1977) EEG theta waves and psychological phenomena: A review and analysis. *Biological Psychology, 5,* 47-82.

Schafer, R. (1964). The clinical analysis of affects.*Journal of American Psychoanalysis Association, 12,* 275-300.

Schafer, R. (1968). *Aspects of internalization.* New York: International Universities Press.

Schafer, R. (1978). *Language and insight: The Sigmund Freud memorial lectures 1975-76, University College London.* New Haven, CT & London: Yale University Press.

Schafer, R. (1979). The appreciative analytic attitude and the construction of multiple histories. *Psychoanalysis and Contemporary Thought, 2,* 3-24.

Schafer, R. (1980). Narration in the psychoanalytic dialogue. *Critical Inquiry, 7,* 29-53

Scheflan, A.E. (1973). *Communicational structure: Analysis of a psychotherapy transaction.* Bloomington, IN: Indiana University Press.

Schetky, D.H., & Green, A.H. (1988). *Child sexual abuse: A handbook for health care and legal professionals.* New York: Bruner/Mazel.

Schimek, J. (1975). The interpretation of the past: Childhood trauma, psychical reality, and historical truth.*Journal of American Psychoanalytic Association, 23,* 845-865.

Schmale, A. (1964). A genetic view of affects. *Psychoanalytic Study Child, 19,* 287-310.

Schneck, J.M. (1966). Hypnoanalytic elucidation of a childhood germ phobia. *International Journal of Clinical and Experimental Hypnosis, 14,* 305-307.

Schneider, J. Smith, C.W., & Whitcher, S. (1983). *The relationship of mental imagery to white blood cell (neutrophil) function: Experimental studies with normal subjects.* Uncirculated mimeograph, Michigan State University College of Medicine, East Lansing, MI.

Schur, M. (1953). The ego in anxiety. In R. Lowerstein (Ed.), *Drives, affects, behavior* (pp. 67-104). New York: International University Press.

Scurfield, R.M. (1985). Post-trauma stress assessment and treatment: Overview and formulations. In C.R. Figley (Ed.), *Trauma and its wake: The study and treatment of post-traumatic stress disorder* (pp. 219-256). New York: Brunner/Mazel.

Sedney, M.A., & Brooks, B. (1984). Factors associated with history of childhood sexual experience in a nonclinical female population. *Journal of the American Association of Child Psychiatry, 23,* 215-218.

Sgroi, S.M. (Ed.). (1982). *Handbook of clinical intervention in child sexual abuse.* Lexington, MA: D.C. Heath.

Sgroi, S.M., Blick L.C., & Porter, F.S. (1982). A conceptual framework for child sexual abuse. In S.M. Sgroi (Ed.), *Handbook of clinical intervention in child sexual abuse* (pp. 9-37). Lexington, MA: D.C. Heath.

Sheehan, D.V., Latta, W.E., Regina, E.G. & Smith, G.M. (1979). Empirical assessment of

Spiegel's Hypnotic Induction Profile and eyeroll hypotheses. *International Journal of Clinical & Experimental Hypnosis, 27,* 103-110.

Sheehan, P.W. (1971). Countering preconceptions about hypnosis: An objective index on involvement with the hypnotist. *Journal of Abnormal Psychology Monograph, 78,* 299-322.

Sheehan, P.W. (1979). Hypnosis and the processes of imagination. In E. Fromm & R Shor (Eds.), *Hypnosis: Developments in research and new perspectives.* (pp. 293-319). New York: Aldine.

Sheehan, P.W. (1980). Factors influencing rapport in hypnosis. *Journal of Abnormal Psychology, 89,* 263-281.

Sheehan, P.W., & Dolby, R.M (1979). Motivated involvement in hypnosis: The illustration of clinical rapport through hypnotic dreams. *Journal of Abnormal Psychology, 88,* 573-583.

Sheehan, P.W., & McConkey, K.M. (1982). *Hypnosis and experience: The exploration of phenomena and process.* Hillsdale, NJ: Lawrence Erlbaum Associates.

Sheehan, P.W., & Orne, M.T. (1968). Some comments on the nature of post-hypnotic behavior. *Journal of Nervous and Mental Disease, 146,* 209-220.

Sheehan, P.W., & Perry, C.W. (1976). *Methodologies of hypnosis. A critical appraisal of contemporary paradigms of hypnosis.* New York: Wiley.

Sheer, D.E. (1984). Focused arousal, 40-Hz EEG, and dysfunction. In T. Albezí Elbert et al. (Eds.), *Self regulation of the brain and behavior* (pp. 64–84). Berlin: Springer Verlag.

Sheikh, A.A., & Jordan, C.S, (1983). Clinical uses of mental imagery. In A.A. Sheikh (Ed.), *Imagery: Current theory, research, and application* (pp. 381-435). New York: Wiley.

Shengold, L (1980). Some reflections on a case of mother/adolescent son incest. *International Journal of Psychoanalysis, 60,* 461-476.

Sherwood, M. (1969). *The logic of explanation in psychoanalysis.* New York: Academic Press.

Shevrin, H., & Dickman, S. (1980). The psychological unconscious: A necessary assumption for all psychology theory? *American Psychologist, 35,* 421-434.

Shor, R.E. (1959). Hypnosis and the concept of the generalized reality orientation. *American Journal of Psychotherapy, 13,* 582-602.

Shor, R.E. (1962). Three dimensions of hypnotic depth. *International Journal of Clinical and Experimental Hypnosis, 10,* 23-38.

Shor, R.E. (1970). *The Inventory of Self-hypnosis: With versions based on breaths and timer.* Unpublished manuscript, Symbolic Processes Laboratory, Durham. NH.

Shor, R.E. (1979). A phenomenological method for the measurement of variables important to an understanding of the nature of hypnosis. In E. Fromm & R.E. Shor (Eds.), *Hypnosis: Developments in research and new perspectives* (2nd ed., pp. 105-138). New York: Aldine.

Shor, R.E., & Orne, E.C. (1962). *Harvard group scale of hypnotic susceptibility.* Palo Alto, CA: Consulting Psychologists' Press.

Shorr, J.E. (1972). *Psycho-imaginative therapy.* New York: Intercontinental Medical Books.

Shostrom, E, (1972). *Manual for the personality orientation inventory (POI). An inventory for the measurement of self-actualization.* San Diego, CA: Educational and Industrial Testing Service.

Sifneos, P. (1972). *Short-term psychotherapy and emotional crisis.* Cambridge, MA: Harvard University Press.

Sifneos, P. (1979). *Short-term dynamic psychotherapy: Evaluation and technique.* New York: Plenum Press.

Sigal, J., Silver, D., Rakoff, V., & Ellin, B. (1973). Some second generation effects of survival of the nazi persecution. *American Journal of Orthopsychiatry, 43,* 320-332.

Silbert, M.H., & Pines, A.M. (1981). Sexual child abuse as an antecedent to prostitution. *Child Abuse & Neglect, 5,* 407-411.

Silver, R.L., Boon, C., & Stones, M.H. (1983). Searching for meaning in misfortune: Making sense of incest. *Journal of Social Issues, 39(2),* 81-102.

Silver, S.M., & Kelly, W.E. (1985). Hypnotherapy of post-traumatic stress disorder in combat veterans from WWII and Vietnam. In W. E. Kelly (Ed.), *Post-traumatic stress disorder and the war veteran patient* (pp. 221-233). New York: Brunner/Mazel.

Simmel, E. (1944). War neurosis. In S. Lorand (Ed.), *Psychoanalysis today* (pp. 227-248). New York: International Universities Press.

Simonton, O.C., Matthews-Simonton, S., & Sparks, T.F.(1980). Psychological intervention in the treatment of cancer. *Psychosomatics. 21,* 226-233.

Simrel, K., Berg, R., & Thomas, J. (1979). Crisis management of sexually abused children. *Pediatric Annals,* 8(5), 317-332

Sloane, P., & Karpinski, E. (1942). Effects of incest on the participants. *American Journal of Orthopsychiatry, 12,* 666-673.

Smith, H., & Israel, E. (1987). Sibling incest: a study of the dynamics of 25 cases. *Child Abuse & Neglect, 11,* 101-108.

Solin, C.A. (1986). Displacement of affect in families following incest disclosure. *American Journal of Orthopsychiatry, 56,* 570-576.

Soll, M.J. (1984/85). Transferable penis and the self representation. *International Journal of Psychoanalytic Psychotherapy, 10,* 473-493.

Spanos, N.P. (1982). Hypnotic behavior: A cognitive-social psychological perspective. *Research Communications in Psychology, Psychiatry and Behavior, 1,* 199-213.

Spanos, N.P. Cross, W.F.,Menary, E., & Smith, J. (1988). Long term effects of cognitive-skill training for the enhancement of hypnotic susceptibility. *British Journal of Experimental & Clinical Hypnosis, 5,* 73-78.

Spanos, N.P., Hodgins, D.C., Stam, H.T. & Gwynn, M.I. (1984)). Suffering for science: The effects of implicit social demands on response to experimentally induced pain. *Journal of Personality and Social Psychology, 46,* 1162-1172.

Spanos, N.P., Kennedy, S.K.,& Gwynn, M.I. (1984). Moderating effects of contextual variables on the relatonship between hypnotic susceptibility and suggested analgesia. *Journal of Abnormal Psychology, 93,* 285-294.

Spanos, N.P., McNeil, C., Gwynn, M.I.,& Stam, H.T. (1984). Effects of suggestion and distraction on reported pain in subjects high and low on hypnotic susceptibility. *Journal of Abnormal Psychology, 93,* 277-284.

Spanos, N.P., Robertson, L.A., Menary, E.P., & Brett, P.J, (1986). Component analysis of cognitive skill training for the enhancement of hypnotic susceptibility. *Journal of Abnormal Psychology, 95,* 350-357.

Spence, D. (1982). *Narrative truth and historical truth: Meaning and interpretation in psychoanalysis.* New York: Norton.

Spencer, J. (1978). Father-daughter incest. *Child Welfare, 57,* 581-589.

Spiegel, D. (1981). Vietnam grief work using hypnosis. *American Journal of Clinical Hypnosis, 24,* 33-40.

Spiegel, D. (1983). Hypnosis with psychotic patients: Comment on Scagnelli-Jobsis. *American Journal of Clinical Hypnosis, 25,* 289-294.

Spiegel, D. (1986). Dissociation, double binds, and posttraumatic stress in multiple personality disorder. In B.G. Braun (Ed.), *Treatment of multiple personality disorder* (pp.61-77). Washington, DC: American Psychiatric Press.

Spiegel, D., Detrick, D., & Frischholz, E. (1982). Hypnotizability and psychopathology. *American Journal of Clinical Hypnosis, 25,* 431-437.

Spiegel, D., Frischholz, E.J., Maruffi, B., & Spiegel, H. (1981). Hypnotic responsivity and the treatment of flying phobia. *American Journal of Clinical Hypnosis, 23,* 239-247.

Spiegel, D., Hunt, T. & Dondershine, H, (1988). Dissociation and hypnotizability in posttraumatic stress disorder. *American Journal of Psychiatry, 145,* 301-305.

Spiegel, H. (1977). The Hypnotic Induction Profile (HIP): A review of its development. *Annals of the New York Academy of Sciences, 296,* 129-142.

Spiegel, H., & Spiegel, D. (1978). *Trance and treatment: Clinical use of hypnosis.* New York: Basic Books.

Spiegelman, J.M., & Vasavada, A.U. (1989). *Hinduism and Jungian psychology.* Phoenix, AZ:

Falcon Press.

Spinhoven, Ph. (1982). Het therapeutisch beland van hypnotiseerbaarheid. *The therapeutic relevance of hypnotizability. Directieve Therapie 2,* 329-365.

Spinhoven, Ph. (1987). Hypnosis and behavior therapy: A review. *International Journal of Clinical and Experimental Hypnosis, 35,* 8-31.

Spinhoven, Ph., Baak, D., Van Dyck, R., & Vermeulen, P. (1988). The effectiveness of an authoritative versus permissive style of hypnotic communication. *International Journal of Clinical and Experimental Hypnosis, 36,* 182-191.

Springer, C.J., Sachs, L.B., & Morrow, J.E. (1977). Group methods of increasing hypnotic susceptibility. *International Journal of Clinical and Experimental Hypnosis, 25,* 184-191.

Springer, S.P., & Deutsch, G. (1989). *Left brain, right brain* (3rd ed.). San Francisco: Freeman.

Steele, B.F. (1986). Notes on the lasting effects of early child abuse throughout the life cycle. *Child Abuse and Neglect, 10,* 283-291.

Stein, C. (1963). The clenched fist technique as a hypnotic procedure in clinical psychotherapy. *American Journal of Clinical Hypnosis, 6,* 113-119.

Stern, D.B., Spiegel, H., & Nee J.C.M. (1979). The Hypnotic Induction Profile: Normative observations, reliability and validity. *American Journal of Clinical Hypnosis, 21,* 109-132.

Stern, D.N. (1985). *The interpersonal world of the infant: A view from psychoanalysis and developmental psychology.* New York: Basic Books.

Stolar, D., & Fromm E. (1973). A further extension of Rapaport's theory of activity and passivity of the ego. *Proceedings of the 81st Annual Convention of the American Psychological Association* (pp. 501-502).

Stolar, D., Fromm, E. (1974). Activity and passivity of the ego in relation to the superego. *International Review of Psychoanalysis, 1,* 297-311.

Stolorow, R.D., & Lachmann, F.M. (1980). *Psychoanalysis of developmental arrests: Theory and treatment.* New York: International Universities Press.

Stone, J.A., & Lundy, R.M. (1985). Behavioral compliance with direct and indirect body movement suggestions. *Journal of Abnormal Psychology, 94,* 256-263.

Stone, M.H. (1981). Borderline syndromes: A consideration of subtypes and an overview, directions for research. *Psychiatric Clinics of North America, 4,* 3-13.

Strauss, B.S. (1986). Dissociative versus integrative hypnotic experience. *American Journal of Clinical Hypnosis, 29,* 132-136.

Stross, L., & Shevrin, H. (1967). A comparison of dream recall in wakefulness and hypnosis. *International Journal of Clinical and Experimental Hypnosis, 15,* 63-71.

Strupp, H.H., & Binder, J.L. (1984). *Psychotherapy in a new key: A guide to time-limited dynamic psychotherapy.* New York: Basic Books.

Stumpf, C. (1965). Drug action in the electrical activity of the hippocampus. *International Reviews of Neurobiology, 8,* 77-138

Stutman, R.K., & Bliss, E.L. (1985). Posttraumatic stresss disorder, hypnotizability and imagery. *American Journal of Psychiatry, 142,* 741-743.

Sullivan, D.S., Johnson, A., & Bratkovitch, J. (1974). Reduction of behavioral deficit in organic brain demage by use of hypnosis. *Journal of Clinical Psychology, 30,* 96-98.

Summit, R. (1982). Beyond belief: The reluctant discovery of incest. In M. Kirkpatrick (Ed.). *Women's sexual experience: Explorations of the dark continent* (pp. 127-150). New York: Plenum.

Summit, R. (1983). The child sexual abuse accommodation syndrome. *Child Abuse and Neglect, 7,* 177-193.

Summit, R., & Kryso, J. (1978). Sexual abuse of children: A clinical spectrum. *American Journal of Orthopsychiatry, 48,* 237-251.

Symonds, M. (1980). The "second injury" to victims [Special issue]. *Evaluation and Change,* 36-38.

Taneli, B., & Krahne, W. (1987). EEG changes of transcendental meditation practitioners. *Neurophysiological correlates of relaxation and psychopathology. Advances in Biological Psychiatry, 16,*

41-71.

Tart, C.T. (1969). *Altered states of consciousness.* New York: Wiley.

Tart, C.T. (1975). *States of consciousness.* New York: Dutton.

Tart, C.T. (1979a). Measuring the depth of an altered state of consciousness, with particular reference to self-report scales of hypnotic depth. In E. Fromm & R.E. Shor (Eds.), *Hypnosis: Developments in research and new perspectives* (pp. 557-604). New York: Aldine.

Tart, C.T. (1979b). Extended North Carolina Scale. In E. Fromm & R.E. Shor (Eds.), *Hypnosis: Developments in research and new perspectives* (2nd ed., pp. 567-601). New York: Aldine.

Tebecis, A.K., Provins, K.A., Farnbach, R.W., & Pentony, P. (1975). Hypnosis and the EEG: A quantitative investigation. *Journal of Nervous and Mental Disease, 161,* 1-17.

Tellegen, A. (1978). On measures and conceptions on hypnosis. *American Journal of Clinical Hypnosis, 21,* 219-237.

Tellegen, A., & Atkinson, G. (1974). Openness to absorbing and self altering experiences ("absorption"), a train related to hypnotic susceptibility. *Journal of Abnormal Psychology, 83,* 268-277.

Terr, L. (1983). Chowchilla revisited: The effects of psychic trauma four years after a school-bus kidnapping. *American Journal of Psychiatry, 140,* 1543-1550.

Terr, L. (1985). Children traumatized in small groups. In S. Eth & R.S. Pynoos (Eds.). *Post-traumatic stress disorder in children.* Washington, DC: American Psychiatric Press.

Thatcher, V.S. (Ed.). (1971). *Webster's new encyclopedic dictionary of the English language.* Chicago: Consolidated Book.

Thorne, D.E., & Hall. H.V. (1963). Hypnotic amnesia revisited. *International Journal of Clinical and Experimental Hypnosis, 11,* 39-47.

Tolpin, M. (1971). On the beginnings of a cohesive self: An application of the concept of transmuting internalization to the study of the transitional object and signal anxiety. *The Psychoanalytic Study of the Child, 26,* 316-353.

Tomkins, S. (1962). *Affect, imagery, consciousness* (Vol. 1). New York: Springer.

Trepper, T.S., & Barrett, M.J. (1986). Vulnerability to Incest: A framework for assessment. *Journal of Psychotherapy and the Family, 2,* 13-26.

Trossman, B. (1968). Adolescent children of concentration camp survivors. *Canadian Psychiatric Association Journal, 13,* 121-123.

Tsai, M., Feldman-Summers, S., & Edgar, M. (1979). Childhood Molestation: Variables related to differential impacts on psychosexual functioning in adult women. *Journal of Abnormal Psychology, 88,* 407-417.

Tsai, M., & Wagner, N. (1978). Therapy groups for women sexually molested as children. *Archives of Sexual Behavior, 7,* 417-427.

Turk, D.C., Meichenbaum, D., & Genest, M. (1983). *Pain and behavioral medicine: A cognitive behavioral perspective.* New York: Guilford.

Udolf, R. (1981). *Handbook of hypnosis for professionals.* New York: Van Nostrand Reinhold.

Ulett, G.A., Akpinar, S., & Itil, T.M. (1972). Hypnosis: Psychological and pharmacological reality. *American Journal of Psychiatry, 128,* 799-805.

Ullman, R.B., & Brothers, D. (1988). *The shattered self: A psychoanalytic stury of trauma.* Hillsdale, NJ: The Analytic Press.

Van Dantzig, A. (1986). De behandeling van trauma [Treatment of trauma]. In J. Dane (Ed.), *Praktijk van de hulpverlening aan oorlogs - en andere geweldsslachtoffers* (pp. 91-102). Lisse, The Netherlands: Swers & Zeitlinger.

Van der Does, A.J.W., Van Dyck, R., Spinhoven, P., & Kloosman, A. (1988). The effectiveness of standardized versus individualized hypnotic suggestions. *International Journal of Clinical & Experimental Hypnosis, 37,* 1-5.

Van der Hart, O (1982). Flexibiliteit van de therapeut versus hypnotiseerbaarheid van de client [Flexibility of the therapist versus hypnotizability of the client]. *Directieve Therapie, 2* (4), 366-373.

Van der Hart, O. (1983). *Rituals in psychotherapy: Transition and continuity.* New York: Irvington.

Van der Hart, O. (1984). *Rituelen in psychotherapie: Overgang en bestendiging. Rituals in psychotheraphy: Transition and continuity* Deventer: Van Loghum slaterus.

Van der Hart, O. (1986). Pierre Janet over hysterie en hypnose [Pierre Janet on hysteria and hypnosis] *Kwartaalschrift voor Directieve Tharapie en Hypnose, 6,* 233-246.

Van der Hart, O. (Ed.) (1987). *Coping with loss: The therapeutic use of leave-taking rituals.* New York: Irvington.

Van der Hart, O. (1985). Metaphoric and symbolic imagery in the hypnotic treatment of an urge to Wander: A case report. *Australian Journal of Clinical and Experimental Hypnosis, 15,* (1), 11-19.

Van der Kolk, B. (1984). *Post-traumatic stress disorder: Psychological and biological sequelae.* Washington, DC: American Psychiatric Press, Inc.

Van der Kolk, B. (1989). The complusion to repeat the trauma. *Psychiatric Clinics of North America, 12,* (2), 389-411.

Van Der Kolk, B., & Kadish, W. (1987). Amnesia, dissociation, and the return of the trauma response. In B. van der Kolk (Ed.), *Psychological trauma* (pp. 173-190). Washington, DC: American Psychiatric Press.

Van Doorn, M., & Aelen, F. (1986). De schrijfopdracht: Van oud zeer nar nieuwe zin [The writing assignment: From old pain to new meaning] *Directieve Therapie, 6* (2), 100-115.

Van Dyck, R. (1986). *Psychotherapie, placebo en suggestie* [Psychotherapy, placebo and suggestion] Lieden: Academisch Proefschrift.

Van Gorp, W.G. Meyer, R.G., & Dunbar, K.D. (1985). The efficacy of direct versus indirect hypnotic induction techniques on reduction of experimental pain. *International Journal of Clinical & Experimental Hypnosis, 33,* 319-328.

Van Nuys, D. (1973). Meditation, attention, and hypnotic susceptibility: A correlational study. *International Journal of Clinical and Experimental Hypnosis, 21,* 59-69.

Vitaliano, P.P., James, J., & Boyer, D, (1981). Sexuality of deviant females: adolescent and adult correlates. *Social Work, 26,* 462-466.

Vogel, W., & Broverman, D.M. (1964). Relationship between EEG and test intelligence: A critical review. *Psychological Bulletin, 62,* 132-144.

Vogel, W., Broverman, D.M., & Klaiber, E.L. (1968). EEG and mental abilities. *Electroencephalography and Clinical Neurophysiology, 24,* 166-175.

Volkan,V. (1968). The introjection and identification with the therapist as an ego-building aspect in the tratment of schizophrenia, *British Journal of Medical Psychology, 41,* 369-380.

Volkan, V. (1976). *Primitive internalized object relations.* New York: International Universities Press.

Volkan, V. (1982). Identification and related psychic events: Their appearance in therapy and their curative value. In S. Slipp (Ed.), *Curative factors in dynamic psychotherapy* (pp. 153-176). New York: McGraw-Hill Books.

Wadden, T.A., & Anderton, Ch. H. (1982). The clinical use of hypnosis. *Psychological Bulletin, 91,* 215-243.

Walker, N.W. Garrett, J.B. Wallace, B. (1976). Restoration of eidetic imagery via hypnotic age regression: A preliminary report. *Journal of Abnormal Psychology 85,* 335-337.

Wallace, B. (1978). Restoration of eidetic imagery via hypnotic age regression: More evidence. *Journal of Abnormal Psychology, 87,* 673-675.

Walsh, C.P. (1986). *The self-concept and sex-role orientation of adult females in therapy with and without incest history.* Unpublished doctoral dissertation, University of Florida, Gainesville, FL.

Ward, E. (1985). *Father–daughter rape.* New York: Grove Press.

Ward, M. (1977). *The brilliant function of pain.* New York: Optimus Books.

Watkins, H.H. (1978). Ego-state therapy. In J.G. Watkins (Ed.), *The therapeutic self* (pp. 360-398). New York: Human Sciences Press.

Watkins, H.H. (1980). The silent abreaction. *International Journal of Clinical and Experimental Hypnosis, 28,* 101-113.

Watkins, J.G. (1949). *Hypnotherapy of war neurosis.* New York: Ronald Press.
Watkins, J.G. (1971). The affect bridge: A hypnoanalytic technique. *International Journal of Clinical and Experimental Hypnosis, 19,* 21-27.
Watkins, J.G. (1977). The psychodynamic manipulation of ego states in hypnotherapy. Paper presented at the American Society of Clinical Hypnosis, Seattle, WA.
Watkins, J.G. (1978a, Winter). Ego states and the problem of responsibility II: The case of Patricia W. *Journal of Psychiatry and Law,* pp. 519-535.
Watkins, J.G. (1978b). Ego state therapy. In J. Watkins (Ed.), *The therapeutic self.* New York: Human Science Press.
Watkins, J.G. (in press). *Clinical hypnosis: Hypnoanalytic techniques* (vol. 2). New York: Irvington.
Watkins, J.G., & Johnson, R.J. (1982). *We the divided self.* New York: Irvington.
Watkins, J.G., & Watkins, H.H. (1978). *Abreactive technique* (audiotape). New York: Psychotherapy Tape Library.
Watkins, J.G., & Watkins, H.H. (1979). The theory and practice of ego state therapy. In H. Grayson (Ed.), *Short-term approaches to psychotherapy* (pp. 176-220). New York: National Institute for the Psychotherapies and Human Science Press.
Watkins, J.G., & Watkins, H.H . (1979-1980). Ego states and hidden observers. *Journal of Altered States of Consciousness, 5,* 3-18.
Watkins, J.G., & Watkins, H.H. (1980). *I. Ego states and hidden observers. II. Ego-state therapy: The woman in black and the lady in white* (Audiotape and transcript). New York: Jeffrey Norton.
Watkins, J.G.,& Watkins, H.H. (1981). Ego-state therapy. In R.J. Corsini (Ed.), *Handbook of innovative therapies* (pp. 252-270). New York: Wiley.
Watkins, J.G., & Watkins, H.H. (1984). Hazards to the therapist in the treatment of multiple personalities. *Psychiatric Clinics of North America, 7,* 11-119.
Watzlawick, P., Weakland, J.H., & Fisch, R. (1974). *Change: Principles of problem formation and problem resolution.* New York: Norton.
Wechsler, D. (1981). *Manual for the Weschler Adult Intelligence Scale-Revised.* New York: The Psychological Corporation.
Weeks, R.B. (1976). The sexually exploited child. *Southern Medical Journal, 69,* 848-850.
Weinberg, K. (1955). *Incest behavior.* New York: Citadel Press
Weiss, E. (Ed.). (1952). *Ego psychology and the psychoses.* New York: Basic Books.
Weitzenhoffer, A.M. (1957). *General Techniques of hypnotism.* New York: Grune & Stratton.
Weitzenhoffer, A.M. (1980). Hypnotic susceptibility revisited. *American Journal of Clinical Hypnosis, 22,* 130-146.
Weitzenhoffer, A.M. (1989). *The practice of hypnotism* (Vol. 1 & 2). New York: Wiley.
Weitzenhoffer, A.M., & Hilgard, E.R. (1959). *Stanford Hypnotic Susceptibility Scale, Forms A and B.* Palo Alto CA: Consulting Psychologists' Press.
Weitzenhoffer, A.M., & Hilgard, E.R. (1962). *Stanford Hypnotic Susceptibility Scale, Form C.* Palo Alto, CA: Consulting Psychologists' Press.
Weitzenhoffer, A.M., & Hilgard, E.R. (1967). *Revised Stanford Profile Scales of Hypnotic Susceptibility, Forms I and II.* Palo Alto, CA: Consulting Psychologists' Press.
Weitzenhoffer, A.M., & Sjoberg, B.M. (1961). Suggestibility with and without "induction of hypnosis," *Journal of Nervous and Mental Diseases, 132,* 205-220.
Wells, L.A. (1981), Family pathology and father-daughter incest: Restricted psychopathology. *Journal of Clinical Psychiatry, 42,* 197-202.
Wertheimer, M. (1945). *Productive thinking.* New York: Harper & Row.
West, L.J., & Deckert, G.H. (1965). Dangers of hypnosis, *Journal of the American Medical Association, 192,* 75-78.
Westermeyer, J. (1978). Incest in psychiatric practice: A description of patients and incestuous relationships. *Journal of Clinical Psychiatry, 39,* 643-648.
Whitaker, C.A., & Malone, T.P. (1981). *The roots of psychotherapy.* New York: Brunner/Mazel. (Original work published, 1953).

White, R.W. (1963). Ego and reality in psychoanalytic theory: A proposal regarding independent ego energies, *Psychological Issues,* 3, Monograph 11.

White, T.H. (1958). *The once and future king.* New York: Putnam.

Wiesel, E. (1969).*Night.* New York: Avon.

Wilson, A., & Fromm, E. (1982). Aftermath of the concentration camp: The second generation. *Journal of American Academy of Psychoanalysis, 10,* 289-313.

Wilson, S.C., & Barber, T.X. (1978). The Creative Imagination Scale as a measure of hypnotic responsiveness: Applications to experimental and clinical hypnosis. *American Journal of Clinical Hypnosis, 20,* 235-243.

Winnicott, D.W. (Ed.). (1965a) *The maturational process and the facilitating environment.* New York: International Universities Press.

Winnicott, D.W. (1965b). The theory of the parent-infant relationship. In D.W. Winnicott (Ed.), *The maturational processes and the facilitating environment* (pp. 37-55). New York: International University Press.

Winnicott, D.W. (1971). The use of an object and relating through identifications. In D.W. Winncott *Playing and reality* (pp. 86-94). New York: Basic Books.

Witztum, E., & Van der Hart, O., & Friedman. B. (1988). The use of metaphors in psychotherapy. *Journal of Contemporary Psychotherapy,* 18, 270-290.

Wolberg, L.R. (1948). *Medical hypnosis* (Vol.1 & 2). New York: Grune & Stratton.

Wolberg, L. (1964). *Hypnoanalysis* (2nd ed.). New York: Grove Press.

Wolberg, L. (1967). Hypnosis in psychoanalytic psychotherapy. In J.E. Gordon (Ed.), *Handbook of clinical and experimental hypnosis* (pp. 260-277). New York: Macmillan.

Wooley, M.J., Vigilanti, M.A. (1984). Psychological separation and the sexual abuse victim. *Psychotherapy: Theory, Research and Practice, 21,* 347-352.

Woolson, D.A. (1986). An experimental comparison of direct and Ericksonian hypnotic induction procedures and the relationship to secondary suggestibility. *American Journal of Clinical Hypnosis, 29,* 23-28.

Wyatt, G. (1985). The sexual abuse of Afro-American and white women in childhood. *Child Abuse & Neglect, 9,* 507-519.

Yates, A. (1982). Children eroticized by incest. *American Journal of Psychiatry, 139,* 482-485.

Zetzel, E. (1970). *The capacity for emotional growth.* New York: International University Press.

AUTHOR INDEX

C

SUBJECT INDEX

N

O

P